Von Willebrand Disease

Von Willebrand Disease
Basic and Clinical Aspects

Edited by

Augusto B. Federici MD
Associate Professor of Hematology
Division of Hematology and Transfusion Medicine
L. Sacco University Hospital
Department of Internal Medicine
University of Milan
Milan, Italy

Christine A. Lee MA, MD, DSc (Med), FRCP, FRCPath, FRCOGad eundem
Emeritus Professor of Haemophilia
University of London
London, UK

Erik E. Berntorp MD, PhD
Professor of Hemophilia
Malmö Centre for Thrombosis and Haemostasis
Lund University
Skåne University Hospital
Malmö, Sweden

David Lillicrap MD
Professor
Department of Pathology and Molecular Medicine
Richardson Laboratory
Queen's University
Kingston, ON, Canada

Robert R. Montgomery MD
Professor of Pediatric Hematology
Department of Pediatrics
Medical College of Wisconsin;
Senior Investigator
Blood Research Institute
Blood Center of Wisconsin
Milwaukee, WI, USA

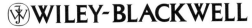

WILEY-BLACKWELL

A John Wiley & Sons, Ltd., Publication

Library of Congress Cataloging-in-Publication Data

Von Willebrand disease : basic and clinical aspects / edited by Augusto B. Federici ... [et al.].
     p. ; cm.
Includes bibliographical references and index.
ISBN 978-1-4051-9512-6 (hardcover : alk. paper)
1. Von Willebrand disease.   I. Federici, Augusto B.
[DNLM:1. von Willebrand Diseases. WH 312]
RC647.V65V66 2011
616.1'57–dc22

2010036377

A catalogue record for this book is available from the British Library.

This book is published in the following electronic formats: ePDF 9781444329933; Wiley Online Library 9781444329926; ePub 9781444329940

Set in 9/11.5 pt Sabon by Toppan Best-set Premedia Limited
Printed and bound in Singapore by Markono Print Media Pte Ltd
01   2011

Contents

Contributors

Thomas C. Abshire MD
Senior Vice President
Medical Services and the Medical Science Institute;
Chief Medical Officer
BloodCenter of Wisconsin
Milwaukee, WI, USA

Luciano Baronciani PhD
Hospital Scientist
Angelo Bianchi Bonomi Haemophilia and
   Thrombosis Centre
Department of Medicine and Medical Specialities
IRCCS Maggiore Policlinico Hospital
Mangiagalli and Regina Elena Foundation and
   University of Milan
Milan, Italy

Jennifer Barr BS
Department of Anatomy and Cell Biology
University of Iowa Carver College of Medicine
Iowa City, IA, USA

Javier Batlle MD
Chairman Servicio de Hematología y Hemoterapia.
INIBIC. C. Hospitalario Universitario A Coruña;
Associate Professor of Department of Medicine
School of Medicine
University of Santiago de Compostela
A Coruña, Spain

Margareta Blombäck MD PhD
Professor Emeritus
Department of Molecular Medicine and Surgery
Division of Clinical Chemistry and Blood
   Coagulation Research
The Karolinska Institute
Karolinska University Hospital
Stockholm, Sweden

Ulrich Budde MD
Director
Department of Hemostaseology
Medilys Laborgesellschaft mbH
c/o Asklepios Klinik Altona
Hamburg, Germany

Giancarlo Castaman MD
Consultant Haematologist
Department of Cell Therapy and Hematology
Hemophilia and Thrombosis Center
San Bortolo Hospital
Vicenza, Italy

Olivier D. Christophe PhD
Senior Researcher
INSERM Unit 770
Le Kremlin-Bicêtre, France

Marinee K.L. Chuah PhD
Professor
Flanders Institute for Biotechnology (VIB)
Vesalius Research Center
University of Leuven
Leuven;
Faculty of Medicine and Pharmacy
University Hospital Campus Jette
Free University of Brussels (VUB)
Brussels, Belgium

Cecile V. Denis PhD
Director of Research
INSERM Unit 770
Le Kremlin-Bicêtre, France

Jorge Di Paola MD
Associate Professor of Pediatrics and Genetics
Postle Family Chair in Pediatric Cancer and Blood
    Disorders
University of Colorado Denver School of Medicine
The Children's Hospital
Aurora, CO, USA

Jeroen C.J. Eikenboom MD, PhD
Associate Professor
Department of Thrombosis and Hemostasis
Leiden University Medical Center
Leiden, the Netherlands

Emmanuel J. Favaloro PhD
Senior Hospital Scientist
Department of Haematology
Institute of Clinical Pathology and Medical
    Research (ICPMR)
Westmead Hospital
Westmead, NSW, Australia

Massimo Franchini MD
Head
Immunohematology and Transfusion Center
Department of Pathology and Laboratory Medicine
University Hospital of Parma
Italy

Edith Fressinaud MD, PhD
Consultant Haematologist
Centre National de Référence de la Maladie de
    Willebrand
Service d'Hématologie biologique
Hôpital Antoine Béclère
Clamart, France

Anne Goodeve BSc, PhD
Reader and Head, Haemostasis Research Group
Department of Cardiovascular Science
Faculty of Medicine, Dentistry and Health
University of Sheffield;
Principal Clinical Scientist
Sheffield Diagnostic Genetics Service
Sheffield Children's NHS Foundation Trust
Sheffield, UK

Sandra L. Haberichter PhD
Associate Professor
Department of Pediatrics – Hematology/Oncology
Medical College of Wisconsin
Milwaukee, WI, USA

Paula D. James MD, FRCPC
Associate Professor, Hematologist
Queen's University
Kingston, ON, Canada

Rezan A. Kadir MD, FRCS (ed), MRCOG, MD
Consultant Obstetrician and Gynaecologist
The Royal Free Hospital
London, UK

Peter A. Kouides MD
Medical and Research Director
Mary M Gooley Hemophilia Center
Rochester General Hospital
Rochester, NY, USA

Peter J. Lenting PhD
Director of Research
INSERM Unit 770
Le Kremlin-Bicêtre, France

Stefan Lethagen MD, PhD
Director of Copenhagen Haemophilia Centre
Thrombosis and Haemostasis Unit
Department of Haematology
Copenhagen University Hospital
Copenhagen, Denmark;
International Medical Director
Director of Medical & Science Haemostasis
    Department
Global Development
Novo Nordisk
Søborg, Denmark

María Fernanda López-Fernández MD
Head, Hemostasis and Thrombosis
Servicio de Hematología y Hemoterapia
Complexo Hospitalario Universitario de A Coruña
A Coruña, Spain

Pier Mannuccio Mannucci MD
Professor of Medicine
Angelo Bianchi Bonomi Haemophilia and
    Thrombosis Centre
University of Milan and IRCCS Maggiore Hospital
Milan, Italy

Claudine Mazurier PhD
Head of Analytical Department, Preclinical
    Development
Laboratoire Français du Fractionnement et des
    Biotechnologies
Lille, France

Dominique Meyer MD
Professor of Haematology
Centre National de Référence de la Maladie de
    Willebrand;
University Paris-Sud
France

David Motto MD, PhD
Assistant Professor
Departments of Internal Medicine and Pediatrics
University of Iowa Carver College of Medicine
Iowa City, IA, USA

Ian Peake BSc, PhD
Sir Edward Mellanby Professor of Molecular
    Medicine
Department of Cardiovascular Science
University of Sheffield Medical School
Sheffield, UK

Almudena Pérez-Rodríguez PhD
Post-doctoral Investigator
Servicio de Hematología y Hemoterapia—INIBIC
Complexo Hospitalario Universitario de A Coruña
A Coruña, Spain

Inge Petrus PhD
Flanders Institute for Biotechnology (VIB)
Vesalius Research Center
University of Leuven
Leuven, Belgium

Jacob H. Rand
Hematology Laboratory
Department of Pathology
Montefiore Center
Bronx, NY, USA

Francesco Rodeghiero MD
Director
Department of Cell Therapy and Hematology
San Bortolo Hospital
Vicenza, Italy

Reinhard Schneppenheim MD, PhD
Director
Department of Pediatric Hematology and Oncology
University Medical Center Hamburg-Eppendorf
Hamburg, Germany

Alberto Tosetto MD
Senior Consultant
Department of Hematology
San Bortolo Hospital
Vicenza, Italy

Thierry VandenDriessche PhD
Group Leader
Flanders Institute for Biotechnology (VIB);
Vesalius Research Center
University of Leuven
Leuven;
Faculty of Medicine and Pharmacy
University Hospital Campus Jette
Free University of Brussels (VUB)
Brussels, Belgium

Foreword

I feel very honored to have been asked to write the foreword to this book on von Willebrand disease (VWD). I am now the oldest living scientist to have experience in this area, and thus it may be of interest for readers to learn about some early experiences that I shared with the late Dr. Inga-Marie Nilsson, which I have described below. Since I started working with VWD in the mid-1950s, there has been enormous progress in the management of the disease in terms of knowledge about mechanisms, treatment, and underlying genetics. We have been able to follow this development in Stockholm because the hemophilia center here is currently responsible for the treatment of 40 patients with type 3 VWD (i.e., the most severe form).

In the 1950s there were only a few known cases of the disease—which was mostly called "pseudohemophilia"—in addition to those cases known in the Åland Islands, where the disease was first identified by Erik von Willebrand. This was probably because most patients with type 3 VWD died young, either *in utero* or, if the patient was female and survived until puberty, as a result of menstrual bleeding. I remember some touching letters written at the end of the 19th century from a businessman to his wife, who was mostly bedridden owing to menstrual bleedings. This woman was an ancestor of a young woman from Stockholm with type 3 VWD, who is currently living a normal family life thanks to therapy in early childhood with the Swedish fraction I-0 (which contained von Willebrand factor [VWF], factor VIII [FVIII], and fibrinogen) and later with commercial VWF-containing concentrates.

When taking a bleeding history for a female in the 1950s, it was useful to ask whether she had been scolded in school for dropping blood onto her handiwork after pricking her finger with a sewing needle. We learned that it was useful to analyze blood groups in family investigations, as we found that a healthy child who showed no sign of having inherited the disease did not share the same father as the sick sibling. We made several mistakes—one girl was transfused with platelets during a severe menstrual bleeding without success but, when treated with fraction I-0, the bleeding stopped. It is possible that the platelet treatment was the reason why she later developed antibodies to VWD. At that time there were no oral contraceptives, which have revolutionized the management of menorrhagia in patients with VWD. In this particular patient, we used testosterone and later hysterectomy (under prophylaxis of fraction I-0) to deal with the menstrual bleedings.

To persuade doctors that a patient had to be treated with a concentrate was a difficult task. I remember the case of a 13-year-old boy who developed severe head trauma as a result of falling from a bicycle. Despite the fact that the boy had a bleeding chart saying that he should be treated immediately in the event of a trauma and the fact that I informed the doctor that the usual signs do not develop in bleeders immediately but sometimes several days later, the doctor refused to treat the boy with concentrates and he died from severe brain hemorrhage.

In 1958 we started prophylactic treatment in patients with hemophilia to avoid joint destruction. However, it was not until many years later that we realized that patients with type 3 VWD also required prophylaxis; therefore, some of them developed joint disabilities. We also did not know that the concentrates with which we treated our patients could contain hepatitis C virus, which has led to the premature death of some patients.

This book has become a very comprehensive and useful work into which many of the authors have put great efforts to make their chapters not only informative but also easy to understand. Progress, difficulties, and alternative ways to diagnose phenotypes and genotypes are described. Molecular diagnosis of type 1, type 2 and its subgroups, and type 3 VWD are presented. In addition, a chapter on gene therapy looking into the future is stimulating to read. Furthermore, many authors have endeavored to include all relevant literature, which is very useful for students.

A problem with regard to historical aspects is that the nomenclature has changed from FVIII-related antigen to VWF antigen. Therefore, some of the early findings with regard to the level of VWF in patients with blood group O or A have not been observed. Nevertheless, the topic of how to proceed in diagnosis when the patient has blood group O or A has been thoroughly discussed. I have the impression that there still are problems with regard to diagnosis of the phenotypes, particularly with regard to the diagnosis of type 1 VWD, even if preanalytic problems are taken into account, for example the quality of methodology and the importance of telling the patient to rest and not to run or be stressed, etc, before blood sampling. I made a serious mistake once when analyzing changes in VWF during the menstrual cycle—the volunteers were not well informed about resting before sampling and we therefore misinterpreted the results; there are not such great variations in FVIII and VWF during the menstrual cycle as initially suggested.

When investigating families with type 3 VWD, we found that the parents and siblings who were genetic carriers of VWD only had a phenotypically mild bleeding disorder and often, but not always, the common analyses of VWD indicated a mild disorder. However, we recorded the usefulness of an increased ratio of FVIII/VWF:Ag for the diagnosis of what we called type 1 VWD in these families.

It must have been an enormous task for the editors to encourage all the authors to write, although possibly some welcomed the opportunity to put together their experience in a comprehensive chapter. The efforts on trying to collate experience in multicenter studies on prophylaxis and diagnostic scores is very valuable and, of course, needs to be supported in order to solve the many difficulties that remain in the diagnosis and management of VWD.

Margareta Blombäck
Professor Emeritus
Karolinska Institutet
Sweden

Preface

Erik von Willebrand described a novel bleeding disorder in 1926 and, in his original publication, he provided an impressive description of the clinical and genetic features of the von Willebrand disease (VWD). In contrast to hemophilia, the epitome of inherited bleeding disorders, both sexes were affected, and mucosal bleeding was the predominant symptom. The history of VWD is fascinating because it demonstrates how good clinical observations, genetic studies, and biochemical skills can improve the basic understanding of a disease and its management. The continuous efforts of scientists and clinicians over the last 85 years have significantly furthered the understanding of the structure and function of von Willebrand factor (VWF), the protein that is absent, reduced, or dysfunctional in patients with VWD. Such basic information about VWF will undoubtedly improve both the diagnosis and the treatment of VWD. Determination of both the phenotype and the genotype is now readily available in many countries, and treatment is becoming more specific and directed by the type and subtype of VWD. Therapeutic agents must correct the dual defect of hemostasis, i.e. the abnormal platelet adhesion due to reduced and/or dysfunctional VWF and the associated low level of factor VIII (FVIII). Desmopressin (DDAVP) is the treatment of choice for type 1 VWD because it induces release of VWF from cellular compartments. VWF concentrates that are virally inactivated, with or without FVIII, are effective and safe in patients unresponsive to DDAVP; a recombinant VWF is currently under evaluation in clinical trials. Retrospective and prospective clinical studies, including bleeding history and laboratory markers for diagnosis, as well as the use of DDAVP and VWF concentrates to treat or prevent bleeding in patients with VWD, have been essential to provide general guidelines for the management of VWD.

This book presents the most important basic and clinical aspects of inherited and acquired defects of VWF, and it includes the many advances that have been made in recent years. The editors hope that a book specifically devoted to VWD can be useful to the hematologists of the 21st century who would like to manage VWD patients in a more comprehensive way using the most updated and evidence-based recommendations.

The editors would like to dedicate this first VWD book to three pioneers on VWD research who made pivotal and original contributions on this field: Arthur Bloom, Inga Maria Nilsson, and Theodore S. Zimmerman. Their life-long devotion to research on VWD and on other bleeding disorders should stimulate further studies on these topics of hematology.

The Editors
Augusto B. Federici
Christine A. Lee
Erik E. Berntorp
David Lillicrap
Robert R. Montgomery
16 January 2011

1

Historical perspective on von Willebrand disease

Erik Berntorp[1] *and Margareta Blombäck*[2]

[1]Malmö Centre for Thrombosis and Haemostasis, Lund University, Skåne University Hospital, Malmö, Sweden

[2]Department of Molecular Medicine and Surgery, Division of Clinical Chemistry and Blood Coagulation Reasearch, The Karolinska Institute, Karolinska University Hospital, Stockholm, Sweden

Introduction

The history of von Willebrand disease (VWD) and its causative factor, the von Willebrand factor (VWF), spans almost a century and was recently comprehensively reviewed by the late professor Birger Blombäck, who described the first publication by Erik von Willebrand [1], the gene cloning in 1985, and the discovery of the specific metalloprotease, ADAMTS13 [2], that degrades VWF. The purpose of this review is to describe the early history of the understanding of the disease and the first steps in the replacement therapy for its severe forms. Also, we describe in greater detail the findings in a group of different families investigated on the Åland Islands.

The scientist of the disease

Erik Adolf von Willebrand (Figure 1.1) was born in Vasa, Finland, in 1870. He qualified as a medical doctor in 1896 and specialized initially in physical therapy and later in internal medicine at Helsinki. Erik von Willebrand devoted much of his professional life to an interest in blood, especially its coagulation properties. In 1899, he defended a doctoral thesis that dealt with his investigation of the changes that occur in blood following a serious hemorrhage. From 1908

Von Willebrand Disease, 1st edition. Edited by Augusto B. Federici, Christine A. Lee, Erik E. Berntorp, David Lillicrap, Robert R. Montgomery. © 2011 Blackwell Publishing Ltd.

until his retirement in 1935, Erik von Willebrand worked at the Deaconess Institute in Helsinki, where he headed the Department of Internal Medicine between 1922 and 1931. Erik von Willebrand was known for his modesty and integrity, and in his obituary it was said that he "usually preferred to discuss his observations of nature rather than his personal achievements." He died in September 1949, at the age of 89 years.

First description of the disease: the Åland family

In 1926, Erik von Willebrand first described the inherited bleeding disorder in *Finska Läkaresällskapets Handlingar* (in Swedish). He identified features that suggested that this disease was distinct from classic hemophilia and other bleeding disorders known at the time, such as anaphylactoid purpura, thrombocytopenic purpura, and the hereditary thrombasthenia described by Glanzmann. What differentiated this bleeding disorder from classic hemophilia was that it was not frequently associated with muscle and joint bleeding, and it affected both women and men. He stressed that a prolonged bleeding time was its most prominent characteristic. He concluded that the condition was a previously unknown form of hemophilia, and called it "hereditary pseudohemophilia." Erik von Willebrand also discussed the pathogenesis of the condition and felt that the bleeding could best be explained by the combined effect of a functional disorder of the platelets and a systemic lesion of the vessel walls.

The original observations leading to this new disease were made in several members of a large family (identified as family S) living on the island of Föglö in the Åland archipelago in the Baltic Sea. The index case was a girl aged 5 years, named Hjördis S, who had marked and recurrent bleeding tendencies and was brought to Helsinki for consultation. Both her mother and father were from families with histo-ries of bleeding. The girl was the ninth of 11 children, of whom seven had experienced bleeding symptoms. Four of her sisters had died from uncontrolled bleeding at an early age. Hjördis herself had experienced several severe episodes of bleeding from the nose and lips and following tooth extractions, as well as bleeding in her ankle. At the age of 3 years she bled for 3 days from a deep wound in her upper lip. The bleeding was so severe that she almost lost consciousness and had to be hospitalized for 10 weeks. At the age of 14 years, Hjördis bled to death during her fourth menstrual period.

Hjördis came from a large family (Figure 1.2). Intrigued by their history, Erik von Willebrand studied the family further with the help of coworkers. He published the pedigree and his clinical and laboratory evaluation in his 1926 paper. He found that 23 of the 66 family members had bleeding problems. The most prominent problem among the affected family members was mucosal bleeding: epistaxis, followed by profuse bleeding from oral lesions, easy bruising, and, in females, excessive bleeding during menstruation and at childbirth. Intestinal bleeding had been the cause of death at early ages in some family members.

In further studies, Erik von Willebrand found two families related to Hjördis S and one unrelated family in whom bleeding symptoms similar to those observed in Hjördis were common [3,4]. In the 1930s, Jürgens, together with von Willebrand [5,6], reinvestigated the patients in Åland and concluded that the disease was due to some impairment of platelet function, including platelet factor 3 deficiency. This observation led to the disease being called von Willebrand–Jürgens thrombopathy, and, although this condition is not officially recognized today, von Willebrand did not dismiss the notion that factors in blood plasma might also be important in the pathogenesis of the disease.

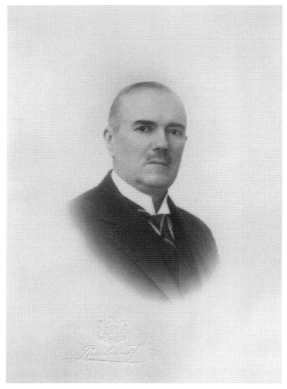

Figure 1.1 Erik von Willebrand.

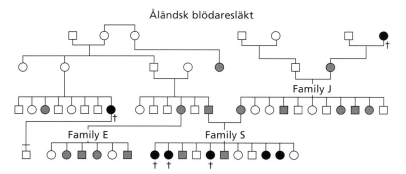

Åländsk blödaresläkt

Family J

Family E

Family S

Figure 1.2 The Åland pedigree as originally described in 1926 [1]. The index case, Hjördis, is the ninth sibling in family S (Fam S). □ unaffected male; ○ unaffected female; ■ male with mild bleeding disease; ⬤ female with mild bleeding disease; ● female with severe bleeding disease; † bled to death.

Other early clinical reports

In 1928, Dr. George R. Minot of Boston described five patients from two families with prolonged bleeding times and symptoms similar to the Åland family members. This may have been one of the first descriptions of VWD [7–9]. In the following years, numerous cases similar to those described by von Willebrand were reported, usually under the name of pseudohemophilia. In 1953, Alexander and Goldstein [10] found a dual defect in two patients with hereditary pseudohemophilia. They confirmed the earlier findings of prolonged bleeding time, normal platelet count and function, and abnormal nail bed capillaries. However, they also found a decreased FVIII level (5–10% of normal) and they observed a prolonged coagulation time that was normalized by normal plasma. The prolonged bleeding time, however, was not normalized and this was later explained by the fact that infusion of a restricted volume of plasma does not provide a sufficient amount of VWF [11]. Larrieu and Soulier [12] also found low FVIII activity and a prolonged bleeding time in pseudohemophilia, but otherwise normal clotting factors and platelet parameters. They proposed the name of von Willebrand syndrome for the condition.

The search for a new factor—the bleeding time factor

The first demonstration of the VWF was during the 1950s through a joint effort by Margareta and Birger Blombäck, working in Stockholm with the purification of fibrinogen, and Inga Marie Nilsson, who had established a clinical coagulation unit in Malmö. It was found that fibrinogen purified from Cohn fraction I of human plasma, when specifically obtained in fraction I-0 (AHF-Kabi), was heavily contaminated with an antihemophilic factor, that is plasma factor VIII (FVIII) [13].

At that time, Dr. Nilsson had a 15-year-old female patient named Birgitta who had a severe hemorrhagic diathesis. When she began to menstruate, the condition worsened and she received frequent blood transfusions. However, Birgitta developed serious side-effects from the transfusions and they were stopped. As a consequence, other treatment options

had to be considered, and a hysterectomy was planned. Her coagulation evaluation had shown a prolonged bleeding time and a somewhat prolonged coagulation time but normal platelet count and function. FVIII activity was low. Since fraction I-0 had a high concentration of FVIII, it was decided that its effects should be tested in Birgitta. To the surprise of the treating physicians, not only did FVIII activity increase as expected but the bleeding time was also normalized [14]. Subsequently, a hysterectomy was successfully performed under the cover of fraction I-0. According to modern classification, this patient had type 3 VWD. She is now well, and has been on regular prophylaxis with VWF concentrate for many years.

In June 1957, Inga Marie Nilsson, Erik Jorpes, Margareta Blombäck, and Stig-Arne Johansson visited Åland and studied 16 patients who had been examined 25–30 years previously by von Willebrand. No patients who had severe forms of the disease were still living. In their investigation they found FVIII activity to be reduced in 15 of 16 cases [15]. The father of Hjördis had a normal level. The Duke bleeding time varied, with two patients having a definite prolongation and three patients a moderate prolongation. Platelet counts were normal and, in contrast to Jürgens' earlier observation, the platelets themselves were normal with respect to platelet factor 3. One of the patients was given fraction I-0, which normalized the FVIII level and the bleeding time. It could be concluded that the Åland family had the same disease described by several other authors in Europe and the USA [16]. At the same time, Jürgens visited the islands (Erik Jorpes had told him of his team's research plan) and took samples from many of the same patients, and confirmed the decreased FVIII levels [17].

The findings by the Swedish group confirmed what had been documented in a number of Swedish families [18]. The observation was also made that FVIII increased during the first 24 h after infusion of fraction I-0 in patients with VWD, in contrast to what is seen in hemophilia [19]. The results of fraction I-0 infusion in a patient with severe VWD are shown in Figure 1.3. The bleeding time is reduced or normalized; factor VIII clotting activity (VIII:C) increases steadily during the first 24 h whereas the VWF (VIIIR:Ag and VIIIR:RC according to old nomenclature) displays a pharmacokinetic profile as expected and as later shown. Control experiments and further studies [11,20,21] revealed that the bleeding time

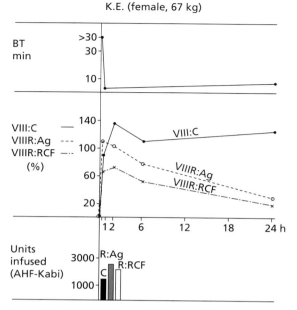

Figure 1.3 VIII:C, VWF:Ag (VIIIR:Ag), VWF:RCo (VIIIR:RCF), and Duke bleeding time (BT) in a patient with severe von Willebrand disease after infusion of human fraction I-0 (AHF-Kabi) [16]. Bleeding time is shortened and VIII:C is successively increased after the initial post-infusion peak during the first 24 h, whereas the von Willebrand factor (VIIIR:Ag and VIIIR:RC) displays a pharmacokinetic profile as expected. Reproduced from Nilson and Holmberg [16].

factor was a plasma factor not earlier described. Fraction I-0 prepared from patients with severe hemophilia A not only corrected the bleeding time in VWD, but also stimulated the production of FVIII activity, whereas fraction I-0 prepared from patients with VWD had no such effect. Purified fibrinogen had no effect on the bleeding time. Still, there was the possibility that the shortening of the bleeding time was due to platelets or platelet factors contaminating fraction I-0. This turned out to be unlikely, since the effect on bleeding time was the same whether the fraction had been prepared from platelet-rich or platelet-poor plasma. Infusion of a platelet suspension from a normal donor to a patient with VWD had no effect on either bleeding time or bleeding tendency, nor did injection of fraction I-0 into a patient with thrombocytopenia. From these findings, it was concluded that the impaired hemostasis in VWD was due to lack of a plasma factor, the bleeding time correcting

factor, or the VWF, which occurs not only in normal plasma but also in hemophilia A plasma. This factor not only corrected the prolonged bleeding time, but apparently increased the level of FVIII. Thus, platelets or platelet factors were not identical with the bleeding time factor, which had been proposed by both Rudolf Jürgens and Erik von Willebrand to be responsible, together with a vascular defect, for the bleeding diathesis. These findings have since been widely confirmed. The claim that a previously unknown factor in plasma had been discovered was communicated at the Congress of the International Society of Hematology in Rome in 1958 (see also [20]).

At first, it was not understood how a plasma factor could affect primary hemostasis and shorten the bleeding time. However, Borchgrevink [22] found decreased platelet adhesiveness *in vivo*, and Salzman [23] demonstrated decreased platelet adhesiveness to glass in VWD. Borchgrevink employed the method suggested by Hellem [24], which used a slow flow and could not discriminate between samples from patients with or without VWD. Salzman modified this method and introduced a higher flow, making it more specific for VWD. It was also shown that normal or hemophilic plasma can normalize the reduced platelet adhesiveness as well as the bleeding time in VWD [23,25,26]. In studies using electron microscopy, Jörgensen and Borchgrevink [27] demonstrated a decreased adhesion of platelets to disrupted endothelium in VWD. This observation indicated that the plasma factor lacking in VWD exerted its action in primary hemostasis via the platelets by enhancing their adhesiveness.

During the 1960s, cases of VWD were reported from several countries. The disease was thought to be uniform and was defined as an autosomal dominant inheritable hemorrhagic disease characterized by a prolonged bleeding time, decreased FVIII clotting activity, decreased platelet adhesiveness as measured by the Salzman method, and progressive increase of FVIII activity after infusion of plasma and FVIII concentrate [16].

However, returning to the earlier papers by Erik von Willebrand and Rudolf Jürgens, the findings on the Åland islands showed what appeared to be a discrepancy between the original family S and some of the others investigated; the original von Willebrand family having "pure" VWD while in other families there were also platelet function defects. Thus, in 1977, Dag Nyman (originally from Åland) and collaborators [28] traveled from Stockholm to Åland to undertake a thorough investigation using new laboratory methods [28]. They found that the families described as having VWD could be divided into four categories: (i) the survivors with a mild disorder from the original family S had the characteristics of type 1 VWD, that is they had similarly decreased levels of VWF:Ag and ristocetin cofactor activity in addition to normal or decreased levels of FVIII, and the platelet aggregation was normal; (ii) one family had a platelet function defect (pure cyclooxygenase defect); (iii) one family had a mixture of VWD and a cyclooxygenase defect; and (iv) one family had a platelet function defect of the aspirin type. These findings, of course, made it easier to investigate the genetic defects of the original VWD (family S).

In the beginning of the 1990s, Zhang and collaborators [29] investigated the DNA sequence from 24 patients with type 3 VWD living in Sweden. They found a cytosine deletion in exon 18 of the *VWF* gene in most of those of Swedish origin and an insertion in exon 28 in those of Finnish origin. Most patients with type 3 VWD were homozygous or double heterozygous for the mutations. Most of the parents had type 1 VWD and were heterozygous. As the Åland population is primarily of Swedish origin, the researchers also investigated family S and found that the surviving members who had type 1 VWD were heterozygous with respect to the mutation in exon 18. There was a small boy with severe VWD whose family was related long ago to another family with VWD from Åland. He was homozygous for the mutation in exon 18 [30].

The end of the beginning

After the publication by Erik von Willebrand in 1926, it took some 30 years until it was clear that a new plasma factor responsible for the hemostatic impairment in VWD had been detected. In that time, a factor concentrate had been produced that was effective in the replacement of VWF: fraction I-0 (or, later, AHF-Kabi). Studies using this concentrate and concentrates purified from different types of bleeding disorders, helped scientists to find and prove the presence of the VWF. This was the end of the beginning.

In 1971, VWF was first detected immunologically and named "FVIII-related antigen" [31]. Since 1985, the VWF has been cloned [32–35], the primary amino-acid sequence has been determined [36], and the complex molecular structure and multiple functions are becoming understood in detail. The metalloprotease ADAMTS13 that cleaves VWF was discovered in 2001 [2]. VWD is no longer a uniform disease [37]. The treatment armamentarium has been developed and includes prophylactic treatment with concentrates in type 3 VWD. It includes desmopressin for most milder cases, new concentrates [38,39], and we are now anticipating development of recombinant VWF for therapeutic use.

References

1 von Willebrand EA. Hereditär pseudohämofili. *Finska Läkaresällskapets Handlingar* 1926; **LXVII**: 87–112.

2 Fujikawa K, Suzuki H, McMullen B, Chung D. Purification of human von Willebrand factor-cleaving protease and its identification as a new member of the metalloproteinase family. *Blood* 2001; **98**: 1662–6.

3 von Willebrand EA. Uber hereditäre pseudohämophilie. *Acta Med Scand* 1931; **76**: 521–50.

4 von Willebrand EA. Uber ein neues vererbbares Blutungsubel: Die konstitutionelle Thrombopathie. *Dtsc Arch Klin Med* 1933; **175**: 453–83.

5 von Willebrand A, Jürgens R. Über eine neues vererbbares Blutungsübel: die konstitutionelle Thrombopathie. *Deutsches Archiv für Klinische Medizin*: München, Leipzig, 1933, vol. 175, pp. 453–483.

6 von Willebrand E, Jürgens R, Dahlberg U. Konstitutionell trombopati, en ny ärftlig blödarsjukdom. *Finska Läkaresällskapets Handlingar* 1934; **LXXVI**: 193–232.

7 Minot GR. A familial hemorrhagic condition associated with prolongation of the bleeding time. *Amer J Med Sci* 1928; **175**: 301.

8 Kasper C. *Von Willebrand Disease. An Introductionary Discussion for Young Physicians*. World Federation of Hemophilia: Montreal, Canada, 2004.

9 Owen JCA, ed. *Inherited coagulation factor deficiencies*. Mayo Foundation for Medical Education and Research: Rochester, 2001.

10 Alexander B, Goldstein R. Dual hemostatic defect in pseudohemophilia. *J Clin Invest* 1953; **32**: 551.

11 Blombäck B. A journey with bleeding time factor. *Compr Biochem* 2007; **45**: 209–55.

12 Larrieu M-J, Soulier J-P. Deficit en facteur antihe'mophilique A, chez une fille associe'a'un trouble du saignement. *Revue d'hematologie* 1953; **8**: 361–70.

13 Blombäck B, Blombäck M. Purification of human and bovine fibrinogen. *Ark Kemi* 1956; **10**: 415–43.

14 Nilsson IM, Blombäck B, Blombäck M, Svennerud S. Kvinnlig hämofili och dess behandling med humant antihämofiliglobulin. *Nordisk Medicin* 1956; **56**: 1654–62.

15 Nilsson IM, Blombäck M, Jorpes E, Blombäck B, Johansson SA. Von Willebrand's disease and its correction with human plasma fraction I-O. *Acta Med Scand* 1957; **159**: 179–88.

16 Nilsson IM, Holmberg L. Von Willebrand's disease today. *Clin Haematol* 1979; **8**: 147–68.

17 Jürgens R, Lehmann W, Wegelius O, Eriksson AW, Hiepler E. Mitteilung uber den Mangel an antihämophilem Globulin (Faktor VIII) bei der Aaländisschen Thrombopatitie (von Willebrand–Jurgens). *Thromb Diath Haemorrh* 1957; **1**: 257–60.

18 Nilsson IM, Blombäck B, von Francken I. On an inherited autosomal hemorrhagic diathesis with antihemophilic globulin (AHG) deficiency and prolonged bleeding time. *Acta Med Scand* 1957; **159**: 35–57.

19 Nilsson IM, Blombäck M, Blombäck B. von Willebrand's disease in Sweden. Its pathogenesis and treatment. *Acta Med Scand* 1959; **164**: 263–78.

20 Blombäck B. Studies on fibrinogen and antihaemophilic globulin, XIIth Conference of the Protein Foundation on blood cells and plasma proteins, Albany, NY, November 1957. *Vox Sang* 1958; **3**: 58.

21 Blombäck M, Blombäck B, Nilsson IM. Response to fractions in von Willebrand's disease. In: Brinkhous KM (ed). *The Haemophilias*, pp. 286–94. University North Carolina Press: Chapel Hill, 1964.

22 Borchgrevink CF. A method for measuring platelet adhesiveness *in vivo*. *Acta Med Scand* 1960; **168**: 157–64.

23 Salzman EW. Measurement of platelet adhesiveness. A simple *in vitro* technique demonstrating an abnormality in von Willebrand's disease. *J Lab Clin Med* 1963; **62**: 724–35.

24 Hellem AJ. The adhesiveness of human blood platelets *in vitro*. *Scand J Clin Lab Invest* 1960; **12** (Suppl. 51): 1–115.

25 Larrieu MJ, Caen JP, Meyer DO, Vainer H, Sultan Y, Bernard J. Congenital bleeding disorders with long bleeding time and normal platelet count. II. von Willebrand's disease (report of thirty-seven patients). *Am J Med* 1968; **45**: 354–72.

26 Meyer DO, Larrieu MJ. von Willebrand's factor and platelet adhesiveness. *J Clin Pathol* 1970; **23**: 228–31.

27 Jörgensen L, Borchgrevink CF. The haemostatic mechanism in patients with haemorrhagic diseases. *Acta Athol Microbiol Scand* 1964; **60**: 55–82.

28 Nyman D, Blombäck M, Lehmann W, Frants RR, Eriksson AW, eds. *Blood Coagulation Studies in Bleeder Families on Åland Islands*. Academic Press: New York and London, 1980.

29 Zhang ZP, Blombäck M, Egberg N, Falk G, Anvret M. Characterization of the von Willebrand factor gene (VWF) in von Willebrand disease type III patients from 24 families of Swedish and Finnish origin. *Genomics* 1994; **21**: 188–93.

30 Zhang ZP, Blombäck M, Nyman D, Anvret M. Mutations of von Willebrand factor gene in families with von Willebrand disease in the Åland Islands. *Proc Natl Acad Sci U S A* 1993; **90**: 7937–40.

31 Zimmerman TS, Ratnoff OD, Powell AE. Immunologic differentiation of classic hemophilia (factor 8 deficiency) and von Willebrand's disease, with observations on combined deficiencies of antihemophilic factor and proaccelerin (factor V) and on an acquired circulating anticoagulant against antihemophilic factor. *J Clin Invest* 1971; **50**: 244–54.

32 Ginsburg D, Handin RI, Bonthron DT, *et al.* Human von Willebrand factor (vWF): isolation of complementary DNA (cDNA) clones and chromosomal localization. *Science* 1985; **228**: 1401–6.

33 Lynch DC, Zimmerman TS, Collins CJ, *et al.* Molecular cloning of cDNA for human von Willebrand factor: authentication by a new method. *Cell* 1985; **41**: 49–56.

34 Sadler JE, Shelton-Inloes BB, Sorace JM, Harlan JM, Titani K, Davie EW. Cloning and characterization of two cDNAs coding for human von Willebrand factor. *Proc Natl Acad Sci U S A* 1985; **82**: 6394–8.

35 Verweij CL, de Vries CJM, Distel B, *et al.* Construction of cDA coding for human von Willebrand factor using antibody probes for colony-screening and mapping of the chromosomal gene. *Nucleic Acids Res* 1985; **13**: 4699.

36 Titani K, Kumar S, Takio K, *et al.* Amino acid sequence of human von Willebrand factor. *Biochemistry* 1986; **25**: 3171–84.

37 Sadler JE, Budde U, Eikenboom JC, *et al.* Update on the pathophysiology and classification of von Willebrand disease: a report of the Subcommittee on von Willebrand Factor. *J Thromb Haemost* 2006; **4**: 2103–14.

38 Mannucci PM. How I treat patients with von Willebrand disease. *Blood* 2001; **97**: 1915–19.

39 Federici AB, Mannucci PM. Management of inherited von Willebrand disease in 2007. *Ann Med* 2007; **39**: 346–58.

2 Biosynthesis and organization of von Willebrand factor

Sandra L. Haberichter
Department of Pediatrics, Medical College of Wisconsin, Milwaukee, WI, USA

Introduction

von Willebrand factor (VWF) is a large multimeric adhesive plasma glycoprotein that is synthesized in megakaryocytes and endothelial cells [1–3]. Decreased levels or defective function of VWF cause the most common inherited bleeding disorder, von Willebrand disease (VWD) [4–10], which has a prevalence estimated by some to be as high as 1% [11,12]. The primary function of VWF is to promote platelet binding to subendothelial tissue at the site of a vascular injury. VWF also mediates platelet–platelet interactions, promoting further clotting. A second critical role for VWF is that it serves as the carrier protein for coagulation factor VIII (FVIII), protecting it from proteolytic degradation in plasma. The biosynthesis and organization of VWF involves a complex intracellular pathway; defects at any point in this pathway may contribute to the decreased plasma VWF level or dysfunction that causes VWD.

Terminology

It was not known until the 1970s that VWF and FVIII are different proteins with distinct functions [13–16]. VWF is the carrier protein for FVIII in plasma; thus, these two proteins are intimately associated with one another and may copurify when isolated from plasma, leading to erroneous identification. Earlier reports referred to VWF as "FVIII-related antigen," and this confusion in terminology occasionally still occurs in texts today [17].

Von Willebrand Disease, 1st edition. Edited by Augusto B. Federici, Christine A. Lee, Erik E. Berntorp, David Lillicrap, Robert R. Montgomery. © 2011 Blackwell Publishing Ltd.

A second antigen is absent from plasma and platelets in patients with severe VWD [18]. This additional antigen was historically called von Willebrand antigen II (VW AgII) but is now termed the VWF propeptide (VWFpp) [18,19]. VWFpp was subsequently found to be synthesized in endothelial cells together with VWF [20]. When the *VWF* gene was later cloned, it was discovered that the N-terminal sequence of pro-VWF was identical to that of VWFpp [19,21]. It is now well established that VWFpp is the 741-amino acid propeptide of VWF that is cleaved from VWF, stored with it in Weibel–Palade bodies of endothelial cells and α-granules in megakaryocytes, and released with VWF into plasma from these storage organelles [19,20,22–25].

Molecular biology of VWF

The *VWF* gene

The coding sequence for VWF was first identified in 1985 by four independent groups [26–29]. The VWF mRNA was shown to be approximately 9 kb in size. After the coding sequence for VWF was identified, the entire *VWF* gene was cloned [30]. The gene has been localized to chromosome 12 [27,31]. The complete intron/exon sequence has been determined, and the 52 exons span approximately 178 kb [30]. The size of exons varies between 40 bp and 1.4 kb for exon 28. A second, partial VWF sequence has been identified on chromosome 22. This pseudogene shows 97% homology with the authentic *VWF* gene on chromosome 12. However, the occurrence of several stop codons within the coding sequence indicates that this gene is not expressed in humans. The presence of this second pseudogene can cause problems in identifying sequence abnormalities in patients with VWD, although this can be overcome with proper design of sequencing primers [32–34].

VWF domain structure

The open reading frame of the VWF cDNA predicts a 2813-amino acid protein as the primary translation product (Figure 2.1a). The transcriptional start site is located 245 nucleotides upstream of the initiator methionine [35]. Using the current numbering system, the initiating methionine codon is defined as nucleotide number one and the corresponding methionine residue is defined as amino acid 1. The N-terminal segment of VWF includes a hydrophobic 22-amino acid signal peptide and a 741-amino acid propeptide (VWFpp) followed by a 2050-amino acid mature VWF molecule (Figure 2.1a). The propeptide is proteolytically removed from the mature VWF protein in the Golgi, presumably by the enzyme furin (PACE). The VWF protein is composed of a series of repeated

homologous domains that are termed A, B, C, and D domains (Figure 2.1b) [25,36–43]. The propeptide contains two D domains, D1 and D2. The mature VWF protein is composed of D′-D3-A1-A2-A3-D4-B1-B2-B3-C1-C2-CK domains. Comparison of VWF domain sequences with other known protein and DNA sequences identifies several sequence homologies. The A domains have been found to be similar to complement factors B and C2, type VI collagen, chicken cartilage matrix protein, and the α-chains of the leukocyte adhesion molecules Mac-1, p150, 95, and LFA-1 [44,45]. A sequence similarity between small segments of the VWF C1 and C2 domains and thrombospondin has also been identified [46,47]. The D domains of VWF show homology to vitellogenins [48]; however, the importance of these homologies to VWF function is unknown.

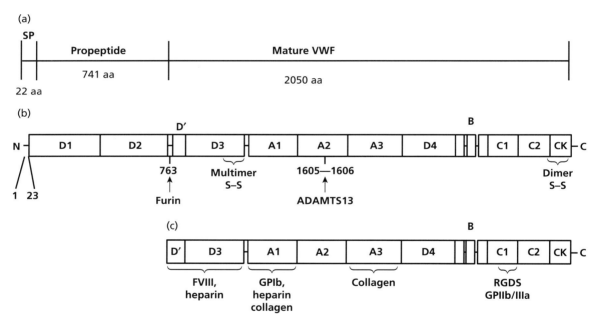

Figure 2.1 Domain structure of von Willebrand factor (VWF). (a) VWF is synthesized as pre-pro-VWF containing a 22-amino acid signal peptide (SP), 741-amino acid propeptide (VWFpp), and 2050-amino acid mature VWF molecule. (b) The VWF protein consists of a series of repeated homologous A, B, C, and D domains. VWFpp consists of the D1 and D2 domains. Mature VWF comprises D1-D3-A1-A2-A3-D4-B1-B2-B3-C1-C2-CK domains. VWFpp is proteolytically cleaved from mature VWF at amino acid 763 by the enzyme furin. The D3 domains contain cysteine residues that participate in the multimerization of VWF. In plasma, VWF is proteolytically cleaved by the ADAMTS13 and the cleavage site is located in the A2 domain, between amino acids 1605 and 1606. The last 150 amino acids of VWF, including the CK domain, are important in the C-terminal dimerization of VWF that precedes multimerization. (c) Various functional domains have been identified in the mature VWF protein and contain sites for interaction with coagulation factor VIII, heparin, platelet glycoprotein GPIb, collagen, and platelet glycoprotein GPIIb/IIIa. This research was originally published in *Blood* [119] © the American Society of Hematology.

Several functions of VWF have been mapped to specific VWF domains (Figure 2.1c). The D′-D3 domains are important in binding FVIII to VWF [49–51]. The VWF A1 domain is essential in binding VWF to platelets through the platelet receptor glycoprotein, GPIbα [52–56], and also contains binding sites for heparin and collagen [52,57–59]. The A2 domain contains the cleavage site for post-secretion processing of VWF by the VWF-cleaving protease, ADAMTS13 [60–65]. The A3 domain has been reported to contain a binding site for collagen [66–69]. The C1 domain contains an Arg-Gly-Asp-Ser (RGDS) sequence that may bind the platelet glycoprotein GPIIb/IIIa [70].

Mutations in these binding domains have been found in patients with VWD. Patients with type 2N VWD have decreased plasma VWF levels as a result of substantially impaired FVIII binding to VWF [8,10]. Mutations have been identified in the D′-D3 domains in several of these individuals [71–77]. Type 2B VWD is characterized by a loss of plasma high-molecular-weight multimers resulting from the spontaneous binding of VWF to platelets. Mutations in patients with type 2B VWD have been identified in the A1 domain, which contains a binding site for the platelet glycoprotein GPIb [78–82]. Other mutations in the A1 domain prevent the binding of VWF to platelets, characteristic of type 2M VWD [83–85]. Individuals with type 2A VWD have decreased high-molecular-weight multimers and a platelet-binding function. Type 2A VWD results from at least two distinct mechanisms, defective multimerization and secretion, or increased susceptibility to proteolysis by ADAMTS13 [86,87]. Mutations causing increased cleavage by ADAMTS13 are likely to be identified in the A2 domain, which contains the cleavage site for ADAMTS13 proteolysis [88–92]. Mutations causing defective multimerization and secretion have been identified in the D1, D2, D′-D3, A1, A2, and CK domains of VWF [93–98]. Mutations associated with impaired binding of VWF to collagen have also been identified [99].

VWF promoter

The VWF promoter is complex, and several upstream regulatory elements controlling VWF expression have been identified. A number of consensus sequences for *cis*-acting elements has been defined in the upstream promoter region and in the first exon, including two GATA-binding sequences [100]. The endothelial cell-specific regulation of VWF expression has been investigated and found to be controlled by a repressor–derepressor mechanism involving an NF1 binding site, an Oct-1 binding site, and Ets transcription factors [35,100–105]. In addition to endothelial cell-specific expression, there are also complex pathways of transcriptional regulation through vascular bed-specific regulation. This vascular bed-specific regulation of the endothelial cell *VWF* gene is controlled by the tissue microenvironment [106]. The E4BP4 transcriptional repressor has also played a role in the cell type-specific regulation of VWF expression [107]. Additionally, single nucleotide polymorphisms (SNPs) in the VWF regulatory region have been identified that are associated with plasma VWF Ag levels, including the nucleotides –1793, –1234, –1185, and –1051. The regulation of VWF expression is complex and controlled by cell-specific and vascular bed-specific regulatory elements.

Cell biology of VWF

von Willebrand factor is synthesized exclusively in endothelial cells and megakaryocytes [108–110]. The processing of VWF involves a very complicated sequence of events. Most of the studies on VWF processing, assembly, and secretion have utilized cultured endothelial cells or transfected mammalian cells, although some studies on VWF expression in megakaryocytes have also been reported [3,19,25,40, 41,108,110,111–124]. The processing of VWF in endothelial cells and megakaryocytes appears to be similar, as VWF from both sources is structurally alike. In both endothelial cells and platelets produced by megakaryocytes, VWF forms high molecular weight multimers and is packaged in secretory vesicles; Weibel–Palade bodies in endothelial cells and α-granules in megakaryocytes [3,122]. Much of our understanding of VWF processing comes from expression studies using a variety of mammalian cells, as summarized in the following paragraphs.

VWF processing and dimerization in the endoplasmic reticulum

When moving through the cell's secretory pathway, VWF undergoes extensive intracellular modifications

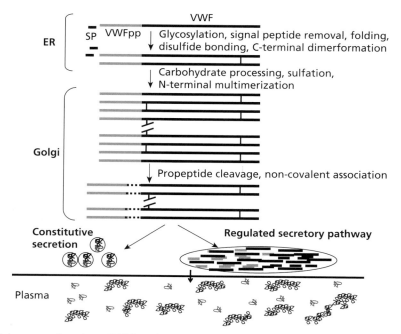

Figure 2.2 Intracellular processing of von Willebrand factor (VWF). The pathway of VWF biosynthesis and organization is depicted in this illustration. The VWF protomer is synthesized as pre-pro-VWF. In the endoplasmic reticulum (ER), VWF is folded, disulfide bonds are formed, glycosylation occurs, the signal peptide is removed, and pro-VWF forms C-terminal dimers. Upon transport to the Golgi apparatus (Golgi), the carbohydrates are processed into complex oligosaccharides, sulfation occurs, and C-terminal pro-VWF dimers are assembled into high molecular weight multimers. Before exiting the Golgi, VWFpp is proteolytically cleaved from VWF, but remains noncovalently associated with the mature VWF multimers. Both VWFpp and mature VWF multimers are either constitutively secreted or routed to regulated secretory granules, Weibel–Palade bodies in endothelial cells, or α-granules in platelets. Once secreted into plasma through either the constitutive or regulated secretory pathway, VWFpp and mature VWF multimers cease to be noncovalently associated and circulate in plasma independently of one another. This research was originally published in *Blood* [119] © the American Society of Hematology.

(Figure 2.2). VWF is initially synthesized as pre-pro-VWF containing a signal peptide, propeptide, and mature VWF polypeptide. In the endoplasmic reticulum, the signal peptide is removed, the pro-VWF protein is folded, and disulfide bonds are formed (Figure 2.2). VWF is a cysteine-rich protein with 64 cysteine residues in VWFpp and 170 cysteines in the mature VWF protein [21]. In the secreted VWF protein all cysteines appear to be involved in disulfide bonds, as historically no free sulfhydryls have been detected. However, some recent studies employing more sensitive techniques suggest that there may indeed be some reactive unpaired cysteines in plasma VWF [112,125]. While the mapping of disulfide bonds has been accomplished for some cysteines in VWF, the majority of disulfide mapping is unre-

solved [126–129]. Given the number of cysteines in the full-length VWF, the process of protein folding and disulfide bonding must be exceptionally complicated.

In the endoplasmic reticulum, the pro-VWF subunits form carboxyl-terminal dimers (Figures 2.2 and 2.3). This dimerization involves the last 151 amino acids of the mature VWF protein [117,130]. Voorberg *et al.* [117] have demonstrated that recombinant VWF which lacks these 151 amino acids fails to dimerize and is proteolytically degraded in the endoplasmic reticulum. Thus, these carboxyl-terminal sequences may serve a role in retaining monomers in the endoplasmic reticulum until they are either dimerized or degraded. The last 90 residues of VWF comprise the CK domain, which contains a sequence

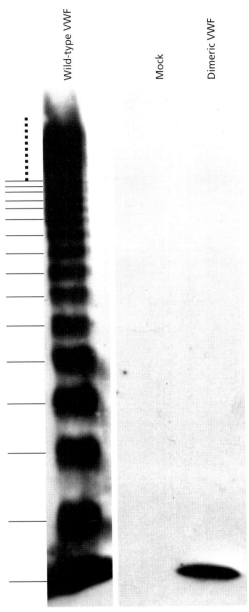

Figure 2.3 von Willebrand factor (VWF) forms high molecular weight multimers. VWF forms a C-terminal dimer in the endoplasmic reticulum, which is generally the smallest form of VWF secreted into plasma. In the Golgi, these C-terminal dimers form N-terminal disulfide bonds to create tetramers, hexamers, octomers, and other such high molecular weight oligomers. The multimeric structure of expressed VWF constructs was analyzed nonreduced on a 2% agarose-SDS gel. Expressed wild-type VWF (lane 2, "Wild-type VWF") shows a full range of multimers. The mock transfected control is shown in lane 2 (Mock). Expression of propeptide-deleted VWF results in loss of multimerization and only a dimeric VWF species is secreted (lane 3, "Dimeric VWF"). The highest molecular weight VWF multimers are the most active in platelet binding and clot formation. This research was originally published in *Blood* [119] © the American Society of Hematology.

homologous to the cysteine knot family of proteins. The common characteristic of this family of proteins is the tendency to dimerize through the formation of disulfide bonds. Further evidence of the importance of this region to VWF dimerization has been provided by an investigation of patients with VWD who have VWF structural abnormalities. Several mutations have been identified in this region of VWF, including C2362F, C2739Y, C2754W, C2773R, and A2801D variants. Expression studies using mutated recombinant VWF variants demonstrated a defective formation of VWF dimers, indicating the critical role of the carboxyl-terminal region in dimerization [97, 131–134]. While the importance of the C-terminal portion of VWF in dimerization is clear, the N-terminal has been found to be less important. The large propeptide VWFpp (pro-VWF) is not necessary for dimerization. Expression of a propeptide-deleted mature VWF (signal peptide sequence followed by mature VWF sequence) results in the secretion of a dimeric VWF protein, indicating that VWFpp is not necessary for the formation of dimers or for exit from the endoplasmic reticulum [41,135,136].

In addition to protein folding, disulfide formation, and dimerization, the large pro-VWF is also extensively modified in the endoplasmic reticulum by addition of high-mannose carbohydrate side chains. The mature VWF protein contains 12 N-linked and 10 O-linked glycosylation sites, and VWFpp contains three potential N-linked sites [137]. The O- and N-linked carbohydrates account for approximately 18–19% of the total VWF protein mass. Interestingly, the N-linked oligosaccharides of the plasma VWF protein contain ABO blood group oligosaccharides [138]. Wagner and colleagues [123] found that when human endothelial cells were metabolically labeled, it took approximately 120 minutes for VWF with complex-type oligosaccharide chains to be detected. As soon as metabolically labeled VWF was detected in the cell, it was also found to be constitutively secreted. The exit of pro-VWF from the endoplasmic reticulum appears to be the rate-limiting step in VWF biosynthesis, as it is for other proteins [139,140]. The exit of VWF from the endoplasmic reticulum is dependent upon both glycosylation and dimerization. When N-linked glycosylation is blocked by the addition of tunicamycin to the culture medium of endothelial cells, as reported by Wagner et al., pro-VWF monomers accumulate in the endoplasmic reticulum. These results also indicate that glycosylation is required for dimerization to occur [111]. In addition to glycosylation and dimerization, exit from the endoplasmic reticulum is also dependent upon proper folding of the VWF protein. Misfolded proteins are selected in the endoplasmic reticulum and targeted for degradation, although many cells may retain misfolded proteins in the endoplasmic reticulum [141,142]. A number of mutations have been identified in patients with VWD that result in impaired VWF secretion or endoplasmic reticulum degradation [143–146]. Defective VWF processing within the endoplasmic reticulum may contribute to the VWD phenotype observed in patients.

VWF processing in the Golgi

When pro-VWF dimers reach the Golgi, the high-mannose glycans are trimmed and galactose and sialic acid are added to form complex-type carbohydrates. Some of the N-linked oligosaccharides are sulfated during transport through the Golgi [147]. Here, the carboxyl-terminal pro-VWF dimers form amino terminal-linked multimers that may exceed 20 million a in size (Figures 2.2 and 2.3). VWF multimerization will be discussed in more detail below. An additional modification that occurs in the Golgi is the proteolytic removal of the 741-amino acid VWFpp (Figure 2.2). Pulse-chase experiments have demonstrated that propeptide cleavage and amino-terminal multimerization of VWF dimers occur at about the same time [123,148]. In a study by Vischer and Wagner [40], both VWFpp cleavage and multimer formation were found to occur after VWF is sulfated. VWFpp is believed to be cleaved from mature VWF by the enzyme furin. The cleavage of VWFpp appears to occur in the Golgi as furin has been found to collocalize with other Golgi resident proteins [149–152]. The site of propeptide cleavage is targeted by the sequence motif Arg-Xxx-Arg/Lys-Arg at the carboxyl-terminal end of the propeptide. The furin-cleaved VWFpp remains associated with the mature VWF multimers until both proteins are eventually secreted from the cell [25,41,113,119,153]. At pH 6.4, in the presence of calcium, mature VWF and VWFpp are associated, while at pH 7.4 this interaction is not sustained [40]. The conditions that promote association are similar to the pH and calcium levels found in the Golgi, which is thought to have a pH near 6.2 and a

10 mmol/L calcium concentration [154,155]. In contrast, VWFpp and mature VWF circulate independently in plasma, which has an approximate pH of 7.4.

VWF multimerization

The unique process of VWF multimerization has been extensively investigated. The compartmentalization of VWF processing steps is best represented by these two distinct VWF polymerization steps. Dimerization of VWF has been shown to be a step that is independent of VWF multimerization [116,132]. The carboxyl-terminal dimerization of VWF discussed above is accomplished in the endoplasmic reticulum, while amino-terminal multimerization of C-terminal VWF dimers is completed in the Golgi. The differential compartmentalization of these two processes implies that different enzymes or mechanisms regulate these two events. The endoplasmic reticulum is the most likely site for disulfide bond formation where the neutral pH and necessary oxidoreductase enzymes, such as protein disulfide isomerase (PDI), promote the process of disulfide bonding [156,157]. The acidic pH, together with the lack of chaperones and oxidoreductases in the Golgi, make for a desolate environment for disulfide bond formation and rearrangement. However, VWF multimers are formed in a head-to-head orientation between adjacent D3 domains within C-terminal dimers to create oligomers that can exceed 20 million Da in size (Figure 2.3). Endoplasmic reticulum to Golgi transport vesicles may not be able to accommodate the excessively large VWF multimers [117,123]. For this reason, VWF has evolved a unique mechanism to accomplish multimerization in the Golgi [158].

The critical role of VWFpp in the multimerization of VWF has been documented by a number of independent studies. Deletion of VWFpp does not affect the secretion of VWF from the cell, but the secreted VWF is in a dimeric form and multimerization is completely abolished [116,135,136]. Multimerization of this dimeric VWFpp-deleted VWF can be restored by coexpression with VWFpp. Expression of VWFpp and VWFpp-deleted mature VWF as two separate expression plasmids results in the formation of a normal spectrum of VWF multimers [136]. VWFpp does not need to be expressed as a contiguous protein with VWF (e.g., pro-VWF) to facilitate VWF multimerization. However, a study by Verweij and col-

leagues [159] demonstrated that VWFpp cleavage from mature VWF is not a prerequisite for multimerization. The introduction of a mutation that prevents furin cleavage, Arg763Gly, still permitted the formation of high molecular weight VWF multimers. VWF multimerization has also been demonstrated using VWF dimers in a cell-free system. A continued presence of an acidic pH was required for multimerization to proceed. However, in this cell-free system, multimerization required VWFpp to be a contiguous part of VWF. Only pro-VWF dimers formed high molecular weight multimers [112]. In sum, these studies indicate that VWFpp can facilitate multimerization of VWF dimers when expressed either as full-length VWF or as two separate proteins. VWFpp is absolutely required for VWF multimerization whether expressed *in cis* or *in trans*.

Both the D1 and D2 domains that comprise VWFpp are necessary to accomplish VWF multimerization. Journet and coworkers [114] demonstrated that the deletion of either domain results in the formation and secretion of VWF dimers. The D domains in VWF are rich in cysteine residues and fairly homologous, with alignment of 23 cysteines between the four D domains [21]. Both the D1 and D2 domains contain vicinal cysteine motifs, CXXC sequences (159-CGLC and 521-CGLC) that are similar to those found at the active site of disulfide isomerases. A study by Mayadas and Wagner [160] showed that insertion of a glycine residue into either of these vicinal cysteine motifs results in the formation of dimers. The dimeric VWF was efficiently transported to the Golgi and secreted from the cell, indicating that the insertion did not have a global structural effect but did abolish multimerization, highlighting the importance of the vicinal cysteines in VWF multimerization.

It has been proposed that VWF may overcome the limitations of the Golgi environment by using its own propeptide to facilitate multimerization by catalyzing disulfide exchange through use of these vicinal cysteines. This mechanism would predict that VWFpp and the mature VWF subunit should form a transient disulfide bond in the cell before multimerization. Recently, this type of intermediate has been identified in the endoplasmic reticulum by expression studies using a recombinant D1-D2-D′-D3 truncated VWF protein and two-dimensional gel electrophoresis [161]. The disulfide-linked intermediate was found to rearrange in the Golgi, and both free VWFpp and

13

D′-D3 dimers were secreted from the cell. This study provided support for the model in which VWFpp functions as an oxidoreductase to facilitate multimerization of VWF in the Golgi. In an extension of this study, two amino acids in the D3 domain of VWF were identified that were important in the multimerization process. Both Cys-1099 and Cys-1142 were found to be oxidized when VWF multimerization succeeds and reduced when it does not [128]. When either cysteine is mutated to an alanine, multimerization did not occur. The exact nature of how these cysteines form intersubunit disulfide bonds is unknown.

Defects in the multimerization of VWF are one cause of type 2A VWD in patients. Patients with type 2A VWD are characterized by decreased high molecular weight multimers and decreased platelet binding function [10]. The lack of high molecular weight multimers in these patients is the result of either increased degradation of plasma multimers by ADAMTS13 or defective multimerization and secretion from the cell [88,93]. In the case of type 2A VWD caused by increased ADAMTS13 cleavage, the VWF undergoes normal multimerization within the cell but is degraded upon secretion into plasma. The majority of mutations in individuals with this type of VWD have been identified

in the A2 domain [92]. Other type 2A VWD mutations cause defects in multimer formation within the cell. Mutations in these patients have been identified in both the D1 and D2 domains of VWFpp, the D3, and CK domains of mature VWF [94,95,97,98,133,162,163]. Not surprisingly, these are the domains that are believed to play a significant role in multimer formation. Defective VWF processing within Golgi may contribute to the VWD phenotype observed in patients.

Regulated storage of VWF in Weibel–Palade bodies and α-granules

von Willebrand factor is synthesized exclusively in endothelial cells and platelets produced by megakaryocytes, and is stored for regulated release in Weibel–Palade bodies and α-granules (Figure 2.4) [108,110,122,164]. Regulated secretion allows for the rapid release of stored proteins at a local site to modulate coagulation, fibrinolysis, and inflammation. The Weibel–Palade body is a rod-shaped organelle (Figure 2.4) that is 1–2 μm in width and up to 4 μm in length [165]. These granules have longitudinal striations comprising closely packed tubules that are composed of VWF multimers. Platelet α-granules appear

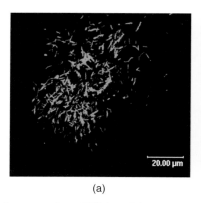
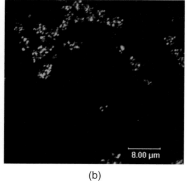

(a) (b)

Figure 2.4 Regulated storage of von Willebrand factor (VWF) in endothelial cells and platelets produced by megakaryocytes. Endothelial cells and platelets store VWF in regulated secretory granules termed Weibel–Palade bodies and α-granules, respectively. (a) VWF in human umbilical vein endothelial cell Weibel–Palade bodies. Weibel–Palade bodies are rod-shaped granules up to 4 μm in length consisting of closely packed tubules of VWF. Human umbilical endothelial cells were cultured on slides, fixed, permeabilized, immunostained for VWF, and examined by confocal microscopy. VWF appears to be package in long rod-like Weibel–Palade bodies. (b) VWF in human platelet α-granules. Platelet α-granules also contain similar tubular structures, but the granules are not elongated or rod-like. Human platelets were spun on slides, fixed, permeabilized, immunostained for VWF and examined by confocal microscopy. VWF is localized in α-granules that are much smaller than Weibel–Palade bodies. This research was originally published in *Blood* [119] © the American Society of Hematology.

to contain similar groups of tubular structures when examined by electron microscopy [164]. The VWF stored in Weibel–Palade bodies and α-granules contains some of the highest molecular weight multimers that are the most efficient for binding to extracellular matrix and to platelets to promote hemostasis [121]. Endothelial cell Weibel–Palade bodies and platelet α-granules also contain the membrane protein P-selectin among other proteins [166,167]. When Weibel–Palade bodies or α-granules undergo exocytosis, VWF is released and P-selectin is expressed on the surface within minutes of exposure to an agonist. *In vivo*, exposure to physiologic stimuli including exercise and epinephrine or administration of DDAVP (1-deamino-8-D-arginine vasopressin) results in a rapid rise in plasma VWF levels, presumably owing to exocytosis from Weibel–Palade bodies [168,169]. The mechanisms controlling the trafficking of VWF to the regulated storage pathway have been extensively investigated. While some studies have examined the storage of VWF in α-granules, the majority of studies on VWF-regulated storage have utilized cultured endothelial cells or transfected mammalian cells.

In addition to VWF, VWFpp is also stored in endothelial cell Weibel–Palade bodies and platelet α-granules [153]. In Weibel–Palade bodies, mature VWF and VWFpp are found in a 1:1 molar ratio [25]. When expressed in a variety of mammalian cells, including AtT-20 mouse pituitary cells, CV-1 monkey kidney cells, MDCK cells, and RIN5F rat insulinoma cells, VWF is trafficked to storage granules [41,113, 118,170]. Expression studies utilizing transfected mammalian cells have shown that VWFpp is required for the targeting of VWF to storage granules [113]. A similar requirement for regulated storage has been documented for the propeptide of prosomatostatin [171]. Expression of mature VWF lacking its propeptide results in the loss of VWF trafficking to storage granules [41,118,122]. Coexpression of mature VWF *in trans* with VWFpp, as two separate expression plasmids, results in the restoration of granular trafficking of VWF, indicating that VWF granular storage does not require VWFpp to be a contiguous part of VWF [41,118]. Both of the D domains have been reported by Journet and coworkers [114] to be necessary for granular trafficking to storage, and deletion of either domain results in loss of VWF granules.

In general, the mechanisms by which proteins are trafficked into storage granules are not completely defined. Secretory granules form in the trans-Golgi network (TGN) initially as immature secretory granules. Subsequent processing events convert these immature secretory granules to mature secretory granules by fusion of vesicles and removal of proteins and membrane proteins. There have been at least two mechanisms proposed for the trafficking of proteins to the regulated secretory pathway [155,172]. The first suggests that specific sorting signals within the stored protein interact with receptors that target the protein to the secretory granule. The second mechanism proposes that secretory proteins condense in the TGN and the selective aggregation of proteins is a key event in the formation of the storage granule. In addition, trafficking to granules involves an association between the protein and lipid rafts in the membrane [173]. Recent studies have suggested that both mechanisms, aggregation and sorting signals, are involved in sorting proteins to regulated storage vesicles, and the relative contribution of these mechanisms may be dependent on the cell type as well as the regulated secretory protein itself [174,175].

Several lines of evidence indicate that VWFpp plays an active role in trafficking VWF to the regulated storage pathway. Propeptide-deleted mature VWF (Δpro) expressed alone in AtT-20 cells does not traffic to granules but instead demonstrates diffuse staining, indicative of endoplasmic reticulum localization (Figure 2.5). In contrast, VWFpp independently traffics to endogenous ACTH-containing storage granules in AtT-20 cells (Figure 2.5) and to Weibel–Palade bodies in endothelial cells [41,42]. When VWFpp was covalently linked to an unrelated, nonsecretory granule protein, C3α, and expressed in bovine aortic endothelial cells, both VWFpp and C3α were trafficked to Weibel–Palade bodies where they underwent regulated release [42]. These studies indicate that VWFpp contains the necessary signal, either a linear sequence or conformation, for sorting to the regulated secretory pathway. When a series of C-terminal and N-terminal truncations of VWFpp were expressed in AtT-20 cells, a truncated VWFpp comprising amino acids 387–545 was found to be co-localized in storage granules with endogenous ACTH [176]. The putative sorting signal may be located in the first 140 amino acids of the D2 domain of VWFpp.

When VWFpp is expressed *in trans* with mature VWF, both proteins are stored in granules (Figure 2.5) [41,118]. Studies suggest that VWFpp functions as an

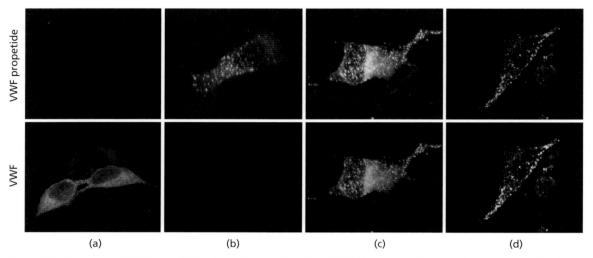

Figure 2.5 Expression of VWF in AtT-20 cells. (a) Propeptide-deleted VWF is not sorted to granules, (b) propeptide alone sorts to granules, (c) propeptide co-expressed with peptide-deleted VWF sorts to granules, (d) full-length VWF sorts to granules.

intracellular chaperone: VWFpp contains the signal for sorting to granules and co-traffics mature VWF [41,118]. In this model, VWFpp and mature VWF remain associated in the Golgi and traffic together to the granule. The low pH and calcium concentration that are found in the Golgi promote this association, while at a plasma pH of 7.4 this association is not maintained [40]. This model requires a site within VWFpp for association with VWF and, conversely, a site within mature VWF for interaction with VWFpp. By using a series of human/canine chimeric VWFpp and mature VWF expression plasmids, and exploiting the differential interspecies storage difference, potential interaction sites have been identified [119]. Amino acid 416 in the D2 domain of VWF and amino acid 869 in the D3 domain of mature VWF were found to be critical for the noncovalent interaction and subsequent storage of VWF. It is not clear whether these two amino acids directly interact or enable a conformation that promotes association. It is very likely that other amino acids are involved in the association of VWFpp and VWF.

Formation of the VWF multimer precedes the formation of Weibel–Palade bodies [40]. However, a number of studies have confirmed that VWF multimerization is not a prerequisite of VWF granular storage. Wagner and colleagues [113] demonstrated that the deletion of a portion of C-terminal VWF

sequence resulted in a dimeric VWF species that was stored in granules. Disruption of either of the vicinal cysteine motifs in VWFpp resulted in a loss of multimerization with normal granular storage [160]. In a study utilizing human/canine chimeric VWFpp and mature VWF expression plasmids, VWF multimerization did not correlate with VWF granular storage: some fully multimerized VWF proteins were not stored in granules while other nonmultimerized VWF proteins were found to be stored in granules [119]. A number of expression studies have been completed characterizing the effects of mutations identified in patients with VWD on VWF multimerization and granular storage. Several mutations including Y87S, R273W, C788R, C1157S, C1225G, and C1234W were found to cause defects in multimerization, yet VWF granular storage was maintained [120,146,162, 177]. These studies suggest that the regions within VWFpp that facilitate VWF multimerization are different from the sites regulating VWF granular storage.

Both multimerization and VWFpp cleavage are thought to be accomplished in the Golgi before the formation of storage granules. Subcellular fractionation of pulse-chased endothelial cells demonstrated that multimerization and cleavage occurred after sulfation but preceded the formation of Weibel–Palade bodies [40]. Furin, the likely VWFpp processing enzyme, has been localized to the TGN [151,178].

Studies exploiting interspecies VWF storage differences also demonstrated that VWFpp was cleaved before the formation of storage granules in AtT-20 cells [41]. When a full-length canine VWFpp-human mature VWF protein with an intact furin cleavage site was expressed, human VWF was not trafficked to storage granules even though normal granular storage of canine VWFpp was maintained. Further evidence was provided in a study utilizing a construct expressing VWFpp linked to the unrelated nonsecretory granule protein C3α with either an intact furin cleavage site or a disrupted cleavage site between the two proteins [42]. When the furin cleavage site was disrupted, both VWFpp and C3α were routed to storage granules. When the furin cleavage site was intact, only VWFpp was trafficked to granules and C3α was endoplasmic reticulum localized. These experiments demonstrated that VWF cleavage is complete before granule formation and that the "proper" sorting of proteins to granules is a fairly efficient process. Two different VWF mutations causing a lack of VWFpp cleavage have been characterized, an Arg763Gly mutation and a splice site mutation causing loss of the furin cleavage site [118,179]. Both variants were trafficked to storage granules, demonstrating that cleavage of VWFpp from mature VWF does not appear to be a prerequisite for granular trafficking.

Weibel–Palade body biogenesis

Expression studies of VWF have utilized several different cell lines, including AtT-20, RIN5F, CV-1, MDCK, HEK-293, COS-1, 3T3, and CHO cells. It was not surprising that cell lines containing endogenous secretory granules, such as AtT-20 and RIN5F cells, were able to traffic VWF into granules and that many cell lines not thought to contain secretory granules, such as COS-1 and CHO cells, did not form VWF-containing granules. However, unexpectedly, expression of VWF induced the formation of VWF-containing granules in HEK293 and MDCK cells which are not thought to have regulated secretory granules [146,170]. Additionally, when VWF is expressed in AtT-20 cells, the VWF-granules that are formed do not co-localize with endogenous ACTH-containing granules, but instead form granules that only contain VWF [180]. These studies indicate that VWF has the ability to induce the formation of its own storage granule.

The biogenesis of the Weibel–Palade body appears to be a VWF-driven event [120,181–183]. Weibel–Palade bodies do not exist in the absence of VWF and cannot be detected in endothelial cells harvested from VWF-deficient dogs (Figure 2.6) and VWF knockout mice [120,184,185]. Neither VWF nor VWFpp expression can be detected in VWD canine aortic endothelial cells (Figure 2.6). In these VWF-null cells, the Weibel–Palade body membrane protein, P-selectin, is redirected to lysosomes. Expression of full-length VWF in VWF-deficient canine endothelial cells (Figure 2.6) and T-24/ECV304 cells resulted in the formation of VWF-containing granules that were morphologically similar to Weibel–Palade bodies [120,186]. In each of these studies, endogenously synthesized P-selectin was redirected from lysosomes to the VWF-containing granule, validating the formation of a Weibel–Palade body. Other expression studies in AtT-20 cells and HEK293 cells have shown that coexpression of VWF and P-selectin results in collocalized granular storage of the two proteins [146, 180]. P-selectin was later found to bind to the D'-D3 domains of VWF [187]. Together, these studies confirm the role of VWF in the biogenesis of the Weibel–Palade body.

Further studies utilizing VWF-deficient endothelial cells from dogs with type 3 VWD demonstrated that both VWFpp and mature VWF were required for the biogenesis of Weibel–Palade bodies [120]. Habericher et al. [120] demonstrated that neither VWFpp nor mature VWF were sufficient for granule formation when expressed independently. By expressing a dimeric VWF variant, Y87S, Haberichter et al. also demonstrated that multimerization was not required for Weibel–Palade body biogenesis, as this variant formed granules that recruited P-selectin. This study suggests that VWFpp may provide the "sorting signal" and mature VWF provides the core of aggregation for granule budding. Expression studies using C-terminal truncations of VWF demonstrated that VWFpp and the D-D3-A1 domains of mature VWF were required to store VWF as tubules that correlate with the elongation of Weibel–Palade bodies [188]. The VWF tubule formation and elongation were both found to be dependent on an acidic pH level. Furthermore, these studies strongly suggested a direct role for VWFpp in compacting VWF into tubules. Most recently, VWF tubule assembly has been recreated in an *in vitro* study using only purified VWFpp

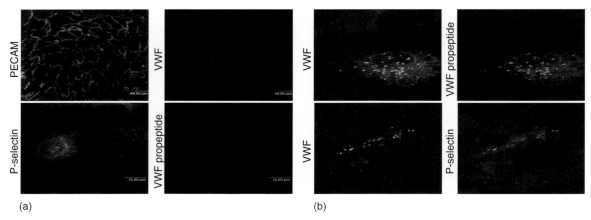

(a) (b)

Figure 2.6 von Willebrand factor (VWF)-dependent Weibel–Palade body biogenesis. (a) VWD endothelial cells. Endothelial cells were harvested from the aortas of dogs with type 3 VWD. Cells were cultured on slides, fixed, permeabilized, immunostained and examined by confocal microscopy. Immunostaining for PECAM (CD31) demonstrated a homogeneous population of endothelial cells. Neither propeptide (VWFpp) nor VWF expression could be detected in these cells. P-selectin staining was found to be mostly diffuse, although several very small granules were detected. VWF-null canine endothelial cells do not appear to contain any Weibel–Palade bodies. (b) VWD endothelial cells transfected with VWF. The VWF-null canine endothelial cells were transfected with full-length wild-type VWF. Staining for VWFpp and VWF revealed collocalized storage of the two proteins in granules. Dual staining for VWF and endogenous P-selectin revealed that P-selectin was recruited to the granule formed by VWF expression. VWF expression induces the formation of a Weibel–Palade-like granule that can recruit P-selectin to the granule membrane. This research was originally published in *Blood* [119] © the American Society of Hematology.

and D′-D3 domains of VWF [189]. Assembly of tubules from these two proteins was found to be dependent upon a low pH and the presence of calcium. A three-dimensional reconstruction of electron microscopy images demonstrated tubules containing a repeating unit of one D′-D3 dimer and two VWFpp molecules. These studies have narrowed the requirements for Weibel–Palade body biogenesis to the D1–D3 domains of VWF. The requirements for VWF trafficking to α-granules in platelets may be similar to Weibel–Palade body trafficking, although mechanisms may not be identical since α-granules are still formed in the absence of VWF.

While VWF is believed to be the most abundant protein in the Weibel–Palade body, several other components have been identified, including P-selectin, the tetraspanin CD63, interleukin 8, osteoprotegerin, α1,3-fucosyltransferase VI, endothelin 1, eotaxin, and tissue plasminogen activator [166,167,190–196]. Although the site of FVIII synthesis has not been unequivocally identified, when expressed together with VWF both proteins traffic to granules together [179,197]. Thus, the loss of Weibel–Palade body formation has substantial biologic implications. Despite the critical role of VWFpp and the D′-D3 domains in Weibel–Palade body formation and the number of mutations identified in these domains in patients with VWD (International Society on Thrombosis and Haemostasis Scientific and Standardization Committee [ISTH SSC] VWF database, http://www.vwf.group.shef.ac.uk/), it remains to be determined whether loss of Weibel–Palade body formation is a common phenomenon in patients with VWF.

Regulated release of VWF

Endothelial cells release VWF and other resident proteins in response to a number of agonists including thrombin, histamine, and several other secretagogues [183]. In patients with VWD, administration of DDAVP results in the release of VWF, presumably from endothelial cell Weibel–Palade bodies [168,169]. The regulated release from Weibel–Palade bodies allows for the very rapid delivery of proteins at a local site of injury. VWF and VWFpp are believed to be the most abundant Weibel–Palade body constituents.

Although earlier studies had suggested that 5–10% of newly synthesized VWF was directed to the regulated secretory pathway, more recent studies estimate that the amount of constitutively secreted VWF is insignificant, and basal release of VWF comes from a post-Golgi storage organelle, presumably the Weibel–Palade body [121,198,199]. The regulated secretion of VWF involves the translocation of Weibel–Palade bodies from the cytoplasm to the plasma membrane and the fusion of these granules with the plasma membrane. The mechanisms controlling the regulated secretion of Weibel–Palade bodies have been investigated by a number of laboratories, and several review articles discuss these mechanisms in detail [183,200–211]. After Weibel–Palade body exocytosis, ultra-long filaments of VWF are released and platelets are captured along the length of the filament [86,188,212]. Platelet activation and aggregation follow, promoting the formation of a platelet plug [213]. While VWF appears to remain associated with the endothelial cell surface following exocytosis, VWFpp rapidly disperses from the site of exocytosis [22]. VWF clearly plays a role in the recruitment of platelets to a site of vascular injury; however, the extracellular function of VWFpp is as yet unresolved.

Interaction of VWF with FVIII

The role of VWF as the carrier protein for FVIII in plasma is well established [8]. It is generally recognized that VWF is synthesized in endothelial cells and megakaryocytes and that FVIII is synthesized in hepatocytes, although expression of FVIII in murine sinusoidal endothelial cells and human microvascular lung endothelial cells has been reported [110,214–218]. When DDAVP is administered to patients with mild VWD or healthy individuals, both VWF and FVIII are released in parallel into plasma, suggesting that the proteins could be synthesized in the same cell. The DDAVP-releasable store of FVIII cannot be restored by the use of VWF or FVIII replacement therapies; instead, it appears that both FVIII and VWF must be endogenously synthesized in the same cell [219,220]. The low levels of FVIII mRNA and protein complicate the identification of cells synthesizing FVIII; thus, the cellular source of DDAVP-releasable FVIII remains controversial. Expression studies using AtT-20 cells have demonstrated that if FVIII and VWF are expressed together, both proteins are stored together in granules [179]. If FVIII is expressed in cells that already synthesize and store VWF in granules, such as endothelial cells and megakaryocytes, the FVIII will be trafficked for storage with VWF [197,221–223]. Two studies have indicated that subsets of endothelial cells synthesize both VWF and FVIII: One identified FVIII expression in murine sinusoidal endothelial cells and the other showed FVIII synthesis by human lung microvascular endothelial cells. Recent studies have demonstrated the utility of targeting FVIII gene therapy to megakaryocytes for the delivery of FVIII and VWF to the site of platelet plug formation [197,222,224–226].

Postsecretion modification of VWF

After secretion, VWF multimers circulate in plasma at a concentration of approximately 10 µg/mL with a half-life of approximately 12 h. The free VWFpp circulates in plasma at a concentration of about 1 µg/mL with a 2–3 h half-life [227,228]. The mechanisms underlying the clearance of VWF and VWFpp from plasma are not well defined. Increased clearance from plasma has recently been identified as a cause of type 1 VWD [229–234]. In this set of patients, VWF has a significantly decreased half-life that results in a substantially decreased level of VWF in plasma. Several mutations have been identified in the VWF D3 and D4 domains of patients with a reduced VWF survival phenotype including C1130R/F/G, W1144G, R1205H, and S2179F [229–231,233]. By using a murine model of VWF clearance, D′-D3 and D4 domains of VWF have been found to contribute to the clearance mechanism [235]. Carbohydrate structure and ABO blood group determinants may also be important in the clearance of VWF from circulation [236–239]. While aberrant mechanisms of VWF clearance may result in a VWD phenotype, much remains to be learned regarding the normal clearance of VWF from circulation.

Once secreted into plasma, VWF multimers may also be degraded by ADAMTS13 [62,63,88,240]. ADAMTS13 is a member of the "disintegrin-like and metalloprotease with thrombospondin repeats" family [62,63,241,242]. VWF is proteolytically cleaved at the Tyr1605–Met1606 bond located within the A2 domain [60,240]. VWF does not appear to be proteolytically processed by ADAMTS13 under static conditions, but is rapidly cleaved when subjected to high shear stress. The ultralarge VWF multimers that are released from endothelial cell Weibel–Palade bodies remain tethered to the endothelial surface by the interaction of VWF with P-selectin or integrin $\alpha_v\beta_3$ [243, 244]. ADAMTS13 rapidly cleaves the tethered ultralarge multimers under flow conditions [245–247]. A number of mutations have been identified in ADAMTS13 that cause thrombotic thrombocytopenic purpura (TTP) [63,248–250]. Conversely, mutations in VWF may cause increased susceptibility of VWF to ADAMTS13 cleavage. These type 2A mutations result in a loss of high molecular weight multimers in plasma and defective platelet binding [88–92,251]. While increased ADAMTS13 cleavage causes type 2A VWD, and lack of ADAMTS13 activity may cause TTP, the role of ADAMTS13 in the normal degradation and processing of VWF is not clear.

In summary, the pathway of VWF biosynthesis is very complex and the secreted protein has undergone a number of intracellular modifications. Defects at any point in the VWF biosynthetic pathway may result in defective secretion, structure, or function of VWF and may result in a VWD phenotype. Defining the molecular defects in patients with VWD may aid in the development of treatment strategies.

References

1 Sadler JE. Biochemistry and genetics of von Willebrand factor. *Annu Rev Biochem* 1998; **67**: 395–424.

2 Wagner DD, Marder VJ. Biosynthesis of von Willebrand protein by human endothelial cells. Identification of a large precursor polypeptide chain. *J Biol Chem* 1983; **258**: 2065–7.

3 Sporn LA, Chavin SI, Marder VJ, Wagner DD. Biosynthesis of von Willebrand protein by human megakaryocytes. *J Clin Invest* 1985; **76**: 1102–6.

4 Federici AB. Diagnosis of inherited von Willebrand disease: a clinical perspective. *Semin Thromb Hemost* 2006; **32**: 555–65.

5 Montgomery RR, Coller BS. von Willebrand disease. In: Colman RW, Hirsh J, Marder VJ, Salzman EW (eds). *Hemostasis and Thrombosis: Basic Principles and Clinical Practice*, pp.134–68. J.B. Lippincott Company: Philadelphia, 1994.

6 Ruggeri ZM. Pathogenesis and classification of von Willebrand disease. *Haemostasis* 1994; **24**: 265–75.

7 Mazurier C, Ribba AS, Gaucher C, Meyer D. Molecular genetics of von Willebrand disease. *Ann Genet* 1998; **41**: 34–43.

8 Sadler JE, Mannucci PM, Berntorp E, *et al.* Impact, diagnosis and treatment of von Willebrand disease. *Thromb Haemost* 2000; **84**: 160–174.

9 Castaman G, Federici AB, Rodeghiero F, Mannucci PM. Von Willebrand's disease in the year 2003: towards the complete identification of gene defects for correct diagnosis and treatment. *Haematologica* 2003; **88**: 94–108.

10 Sadler JE, Budde U, Eikenboom JC, *et al.* Update on the pathophysiology and classification of von Willebrand disease: a report of the Subcommittee on von Willebrand Factor. *J Thromb Haemost* 2006; **4**: 2103–14.

11 Rodeghiero F, Castaman G, Dini E. Epidemiological investigation of the prevalence of von Willebrand's disease. *Blood* 1987; **69**: 454–9.

12 Werner EJ, Broxson EH, Tucker EL, *et al.* Prevalence of von Willebrand disease in children: a multiethnic study. *J Pediatr* 1993; **123**: 893–8.

13 Howard MA, Sawers RJ, Firkin BG. Ristocetin: a means of differentiating von Willebrand's disease into two groups. *Blood* 1973; **41**: 687–90.

14 Bennett B, Forman WB, Ratnoff OD. Studies on the nature of antihemophilic factor (factor VIII). Further evidence relating the AHF-like antigens in normal and hemophilic plasmas. *J Clin Invest* 1973; **52**: 2191–7.

15 Zimmerman TS, Edgington TS. Factor VIII coagulant activity and factor VIII-like antigen: independent molecular entities. *J Exp Med* 1973; **138**: 1015–20.

16 Bouma BN, van Mourik JA, Wiegerinck Y, Sixma JJ, Mochtar IA. Immunological characterization of antihaemophilic factor A related antigen in haemophilia A. *Scand J Haematol* 1973; **11**: 184–7.

17 Zimmerman TS, Roberts J, Edgington TS. Factor-VIII-related antigen: multiple molecular forms in human plasma. *Proc Natl Acad Sci U S A* 1975; **72**: 5121–5.

18 Montgomery RR, Zimmerman TS. von Willebrand's disease antigen II. A new plasma and platelet antigen deficient in severe von Willebrand's disease. *J Clin Invest* 1978; **61**: 1498–507.

19 Fay PJ, Kawai Y, Wagner DD, *et al.* Propolypeptide of von Willebrand factor circulates in blood and is identical to von Willebrand antigen II. *Science* 1986; **232**: 995–8.

20 McCarroll DR, Levin EG, Montgomery RR. Endothelial cell synthesis of von Willebrand antigen II, von Willebrand factor, and von Willebrand factor/von Willebrand antigen II complex. *J Clin Invest* 1985; **75**: 1089–95.

21 Verweij CL, Diergaarde PJ, Hart M, Pannekoek H. Full-length von Willebrand factor (vWF) cDNA encodes a highly repetitive protein considerably larger than the mature vWF subunit. *EMBO J* 1986; **5**: 1839–47, erratum in *EMBO J* 1986; **5**: 3074.

22 Hannah MJ, Skehel P, Erent M, *et al*. Differential kinetics of cell surface loss of von Willebrand factor and its propolypeptide after secretion from Weibel–Palade bodies in living human endothelial cells. *J Biol Chem* 2005; **280**: 22827–30.

23 McCarroll DR, Ruggeri ZM, Montgomery RR. The effect of DDAVP on plasma levels of von Willebrand antigen II in normal individuals and patients with von Willebrand's disease. *Blood* 1984; **63**: 532–5.

24 Scott JP, Montgomery RR. Platelet von Willebrand's antigen II: active release by aggregating agents and a marker of platelet release reaction *in vivo*. *Blood* 1981; **58**: 1075–80.

25 Wagner DD, Fay PJ, Sporn LA, *et al*. Divergent fates of von Willebrand factor and its propolypeptide (von Willebrand antigen II) after secretion from endothelial cells. *Proc Natl Acad Sci U S A* 1987; **84**: 1955–9.

26 Lynch DC, Zimmerman TS, Collins CJ, *et al*. Molecular cloning of cDNA for human von Willebrand factor: authentication by a new method. *Cell* 1985; **41**: 49–56.

27 Ginsburg D, Handin RI, Bonthron DT, *et al*. Human von Willebrand factor (vWF): isolation of complementary DNA (cDNA) clones and chromosomal localization. *Science* 1985; **228**: 1401–6.

28 Sadler JE, Shelton-Inloes BB, Sorace JM, *et al*. Cloning and characterization of two cDNAs coding for human von Willebrand factor. *Proc Natl Acad Sci U S A* 1985; **82**: 6394–8.

29 Verweij CL, Hofker M, Quadt R, Briet E, Pannekoek H. RFLP for a human von Willebrand factor (vWF) cDNA clone, pvWF1100. *Nucleic Acids Res* 1985; **13**: 8289, erratum in *Nucleic Acid Res* 1986; **14**: 1930.

30 Mancuso DJ, Tuley EA, Westfield LA, *et al*. Structure of the gene for human von Willebrand factor. *J Biol Chem* 1989; **264**: 19514–27.

31 Verweij CL, de Vries CJ, Distel B, *et al*. Construction of cDNA coding for human von Willebrand factor using antibody probes for colony-screening and mapping of the chromosomal gene. *Nucleic Acids Res* 1985; **13**: 4699–717.

32 Shelton-Inloes BB, Chehab FF, Mannucci PM, Federici AB, Sadler JE. Gene deletions correlate with the development of alloantibodies in von Willebrand disease. *J Clin Invest* 1987; **79**: 1459–65.

33 Mancuso DJ, Tuley EA, Westfield LA, *et al*. Human von Willebrand factor gene and pseudogene: structural analysis and differentiation by polymerase chain reaction. *Biochemistry* 1991; **30**: 253–69.

34 Ginsburg D, Konkle BA, Gill JC, *et al*. Molecular basis of human von Willebrand disease: analysis of platelet von Willebrand factor mRNA. *Proc Natl Acad Sci U S A* 1989; **86**: 3723–7.

35 Collins CJ, Underdahl JP, Levene RB, *et al*. Molecular cloning of the human gene for von Willebrand factor and identification of the transcription initiation site. *Proc Natl Acad Sci U S A* 1987; **84**: 4393–7.

36 Ruggeri ZM, Ware J. The structure and function of von Willebrand factor. *Thromb Haemost* 1992; **67**: 594–9.

37 Shelton-Inloes BB, Broze GJ, Jr., Miletich JP, Sadler JE. Evolution of human von Willebrand factor: cDNA sequence polymorphisms, repeated domains, and relationship to von Willebrand antigen II. *Biochem Biophys Res Commun* 1987; **144**: 657–65.

38 Shelton-Inloes BB, Titani K, Sadler JE. cDNA sequences for human von Willebrand factor reveal five types of repeated domains and five possible protein sequence polymorphisms. *Biochemistry* 1986; **25**: 3164–71.

39 van de Ven WJ, Voorberg J, Fontijn R, *et al*. Furin is a subtilisin-like proprotein processing enzyme in higher eukaryotes. *Mol Biol Rep* 1990; **14**: 265–75.

40 Vischer UM, Wagner DD. von Willebrand factor proteolytic processing and multimerization precede the formation of Weibel–Palade bodies. *Blood* 1994; **83**: 3536–44.

41 Haberichter SL, Fahs SA, Montgomery RR. Von Willebrand factor storage and multimerization: 2 independent intracellular processes. *Blood* 2000; **96**: 1808–15.

42 Haberichter SL, Jozwiak MA, Rosenberg JB, Christopherson PA, Montgomery RR. The von Willebrand factor propeptide (VWFpp) traffics an unrelated protein to storage. *Arterioscler Thromb Vasc Biol* 2002; **22**: 921–6.

43 Casonato A, Sartorello F, Cattini MG, *et al*. An Arg760Cys mutation in the consensus sequence of the von Willebrand factor propeptide cleavage site is responsible for a new von Willebrand disease variant. *Blood* 2003; **101**: 151–6.

44 Sadler JE, Mancuso DJ, Randi AM, Tuley EA, Westfield LA. Molecular biology of von Willebrand factor. *Ann N Y Acad Sci* 1991; **614**: 114–24.

45 Koller E, Winterhalter KH, Trueb B. The globular domains of type VI collagen are related to the collagen-binding domains of cartilage matrix protein and von Willebrand factor. *EMBO J* 1989; **8**: 1073–7.

46 Hunt LT, Barker WC. von Willebrand factor shares a distinctive cysteine-rich domain with thrombospondin and procollagen. *Biochem Biophys Res Commun* 1987; **144**: 876–82.

47 Lawler J, Hynes RO. An integrin receptor on normal and thrombasthenic platelets that binds thrombospondin. *Blood* 1989; **74**: 2022–7.

48 Baker ME. Invertebrate vitellogenin is homologous to human von Willebrand factor. *Biochem J* 1988; **256**: 1059–61.

49 Foster PA, Fulcher CA, Marti T, Titani K, Zimmerman TS. A major factor VIII binding domain resides within the amino-terminal 272 amino acid residues of von Willebrand factor. *J Biol Chem* 1987; **262**: 8443–6.

50 Lavergne JM, Piao YC, Ferreira V, *et al*. Primary structure of the factor VIII binding domain of human, porcine and rabbit von Willebrand factor. *Biochem Biophys Res Commun* 1993; **194**: 1019–24.

51 Takahashi Y, Kalafatis M, Girma JP, *et al*. Localization of a factor VIII binding domain on a 34 kilodalton fragment of the N-terminal portion of von Willebrand factor. *Blood* 1987; **70**: 1679–82.

52 Adachi T, Matsushita T, Dong Z, *et al*. Identification of amino acid residues essential for heparin binding by the A1 domain of human von Willebrand factor. *Biochem Biophys Res Commun* 2006; **339**: 1178–83.

53 Ruggeri ZM, Zimmerman TS, Russell S, Bader R, De Marco L. von Willebrand factor binding to platelet glycoprotein Ib complex. *Methods Enzymol* 1992; **215**: 263–75.

54 Girma JP, Ribba AS, Meyer D. Structure–function relationship of the A1 domain of von Willebrand factor. *Thromb Haemost* 1995; **74**: 156–60.

55 Huizinga EG, Tsuji S, Romijn RA, *et al*. Structures of glycoprotein Ibalpha and its complex with von Willebrand factor A1 domain. *Science* 2002; **297**: 1176–9.

56 Kroner PA, Frey AB. Analysis of the structure and function of the von Willebrand factor A1 domain using targeted deletions and alanine-scanning mutagenesis. *Biochemistry* 1996; **35**: 13460–8.

57 Fujimura Y, Titani K, Holland LZ, *et al*. A heparin-binding domain of human von Willebrand factor. Characterization and localization to a tryptic fragment extending from amino acid residue Val-449 to Lys-728. *J Biol Chem* 1987; **262**: 1734–9.

58 Mohri H, Yoshioka A, Zimmerman TS, Ruggeri ZM. Isolation of the von Willebrand factor domain interacting with platelet glycoprotein Ib, heparin, and collagen and characterization of its three distinct functional sites. *J Biol Chem* 1989; **264**: 17361–7.

59 Pareti FI, Niiya K, McPherson JM, Ruggeri ZM. Isolation and characterization of two domains of human von Willebrand factor that interact with fibrillar collagen types I and III. *J Biol Chem* 1987; **262**: 13835–41.

60 Furlan M, Robles R, Lamie B. Partial purification and characterization of a protease from human plasma cleaving von Willebrand factor to fragments produced by *in vivo* proteolysis. *Blood* 1996; **87**: 4223–34.

61 Tsai HM, Lian EC. Antibodies to von Willebrand factor-cleaving protease in acute thrombotic thrombocytopenic purpura. *N Engl J Med* 1998; **339**: 1585–94.

62 Zheng X, Chung D, Takayama TK, *et al*. Structure of von Willebrand factor-cleaving protease (ADAMTS13), a metalloprotease involved in thrombotic thrombocytopenic purpura. *J Biol Chem* 2001; **276**: 41059–63.

63 Levy GG, Nichols WC, Lian EC, *et al*. Mutations in a member of the ADAMTS gene family cause thrombotic thrombocytopenic purpura. *Nature* 2001; **413**: 488–94.

64 Zheng X, Majerus EM, Sadler JE. ADAMTS13 and TTP. *Curr Opin Hematol* 2002; **9**: 389–94.

65 Tsai HM. Deficiency of ADAMTS13 in thrombotic thrombocytopenic purpura. *Int J Hematol* 2002; **76** (Suppl. 2): 132–8.

66 Huizinga EG, Martijn van der Plas R, Kroon J, Sixma JJ, Gros P. Crystal structure of the A3 domain of human von Willebrand factor: implications for collagen binding. *Structure* 1997; **5**: 1147–56.

67 Lankhof H, van Hoeij M, Schiphorst ME, *et al*. A3 domain is essential for interaction of von Willebrand factor with collagen type III. *Thromb Haemost* 1996; **75**: 950–8.

68 Romijn RA, Westein E, Bouma B, *et al*. Mapping the collagen-binding site in the von Willebrand factor-A3 domain. *J Biol Chem* 2003; **278**: 15035–9.

69 Romijn RA, Bouma B, Wuyster W, *et al*. Identification of the collagen-binding site of the von Willebrand factor A3-domain. *J Biol Chem* 2001; **276**: 9985–91.

70 Girma JP, Kalafatis M, Pietu G, *et al*. Mapping of distinct von Willebrand factor domains interacting with platelet GPIb and GPIIb/IIIa and with collagen using monoclonal antibodies. *Blood* 1986; **67**: 1356–66.

71 Perez-Casal M, Daly M, Peake I, Batlle J. A case of recessive type 2N von Willebrand's disease due to Arg 53 Trp substitution. *Am J Hematol* 1995; **48**: 140.

72 Kroner PA, Friedman KD, Fahs SA, Scott JP, Montgomery RR. Abnormal binding of factor VIII is linked with the substitution of glutamine for arginine 91 in von Willebrand factor in a variant form of von Willebrand disease. *J Biol Chem* 1991; **266**: 19146–9.

73 Gu J, Jorieux S, Lavergne JM, *et al*. A patient with type 2N von Willebrand disease is heterozygous for a new mutation: Gly22Glu. Demonstration of a defective expression of the second allele by the use of monoclonal antibodies. *Blood* 1997; **89**: 3263–9.

74 Casonato A, Gaucher C, Pontara E, *et al*. Type 2N von Willebrand disease due to Arg91Gln substitution and a cytosine deletion in exon 18 of the von Willebrand factor gene. *Br J Haematol* 1998; **103**: 39–41.

75 Allen S, Abuzenadah AM, Blagg JL, *et al*. Two novel type 2N von Willebrand disease-causing mutations that result in defective factor VIII binding, multimerization,

and secretion of von Willebrand factor. *Blood* 2000; **95**: 2000–7.

76 Hilbert L, d'Oiron R, Fressinaud E, Meyer D, Mazurier C. First identification and expression of a type 2N von Willebrand disease mutation (E1078K) located in exon 25 of von Willebrand factor gene. *J Thromb Haemost* 2004; **2**: 2271–3.

77 Hilbert L, Jorieux S, Fontenay-Roupie M, *et al*. Expression of two type 2N von Willebrand disease mutations identified in exon 18 of von Willebrand factor gene. *Br J Haematol* 2004; **127**: 184–9.

78 Wood N, Standen GR, Bowen DJ, *et al*. UHG-based mutation screening in type 2B von Willebrand's disease: detection of a candidate mutation Ser547Phe. *Thromb Haemost* 1996; **75**: 363–7.

79 Federici AB, Mannucci PM, Stabile F, *et al*. A type 2b von Willebrand disease mutation (Ile546→Val) associated with an unusual phenotype. *Thromb Haemost* 1997; **78**: 1132–7.

80 Lankhof H, Damas C, Schiphorst ME, *et al*. Functional studies on platelet adhesion with recombinant von Willebrand factor type 2B mutants R543Q and R543W under conditions of flow. *Blood* 1997; **89**: 2766–72.

81 Casana P, Martinez F, Espinos C, *et al*. Search for mutations in a segment of the exon 28 of the human von Willebrand factor gene: new mutations, R1315C and R1341W, associated with type 2M and 2B variants. *Am J Hematol* 1998; **59**: 57–63.

82 Hilbert L, Gaucher C, Abgrall JF, *et al*. Identification of new type 2B von Willebrand disease mutations: Arg543Gln, Arg545Pro and Arg578Leu. *Br J Haematol* 1998; **103**: 877–84.

83 Mancuso DJ, Kroner PA, Christopherson PA, *et al*. Type 2M:Milwaukee-1 von Willebrand disease: an in-frame deletion in the Cys509-Cys695 loop of the von Willebrand factor A1 domain causes deficient binding of von Willebrand factor to platelets. *Blood* 1996; **88**: 2559–68.

84 Hillery CA, Mancuso DJ, Evan SJ, *et al*. Type 2M von Willebrand disease: F606I and I662F mutations in the glycoprotein Ib binding domain selectively impair ristocetin- but not botrocetin-mediated binding of von Willebrand factor to platelets. *Blood* 1998; **91**: 1572–81.

85 Hilbert L, Jenkins PV, Gaucher C, *et al*. Type 2M vWD resulting from a lysine deletion within a four lysine residue repeat in the A1 loop of von Willebrand factor. *Thromb Haemost* 2000; **84**: 188–94.

86 Dong JF, Moake JL, Nolasco L, *et al*. ADAMTS-13 rapidly cleaves newly secreted ultralarge von Willebrand factor multimers on the endothelial surface under flowing conditions. *Blood* 2002; **100**: 4033–9.

87 Tsai HM. Type 2 A (group II) von Willebrand disease mutations increase the susceptibility of VWF to ADAMTS-13. *J Thromb Haemost* 2004; **2**: 2057.

88 Tsai HM, Sussman II, Ginsburg D, *et al*. Proteolytic cleavage of recombinant type 2A von Willebrand factor mutants R834W and R834Q: inhibition by doxycycline and by monoclonal antibody VP-1. *Blood* 1997; **89**: 1954–62.

89 Sutherland JJ, O'Brien LA, Lillicrap D, Weaver DF. Molecular modeling of the von Willebrand factor A2 domain and the effects of associated type 2A von Willebrand disease mutations. *J Mol Model* 2004; **10**: 259–70.

90 O'Brien LA, Sutherland JJ, Hegadorn C, *et al*. A novel type 2A (Group II) von Willebrand disease mutation (L1503Q) associated with loss of the highest molecular weight von Willebrand factor multimers. *J Thromb Haemost* 2004; **2**: 1135–42.

91 O'Brien LA, Sutherland JJ, Weaver DF, Lillicrap D. Theoretical structural explanation for Group I and Group II, type 2A von Willebrand disease mutations. *J Thromb Haemost* 2005; **3**: 796–7.

92 Hassenpflug WA, Budde U, Obser T, *et al*. Impact of mutations in the von Willebrand factor A2 domain on ADAMTS13-dependent proteolysis. *Blood* 2006; **107**: 2339–45.

93 Lyons SE, Bruck ME, Bowie EJ, Ginsburg D. Impaired intracellular transport produced by a subset of type IIA von Willebrand disease mutations. *J Biol Chem* 1992; **267**: 4424–30.

94 Allen S, Abuzenadah AM, Hinks J, *et al*. A novel von Willebrand disease-causing mutation (Arg273Trp) in the von Willebrand factor propeptide that results in defective multimerization and secretion. *Blood* 2000; **96**: 560–8.

95 Holmberg L, Karpman D, Isaksson C, *et al*. Ins405AsnPro mutation in the von Willebrand factor propeptide in recessive type 2A (IIC) von Willebrand's disease. *Thromb Haemost* 1998; **79**: 718–22.

96 James PD, O'Brien LA, Hegadorn CA, *et al*. A novel type 2A von Willebrand factor mutation located at the last nucleotide of exon 26 (3538G>A) causes skipping of 2 nonadjacent exons. *Blood* 2004; **104**: 2739–45.

97 Hommais A, Stepanian A, Fressinaud E, *et al*. Impaired dimerization of von Willebrand factor subunit due to mutation A2801D in the CK domain results in a recessive type 2A subtype IID von Willebrand disease. *Thromb Haemost* 2006; **95**: 776–81.

98 Ribba AN, Hilbert L, Lavergne JM, *et al*. The arginine-552-cysteine (R1315C) mutation within the A1 loop of von Willebrand factor induces an abnormal folding with a loss of function resulting in type 2A-like phenotype of von Willebrand disease: study of 10 patients

and mutated recombinant von Willebrand factor. *Blood* 2001; **97**: 952–9.

99 Ribba AS, Loisel I, Lavergne JM, *et al.* Ser968Thr mutation within the A3 domain of von Willebrand factor (VWF) in two related patients leads to a defective binding of VWF to collagen. *Thromb Haemost* 2001; **86**: 848–54.

100 Guan J, Guillot PV, Aird WC. Characterization of the mouse von Willebrand factor promoter. *Blood* 1999; **94**: 3405–12.

101 Jahroudi N, Lynch DC. Endothelial-cell-specific regulation of von Willebrand factor gene expression. *Mol Cell Biol* 1994; **14**: 999–1008.

102 Ferreira V, Assouline Z, Schwachtgen JL, *et al.* The role of the 5′-flanking region in the cell-specific transcription of the human von Willebrand factor gene. *Biochem J* 1993; **293**: 641–8.

103 Schwachtgen JL, Remacle JE, Janel N, *et al.* Oct-1 is involved in the transcriptional repression of the von Willebrand factor gene promoter. *Blood* 1998; **92**: 1247–58.

104 Schwachtgen JL, Janel N, Barek L, *et al.* Ets transcription factors bind and transactivate the core promoter of the von Willebrand factor gene. *Oncogene* 1997; **15**: 3091–102.

105 Ardekani AM, Greenberger JS, Jahroudi N. Two repressor elements inhibit expression of the von Willebrand factor gene promoter *in vitro*. *Thromb Haemost* 1998; **80**: 488–94.

106 Aird WC, Edelberg JM, Weiler-Guettler H, *et al.* Vascular bed-specific expression of an endothelial cell gene is programmed by the tissue microenvironment. *J Cell Biol* 1997; **138**: 1117–24.

107 Hough C, Cuthbert CD, Notley C, *et al.* Cell type-specific regulation of von Willebrand factor expression by the E4BP4 transcriptional repressor. *Blood* 2005; **105**: 1531–9.

108 Jaffe EA, Hoyer LW, Nachman RL. Synthesis of von Willebrand factor by cultured human endothelial cells. *Proc Natl Acad Sci U S A* 1974; **71**: 1906–9.

109 Jaffe EA. Synthesis of factor VIII antigen by cultured human endothelial cells. *Ann N Y Acad Sci* 1975; **240**: 62–9.

110 Nachman R, Levine R, Jaffe EA. Synthesis of factor VIII antigen by cultured guinea pig megakaryocytes. *J Clin Invest* 1977; **60**: 914–21.

111 Wagner DD, Mayadas T, Marder VJ. Initial glycosylation and acidic pH in the Golgi apparatus are required for multimerization of von Willebrand factor. *J Cell Biol* 1986; **102**: 1320–4.

112 Mayadas TN, Wagner DD. In vitro multimerization of von Willebrand factor is triggered by low pH. Importance of the propolypeptide and free sulfhydryls. *J Biol Chem* 1989; **264**: 13497–503.

113 Wagner DD, Saffaripour S, Bonfanti R, *et al.* Induction of specific storage organelles by von Willebrand factor propolypeptide. *Cell* 1991; **64**: 403–13.

114 Journet AM, Saffaripour S, Wagner DD. Requirement for both D domains of the propolypeptide in von Willebrand factor multimerization and storage. *Thromb Haemost* 1993; **70**: 1053–7.

115 Journet AM, Saffaripour S, Cramer EM, Tenza D, Wagner DD. von Willebrand factor storage requires intact prosequence cleavage site. *Eur J Cell Biol* 1993; **60**: 31–41.

116 Voorberg J, Fontijn R, van Mourik JA, Pannekoek H. Domains involved in multimer assembly of von Willebrand factor (vWF): multimerization is independent of dimerization. *EMBO J* 1990; **9**: 797–803.

117 Voorberg J, Fontijn R, Calafat J, *et al.* Assembly and routing of von Willebrand factor variants: the requirements for disulfide-linked dimerization reside within the carboxy-terminal 151 amino acids. *J Cell Biol* 1991; **113**: 195–205.

118 Voorberg J, Fontijn R, Calafat J, *et al.* Biogenesis of von Willebrand factor-containing organelles in heterologous transfected CV-1 cells. *EMBO J* 1993; **12**: 749–58.

119 Haberichter SL, Jacobi P, Montgomery RR. Critical independent regions in the VWF propeptide and mature VWF that enable normal VWF storage. *Blood* 2003; **101**: 1384–91.

120 Haberichter SL, Merricks EP, Fahs SA, *et al.* Re-establishment of VWF-dependent Weibel–Palade bodies in VWD endothelial cells. *Blood* 2005; **105**: 145–52.

121 Sporn LA, Marder VJ, Wagner DD. Inducible secretion of large, biologically potent von Willebrand factor multimers. *Cell* 1986; **46**: 185–90.

122 Wagner DD, Olmsted JB, Marder VJ. Immunolocalization of von Willebrand protein in Weibel–Palade bodies of human endothelial cells. *J Cell Biol* 1982; **95**: 355–60.

123 Wagner DD, Marder VJ. Biosynthesis of von Willebrand protein by human endothelial cells: processing steps and their intracellular localization. *J Cell Biol* 1984; **99**: 2123–30.

124 Jaffe EA, Nachman RL. Subunit structure of factor VIII antigen synthesized by cultured human endothelial cells. *J Clin Invest* 1975; **56**: 698–702.

125 Li Y, Choi H, Zhou Z, *et al.* Covalent regulation of ULVWF string formation and elongation on endothelial cells under flow conditions. *J Thromb Haemost* 2008; **6**: 1135–43.

126 Dong Z, Thoma RS, Crimmins DL, *et al.* Disulfide bonds required to assemble functional von Willebrand factor multimers. *J Biol Chem* 1994; **269**: 6753–8.

127 Katsumi A, Tuley EA, Bodo I, Sadler JE. Localization of disulfide bonds in the cystine knot domain of human

von Willebrand factor. *J Biol Chem* 2000; **275**: 25585–94.

128 Purvis AR, Gross J, Dang LT, *et al*. Two Cys residues essential for von Willebrand factor multimer assembly in the Golgi. *Proc Natl Acad Sci U S A* 2007; **104**: 15647–52.

129 Tjernberg P, Vos HL, Spaargaren-van Riel CC, *et al*. Differential effects of the loss of intrachain- versus interchain–disulfide bonds in the cystine-knot domain of von Willebrand factor on the clinical phenotype of von Willebrand disease. *Thromb Haemost* 2006; **96**: 717–24.

130 Marti T, Rosselet SJ, Titani K, Walsh KA. Identification of disulfide-bridged substructures within human von Willebrand factor. *Biochemistry* 1987; **26**: 8099–109.

131 Schneppenheim R, Brassard J, Krey S, *et al*. Defective dimerization of von Willebrand factor subunits due to a Cys->Arg mutation in type IID von Willebrand disease. *Proc Natl Acad Sci U S A* 1996; **93**: 3581–6.

132 Schneppenheim R, Budde U, Obser T, *et al*. Expression and characterization of von Willebrand factor dimerization defects in different types of von Willebrand disease. *Blood* 2001; **97**: 2059–66.

133 Tjernberg P, Vos HL, Castaman G, Bertina RM, Eikenboom JC. Dimerization and multimerization defects of von Willebrand factor due to mutated cysteine residues. *J Thromb Haemost* 2004; **2**: 257–65.

134 Tjernberg P, Castaman G, Vos HL, Bertina RM, Eikenboom JC. Homozygous C2362F von Willebrand factor induces intracellular retention of mutant von Willebrand factor resulting in autosomal recessive severe von Willebrand disease. *Br J Haematol* 2006; **133**: 409–18.

135 Verweij CL, Hart M, Pannekoek H. Expression of variant von Willebrand factor (vWF) cDNA in heterologous cells: requirement of the pro-polypeptide in vWF multimer formation. *EMBO J* 1987; **6**: 2885–90.

136 Wise RJ, Pittman DD, Handin RI, Kaufman RJ, Orkin SH. The propeptide of von Willebrand factor independently mediates the assembly of von Willebrand multimers. *Cell* 1988; **52**: 229–36.

137 Titani K, Kumar S, Takio K, *et al*. Amino acid sequence of human von Willebrand factor. *Biochemistry* 1986; **25**: 3171–84.

138 Matsui T, Titani K, Mizuochi T. Structures of the asparagine-linked oligosaccharide chains of human von Willebrand factor. Occurrence of blood group A, B, and H(O) structures. *J Biol Chem* 1992; **267**: 8723–31.

139 Wittrup KD. Disulfide bond formation and eukaryotic secretory productivity. *Curr Opin Biotechnol* 1995; **6**: 203–8.

140 Lodish HF, Kong N, Snider M, Strous GJ. Hepatoma secretory proteins migrate from rough endoplasmic reticulum to Golgi at characteristic rates. *Nature* 1983; **304**: 80–3.

141 Hampton RY. ER-associated degradation in protein quality control and cellular regulation. *Curr Opin Cell Biol* 2002; **14**: 476–82.

142 Bonifacino JS, Lippincott-Schwartz J. Degradation of proteins within the endoplasmic reticulum. *Curr Opin Cell Biol* 1991; **3**: 592–600.

143 Bodo I, Katsumi A, Tuley EA, *et al*. Type 1 von Willebrand disease mutation Cys1149Arg causes intracellular retention and degradation of heterodimers: a possible general mechanism for dominant mutations of oligomeric proteins. *Blood* 2001; **98**: 2973–9.

144 Eikenboom JC, Matsushita T, Reitsma PH, *et al*. Dominant type 1 von Willebrand disease caused by mutated cysteine residues in the D3 domain of von Willebrand factor. *Blood* 1996; **88**: 2433–41.

145 Castaman G, Eikenboom JC, Missiaglia E, Rodeghiero F. Autosomal dominant type 1 von Willebrand disease due to G3639T mutation (C1130F) in exon 26 of von Willebrand factor gene: description of five Italian families and evidence for a founder effect. *Br J Haematol* 2000; **108**: 876–9.

146 Michaux G, Hewlett LJ, Messenger SL, *et al*. Analysis of intracellular storage and regulated secretion of 3 von Willebrand disease-causing variants of von Willebrand factor. *Blood* 2003; **102**: 2452–8.

147 Carew JA, Browning PJ, Lynch DC. Sulfation of von Willebrand factor. *Blood* 1990; **76**: 2530–9.

148 Lynch DC, Zimmerman TS, Kirby EP, Livingston DM. Subunit composition of oligomeric human von Willebrand factor. *J Biol Chem* 1983; **258**: 12757–60.

149 Bosshart H, Humphrey J, Deignan E, *et al*. The cytoplasmic domain mediates localization of furin to the trans–Golgi network en route to the endosomal/lysosomal system. *J Cell Biol* 1994; **126**: 1157–72.

150 Shapiro J, Sciaky N, Lee J, *et al*. Localization of endogenous furin in cultured cell lines. *J Histochem Cytochem* 1997; **45**: 3–12.

151 Rehemtulla A, Kaufman RJ. Preferred sequence requirements for cleavage of pro-von Willebrand factor by propeptide-processing enzymes. *Blood* 1992; **79**: 2349–55.

152 Wise RJ, Barr PJ, Wong PA, *et al*. Expression of a human proprotein processing enzyme: correct cleavage of the von Willebrand factor precursor at a paired basic amino acid site. *Proc Natl Acad Sci U S A* 1990; **87**: 9378–82.

153 Ewenstein BM, Warhol MJ, Handin RI, Pober JS. Composition of the von Willebrand factor storage organelle (Weibel–Palade body) isolated from cultured

human umbilical vein endothelial cells. *J Cell Biol* 1987; **104**: 1423–33.

154 Halban PA, Irminger JC. Sorting and processing of secretory proteins. *Biochem J* 1994; **299**: 1–18.

155 Tooze SA. Biogenesis of secretory granules in the trans–Golgi network of neuroendocrine and endocrine cells. *Biochim Biophys Acta* 1998; **1404**: 231–44.

156 Frand AR, Cuozzo JW, Kaiser CA. Pathways for protein disulphide bond formation. *Trends Cell Biol* 2000; **10**: 203–10.

157 Akagi S, Yamamoto A, Yoshimori T, *et al*. Distribution of protein disulfide isomerase in rat hepatocytes. *J Histochem Cytochem* 1988; **36**: 1533–42.

158 Rivera VM, Wang X, Wardwell S, *et al*. Regulation of protein secretion through controlled aggregation in the endoplasmic reticulum. *Science* 2000; **287**: 826–30.

159 Verweij CL, Hart M, Pannekoek H. Proteolytic cleavage of the precursor of von Willebrand factor is not essential for multimer formation. *J Biol Chem* 1988; **263**: 7921–4.

160 Mayadas TN, Wagner DD. Vicinal cysteines in the prosequence play a role in von Willebrand factor multimer assembly. *Proc Natl Acad Sci U S A* 1992; **89**: 3531–5.

161 Purvis AR, Sadler JE. A covalent oxidoreductase intermediate in propeptide-dependent von Willebrand factor multimerization. *J Biol Chem* 2004; **279**: 49982–8.

162 Rosenberg JB, Haberichter SL, Jozwiak MA, *et al*. The role of the D1 domain of the von Willebrand factor propeptide in multimerization of VWF. *Blood* 2002; **100**: 1699–706.

163 Gaucher C, Dieval J, Mazurier C. Characterization of von Willebrand factor gene defects in two unrelated patients with type IIC von Willebrand disease. *Blood* 1994; **84**: 1024–30.

164 Cramer EM, Meyer D, le Menn R, Breton-Gorius J. Eccentric localization of von Willebrand factor in an internal structure of platelet alpha-granule resembling that of Weibel–Palade bodies. *Blood* 1985; **66**: 710–13.

165 Weibel ER, Palade GE. New cytoplasmic components in arterial endothelia. *J Cell Biol* 1964; **23**: 101–12.

166 Bonfanti R, Furie BC, Furie B, Wagner DD. PADGEM (GMP140) is a component of Weibel–Palade bodies of human endothelial cells. *Blood* 1989; **73**: 1109–12.

167 McEver RP, Beckstead JH, Moore KL, Marshall-Carlson L, Bainton DF. GMP-140, a platelet alpha-granule membrane protein, is also synthesized by vascular endothelial cells and is localized in Weibel–Palade bodies. *J Clin Invest* 1989; **84**: 92–9.

168 Kaufmann JE, Oksche A, Wollheim CB, *et al*. Vasopressin-induced von Willebrand factor secretion from endothelial cells involves V2 receptors and cAMP. *J Clin Invest* 2000; **106**: 107–16.

169 Mannucci PM, Canciani MT, Rota L, Donovan BS. Response of factor VIII/von Willebrand factor to DDAVP in healthy subjects and patients with haemophilia A and von Willebrand's disease. *Br J Haematol* 1981; **47**: 283–93.

170 Hop C, Fontijn R, van Mourik JA, Pannekoek H. Polarity of constitutive and regulated von Willebrand factor secretion by transfected MDCK-II cells. *Exp Cell Res* 1997; **230**: 352–61.

171 Sevarino KA, Stork P, Ventimiglia R, Mandel G, Goodman RH. Amino-terminal sequences of prosomatostatin direct intracellular targeting but not processing specificity. *Cell* 1989; **57**: 11–19.

172 Arvan P, Castle D. Sorting and storage during secretory granule biogenesis: looking backward and looking forward. *Biochem J* 1998; **332**: 593–610.

173 Tooze SA, Martens GJ, Huttner WB. Secretory granule biogenesis: rafting to the SNARE. *Trends Cell Biol* 2001; **11**: 116–22.

174 Gerdes HH, Glombik MM. Signal-mediated sorting to the regulated pathway of protein secretion. *Ann Anat* 1999; **181**: 447–53.

175 Gorr SU, Moore YR. Sorting of a constitutive secretory protein to the regulated secretory pathway of exocrine cells. *Biochem Biophys Res Commun* 1999; **257**: 545–8.

176 Haberichter SL, Fahs SA, Jozwiak MA, Retzlaff KL, Montgomery RR. The sorting signal for von Willebrand factor (VWF) granular storage lies within the first 140 amino acids of the D2 domain of the VWF propeptide (VWFpp). *J Thromb Haemost* 2003; **1** (Suppl. 1): OC401.

177 Hommais A, Stepanian A, Fressinaud E, *et al*. Mutations C1157F and C1234W of von Willebrand factor cause intracellular retention with defective multimerization and secretion. *J Thromb Haemost* 2006; **4**: 148–57.

178 Rehemtulla A, Dorner AJ, Kaufman RJ. Regulation of PACE propeptide-processing activity: requirement for a post-endoplasmic reticulum compartment and autoproteolytic activation. *Proc Natl Acad Sci U S A* 1992; **89**: 8235–9.

179 Rosenberg JB, Foster PA, Kaufman RJ, *et al*. Intracellular trafficking of factor VIII to von Willebrand factor storage granules. *J Clin Invest* 1998; **101**: 613–24.

180 Blagoveshchenskaya AD, Hannah MJ, Allen S, Cutler DF. Selective and signal-dependent recruitment of membrane proteins to secretory granules formed by heterologously expressed von Willebrand factor. *Mol Biol Cell* 2002; **13**: 1582–93.

181 Hannah MJ, Williams R, Kaur J, Hewlett LJ, Cutler DF. Biogenesis of Weibel–Palade bodies. *Semin Cell Dev Biol* 2002; **13**: 313–24.

182 Wagner DD. The Weibel–Palade body: the storage granule for von Willebrand factor and P-selectin. *Thromb Haemost* 1993; **70**: 105–10.

183 van Mourik JA, Romani DW, Voorberg J. Biogenesis and exocytosis of Weibel–Palade bodies. *Histochem Cell Biol* 2002; **117**: 113–22.

184 Denis C, Methia N, Frenette PS, *et al*. A mouse model of severe von Willebrand disease: defects in hemostasis and thrombosis. *Proc Natl Acad Sci U S A* 1998; **95**: 9524–9.

185 Denis CV, Andre P, Saffaripour S, Wagner DD. Defect in regulated secretion of P-selectin affects leukocyte recruitment in von Willebrand factor-deficient mice. *Proc Natl Acad Sci U S A* 2001; **98**: 4072–7.

186 Hop C, Guilliatt A, Daly M, *et al*. Assembly of multimeric von Willebrand factor directs sorting of P-selectin. *Arterioscler Thromb Vasc Biol* 2000; **20**: 1763–8.

187 Michaux G, Pullen TJ, Haberichter SL, Cutler DF. P-selectin binds to the D′-D3 domains of von Willebrand factor in Weibel–Palade bodies. *Blood* 2006; **107**: 3922–4.

188 Michaux G, Abbitt KB, Collinson LM, *et al*. The physiological function of von Willebrand's factor depends on its tubular storage in endothelial Weibel–Palade bodies. *Dev Cell* 2006; **10**: 223–32.

189 Huang RH, Wang Y, Roth R, *et al*. Assembly of Weibel–Palade body-like tubules from N-terminal domains of von Willebrand factor. *Proc Natl Acad Sci U S A* 2008; **105**: 482–7.

190 Oynebraten I, Barois N, Hagelsteen K, *et al*. Characterization of a novel chemokine-containing storage granule in endothelial cells: evidence for preferential exocytosis mediated by protein kinase A and diacylglycerol. *J Immunol* 2005; **175**: 5358–69.

191 Ozaka T, Doi Y, Kayashima K, Fujimoto S. Weibel–Palade bodies as a storage site of calcitonin gene-related peptide and endothelin-1 in blood vessels of the rat carotid body. *Anat Rec* 1997; **247**: 388–94.

192 Vischer UM, Wagner DD. CD63 is a component of Weibel–Palade bodies of human endothelial cells. *Blood* 1993; **82**: 1184–91.

193 Wolff B, Burns AR, Middleton J, Rot A. Endothelial cell 'memory' of inflammatory stimulation: human venular endothelial cells store interleukin 8 in Weibel–Palade bodies. *J Exp Med* 1998; **188**: 1757–62.

194 Shahbazi S, Lenting PJ, Fribourg C, *et al*. Characterization of the interaction between von Willebrand factor and osteoprotegerin. *J Thromb Haemost* 2007; **5**: 1956–62.

195 Schnyder-Candrian S, Borsig L, Moser R, Berger EG. Localization of alpha 1,3-fucosyltransferase VI in Weibel–Palade bodies of human endothelial cells. *Proc Natl Acad Sci U S A* 2000; **97**: 8369–74.

196 Rosnoblet C, Vischer UM, Gerard RD, *et al*. Storage of tissue-type plasminogen activator in Weibel–Palade bodies of human endothelial cells. *Arterioscler Thromb Vasc Biol* 1999; **19**: 1796–803.

197 Wilcox DA, Shi Q, Nurden P, *et al*. Induction of megakaryocytes to synthesize and store a releasable pool of human factor VIII. *J Thromb Haemost* 2003; **1**: 2477–89.

198 Tsai HM, Nagel RL, Hatcher VB, Seaton AC, Sussman II. The high molecular weight form of endothelial cell von Willebrand factor is released by the regulated pathway. *Br J Haematol* 1991; **79**: 239–45.

199 Giblin JP, Hewlett LJ, Hannah MJ. Basal secretion of von Willebrand factor from human endothelial cells. *Blood* 2008; **112**: 957–64.

200 de Leeuw HP, Fernandez-Borja M, Reits EA, *et al*. Small GTP-binding protein Ral modulates regulated exocytosis of von Willebrand factor by endothelial cells. *Arterioscler Thromb Vasc Biol* 2001; **21**: 899–904.

201 Pinsky DJ, Naka Y, Liao H, *et al*. Hypoxia-induced exocytosis of endothelial cell Weibel–Palade bodies. A mechanism for rapid neutrophil recruitment after cardiac preservation. *J Clin Invest* 1996; **97**: 493–500.

202 Doi Y, Ozaka T, Fukushige H, *et al*. Increase in number of Weibel–Palade bodies and endothelin-1 release from endothelial cells in the cadmium-treated rat thoracic aorta. *Virchows Arch* 1996; **428**: 367–73.

203 Arribas M, Cutler DF. Weibel–Palade body membrane proteins exhibit differential trafficking after exocytosis in endothelial cells. *Traffic* 2000; **1**: 783–93.

204 Datta YH, Ewenstein BM. Regulated secretion in endothelial cells: biology and clinical implications. *Thromb Haemost* 2001; **86**: 1148–55.

205 Zupancic G, Ogden D, Magnus CJ, Wheeler-Jones C, Carter TD. Differential exocytosis from human endothelial cells evoked by high intracellular Ca(2+) concentration. *J Physiol* 2002; **544**: 741–55.

206 Matsushita K, Morrell CN, Cambien B, *et al*. Nitric oxide regulates exocytosis by S-nitrosylation of N-ethylmaleimide-sensitive factor. *Cell* 2003; **115**: 139–50.

207 Erent M, Meli A, Moisoi N, *et al*. Rate, extent and concentration dependence of histamine-evoked Weibel–Palade body exocytosis determined from individual fusion events in human endothelial cells. *J Physiol* 2007; **583**: 195–212.

208 Babich V, Meli A, Knipe L, *et al*. Selective release of molecules from Weibel–Palade bodies during a lingering kiss. *Blood* 2008; **111**: 5282–90.

209 Romani DW, Rondaij MG, Hordijk PL, Voorberg J, van Mourik JA. Real-time imaging of the dynamics and secretory behavior of Weibel–Palade bodies. *Arterioscler Thromb Vasc Biol* 2003; **23**: 755–61.

210 Rondaij MG, Bierings R, Kragt A, van Mourik JA, Voorberg J. Dynamics and plasticity of Weibel–Palade

bodies in endothelial cells. *Arterioscler Thromb Vasc Biol* 2006; **26**: 1002–7.

211 Rondaij MG, Bierings R, van Agtmaal EL, *et al.* Guanine exchange factor RalGDS mediates exocytosis of Weibel–Palade bodies from endothelial cells. *Blood* 2008; **112**: 56–63.

212 Andre P, Denis CV, Ware J, *et al.* Platelets adhere to and translocate on von Willebrand factor presented by endothelium in stimulated veins. *Blood* 2000; **96**: 3322–8.

213 Ruggeri ZM. Von Willebrand factor, platelets and endothelial cell interactions. *J Thromb Haemost* 2003; **1**: 1335–42.

214 Jaffe EA, Hoyer LW, Nachman RL. Synthesis of antihemophilic factor antigen by cultured human endothelial cells. *J Clin Invest* 1973; **52**: 2757–64.

215 Jacquemin M, Neyrinck A, Hermanns MI, *et al.* FVIII production by human lung microvascular endothelial cells. *Blood* 2006; **108**: 515–17.

216 Gibson-D'Ambrosio RE, Crowe DL, Shuler CE, D'Ambrosio SM. The establishment and continuous subculturing of normal human adult hepatocytes: expression of differentiated liver functions. *Cell Biol Toxicol* 1993; **9**: 385–403.

217 Ingerslev J, Christiansen BS, Heickendorff L, Munck PC. Synthesis of factor VIII in human hepatocytes in culture. *Thromb Haemost* 1988; **60**: 387–91.

218 Do H, Healey JF, Waller EK, Lollar P. Expression of factor VIII by murine liver sinusoidal endothelial cells. *J Biol Chem* 1999; **274**: 19587–92.

219 Montgomery RR, Gill JC. Interactions between von Willebrand factor and Factor VIII: where did they first meet. *J Pediatr Hematol Oncol* 2000; **22**: 269–75.

220 Haberichter SL, Shi Q, Montgomery RR. Regulated release of VWF and FVIII and the biologic implications. *Pediatr Blood Cancer* 2006; **46**: 547–53.

221 Rosenberg JB, Greengard JS, Montgomery RR. Genetic induction of a releasable pool of factor VIII in human endothelial cells. *Arterioscler Thromb Vasc Biol* 2000; **20**: 2689–95.

222 Yarovoi HV, Kufrin D, Eslin DE, *et al.* Factor VIII ectopically expressed in platelets: efficacy in hemophilia A treatment. *Blood* 2003; **102**: 4006–13.

223 Shi Q, Wilcox DA, Fahs SA, Kroner PA, Montgomery RR. Expression of human factor VIII under control of the platelet-specific alphaIIb promoter in megakaryocytic cell line as well as storage together with VWF. *Mol Genet Metab* 2003; **79**: 25–33.

224 Shi Q, Fahs SA, Wilcox DA, *et al.* Syngeneic transplantation of hematopoietic stem cells that are genetically modified to express factor VIII in platelets restores hemostasis to hemophilia A mice with preexisting FVIII immunity. *Blood* 2008; **112**: 2713–21.

225 Yarovoi H, Nurden AT, Montgomery RR, Nurden P, Poncz M. Intracellular interaction of von Willebrand factor and factor VIII depends on cellular context: lessons from platelet-expressed factor VIII. *Blood* 2005; **105**: 4674–6.

226 Shi Q, Wilcox DA, Fahs SA, *et al.* Factor VIII ectopically targeted to platelets is therapeutic in hemophilia A with high-titer inhibitory antibodies. *J Clin Invest* 2006; **116**: 1974–82.

227 Borchiellini A, Fijnvandraat K, ten Cate JW, *et al.* Quantitative analysis of von Willebrand factor propeptide release in vivo: effect of experimental endotoxemia and administration of 1-deamino-8-D-arginine vasopressin in humans. *Blood* 1996; **88**: 2951–8.

228 van Mourik JA, Boertjes R, Huisveld IA, *et al.* von Willebrand factor propeptide in vascular disorders: A tool to distinguish between acute and chronic endothelial cell perturbation. *Blood* 1999; **94**: 179–85.

229 Casonato A, Pontara E, Sartorello F, *et al.* Reduced von Willebrand factor survival in type Vicenza von Willebrand disease. *Blood* 2002; **99**: 180–4.

230 Haberichter SL, Balistreri M, Christopherson P, *et al.* Assay of the von Willebrand factor (VWF) propeptide to identify patients with type 1 von Willebrand disease with decreased VWF survival. *Blood* 2006; **108**: 3344–51.

231 Haberichter SL, Castaman G, Budde U, *et al.* Identification of type 1 von Willebrand disease patients with reduced von Willebrand factor survival by assay of the VWF propeptide in the European study: molecular and clinical markers for the diagnosis and management of type 1 VWD (MCMDM-1VWD). *Blood* 2008; **111**: 4979–85.

232 Brown SA, Eldridge A, Collins PW, Bowen DJ. Increased clearance of von Willebrand factor antigen post-DDAVP in Type 1 von Willebrand disease: is it a potential pathogenic process? *J Thromb Haemost* 2003; **1**: 1714–17.

233 Schooten CJ, Tjernberg P, Westein E, *et al.* Cysteine-mutations in von Willebrand factor associated with increased clearance. *J Thromb Haemost* 2005; **3**: 2228–37.

234 Lenting PJ, van Schooten CJ, Denis CV. Clearance mechanisms of von Willebrand factor and factor VIII. *J Thromb Haemost* 2007; **5**: 1353–60.

235 Lenting PJ, Westein E, Terraube V, *et al.* An experimental model to study the in vivo survival of von Willebrand factor. Basic aspects and application to the R1205H mutation. *J Biol Chem* 2004; **279**: 12102–9.

236 van Schooten CJ, Denis CV, Lisman T, *et al.* Variations in glycosylation of von Willebrand factor with O-linked sialylated T antigen are associated with its plasma levels. *Blood* 2007; **109**: 2430–7.

237 Gallinaro L, Cattini MG, Sztukowska M, *et al*. A shorter von Willebrand factor survival in O blood group subjects explains how ABO determinants influence plasma von Willebrand factor. *Blood* 2008; **111**: 3540–5.

238 Ellies LG, Ditto D, Levy GG, *et al*. Sialyltransferase ST3Gal-IV operates as a dominant modifier of hemostasis by concealing asialoglycoprotein receptor ligands. *Proc Natl Acad Sci U S A* 2002; **99**: 10042–7.

239 Mohlke KL, Purkayastha AA, Westrick RJ, *et al*. Mvwf, a dominant modifier of murine von Willebrand factor, results from altered lineage-specific expression of a glycosyltransferase. *Cell* 1999; **96**: 111–20.

240 Tsai HM. Physiologic cleavage of von Willebrand factor by a plasma protease is dependent on its conformation and requires calcium ion. *Blood* 1996; **87**: 4235–44.

241 Gerritsen HE, Robles R, Lammle B, Furlan M. Partial amino acid sequence of purified von Willebrand factor-cleaving protease. *Blood* 2001; **98**: 1654–61.

242 Fujikawa K, Suzuki H, McMullen B, Chung D. Purification of human von Willebrand factor-cleaving protease and its identification as a new member of the metalloproteinase family. *Blood* 2001; **98**: 1662–6.

243 Padilla A, Moake JL, Bernardo A, *et al*. P-selectin anchors newly released ultralarge von Willebrand factor multimers to the endothelial cell surface. *Blood* 2004; **103**: 2150–6.

244 Huang J, Roth R, Heuser JE, Sadler JE. Integrin alpha(v)beta(3) on human endothelial cells binds von Willebrand factor strings under fluid shear stress. *Blood* 2008; **113**: 1589–97.

245 Dong JF, Moake JL, Bernardo A, *et al*. ADAMTS-13 metalloprotease interacts with the endothelial cell-derived ultra-large von Willebrand factor. *J Biol Chem* 2003; **278**: 29633–9.

246 Lopez JA, Dong JF. Cleavage of von Willebrand factor by ADAMTS-13 on endothelial cells. *Semin Hematol* 2004; **41**: 15–23.

247 Dong JF. Cleavage of ultra-large von Willebrand factor by ADAMTS-13 under flow conditions. *J Thromb Haemost* 2005; **3**: 1710–16.

248 Schneppenheim R, Budde U, Oyen F, *et al*. von Willebrand factor cleaving protease and ADAMTS13 mutations in childhood TTP. *Blood* 2003; **101**: 1845–50.

249 Veyradier A, Lavergne JM, Ribba AS, *et al*. Ten candidate ADAMTS13 mutations in six French families with congenital thrombotic thrombocytopenic purpura (Upshaw–Schulman syndrome). *J Thromb Haemost* 2004; **2**: 424–9.

250 Licht C, Stapenhorst L, Simon T, *et al*. Two novel ADAMTS13 gene mutations in thrombotic thrombocytopenic purpura/hemolytic-uremic syndrome (TTP/HUS). *Kidney Int* 2004; **66**: 955–8.

251 Hilbert L, Federici AB, Baronciani L, Dallagiovanna S, Mazurier C. A new candidate mutation, G1629R, in a patient with type 2A von Willebrand's disease: basic mechanisms and clinical implications. *Haematologica* 2004; **89**: 1128–33.

3

von Willebrand factor structure and function

Robert R. Montgomery[1] *and Sandra L. Haberichter*[2]

[1]Blood Research Institute, The Blood Center of Southeastern Wisconsin, Milwaukee, WI, USA

[2]Department of Pediatrics, Medical College of Wisconsin, Milwaukee, WI, USA

Introduction

The structure of von Willebrand factor (VWF) is primarily established through intracellular synthesis and processing that has been discussed in detail in Chapter 2 on VWF biosynthesis. This chapter will only briefly discuss this synthesis in the context of how it relates to functional modification, particularly those modifications that result in variant von Willebrand disease (VWD). Before the use of recombinant molecular techniques, most of the functions of VWF were recognized, and their structural correlates identified, through biochemical studies and through cell biology. This chapter will refer to many of these pioneering efforts, but it will not be an exhaustive review except where necessary. For example, if one does a literature search on VWF, many of the early references will not be identified because at that time (early 1970s) it was known as factor VIII (FVIII)-related antigen (FVIIIR:Ag or FVIII:Ag), high molecular weight FVIII antigen, or antihemophilic factor-like antigen (AHF-like antigen). The functions of VWF and the critical structural requisites will initially be summarized and then their structure–function relationships to one another will be discussed in greater detail. Some of the defects in function will result in variant forms of VWF that are responsible for variant VWD, which will be discussed in greater detail in Chapters 6, 9, and 12.

Von Willebrand Disease, 1st edition. Edited by Augusto B. Federici, Christine A. Lee, Erik E. Berntorp, David Lillicrap, Robert R. Montgomery. © 2011 Blackwell Publishing Ltd.

Four functions of VWF

There are at least four functions of VWF. Two of these functions are related to the initiation of hemostasis, firstly where VWF adheres to subendothelial matrix proteins (e.g., collagen) exposed during vascular injury [1–3] and, secondly, where this tethered VWF binds circulating platelets to initiate platelet adhesion through the glycoprotein Ib receptor (GPIb) [4–7]. Following adhesion, platelets are activated and undergo platelet aggregation, a process that primarily uses fibrinogen binding. A third function of VWF is to support platelet aggregation through binding to GPIIb/IIIa if fibrinogen levels are reduced or if the local concentration of VWF is sufficiently high to participate in that process [8–11]. The fourth function of VWF is to serve as a carrier protein for plasma FVIII. It was this process that resulted in the initial thinking that FVIII and VWF were part of the same protein, and explains why VWF was initially called FVIII-related antigen. Since activated FVIII ultimately must bind to the activated platelet's exposed phosphotidyl serine for its procoagulant activity, teleologically one might predict that the binding of VWF would facilitate the delivery of FVIII, but that function has not been fully defined.

Structure of VWF

The sequence of VWF was determined by classic protein sequencing at about the same time as the sequence was deduced from DNA sequencing [12–15], although the latter enabled the recognition of a large propeptide that was subsequently shown to be identical to the previously reported von Willebrand antigen II (VW:AgII) [16,17]. Each of these will be discussed in greater detail below.

Perhaps the most unique feature of VWF is its multimeric structure, which is responsible for VWF multimers in plasma that range from approximately 600,000 Da to >20 million Da [18–20]. As discussed in Chapter 2, these are the result of N-terminal disulfide bond multimerization of C-terminal disulfide-bonded dimers [21–23]. They form a long string of head-to-head and tail-to-tail bound monomers, yet the circulating resting structure has been described as a random coil or a ball of yarn [24–26]. It is this coiled structure that helps to keep VWF in a nonactive conformation until it is bound to the subendothelial matrix and unraveled by the shear stress of circulating blood. Both the binding of VWF to collagen and the binding of VWF to platelet GPIb are enhanced by large multimer size [27–29]. The binding of VWF to FVIII and to GPIIb/IIIa (integrin $\alpha_{IIb}\beta_3$) are not necessarily enhanced by the larger multimers.

In cell culture, VWF is secreted primarily through the regulated secretory pathway in cells with regulated storage, but some constitutive secretion also appears to occur [30,31]. With constitutive secretion, the multimers may not be fully processed and may consist of variably multimerized pro-VWF with a lack of VWF propeptide (VWFpp) cleavage [32–34]. *In vivo* it is not clear how much constitutive secretion occurs, since pro-VWF is not normally detected in plasma. After DDAVP (1-deamino-8-D-arginine vasopressin)-stimulated release of VWF, both the VWFpp and VWF are released, but there is no evidence of pro-VWF in plasma. Studies in dogs with type 3 VWD infused with pro-VWF synthesized in CHO cells demonstrated rapid cleavage of the VWFpp from pro-VWF in plasma [35,36]. Thus, if small amounts of pro-VWF are released normally by constitutive secretion into plasma, they might go undetected because of this enzymatic processing.

Plasma VWF is also processed by ADAMTS13, which cleaves VWF between Tyr[1605] and Met[1606] and will be discussed in greater detail in Chapter 4 [37–39]. This results in VWF multimer cleavage *in vivo* and is responsible, in part, for some of the variable-length multimers detected by high-resolution gel electrophoresis of VWF (see Chapter 9) and the presence of the "triplet structure" of VWF multimers analyzed by that

method [20,40–43]. Multimers cleaved by ADAMTS13 will be truncated on either the N-terminal or C-terminal end and migrate differently from the unprocessed multimer (normal C- and N-terminus) of approximately the same length. Using low-resolution gels, the individual multimers do not reveal these triplets.

In the late 1970s a second antigen was reported as missing from the plasma of patients with type 3 VWD which was referred to as VW:AgII [16]. Early studies demonstrated its release from endothelial cells and platelets, and its increased concentration in variant forms of VWD plasma [44–47]. Cellular studies demonstrated that VW:AgII (VWFpp) and VWF were distinct from one another, but within endothelial cells there appeared to be a common precursor that shared epitopes with both antigens (subsequently demonstrated to be pro-VWF) [47]. After the pro-VWF gene was sequenced, VW:AgII was demonstrated to be the propeptide of VWF, and therefore will be referred to as VWFpp [17].

VWF domain structure

After VWF was sequenced and analyzed, it became evident that it consisted of several homologous domains that shared structural features with one another. Figure 3.3 illustrates this domain structure and how it relates to biochemical and functional activities. There are three A domains, three B domains, two C domains, four D domains and a partial D domain referred to as D' [12,51–53].

The 22-amino acid signal peptide is responsible for directing VWF to the intracellular secretory pathway; it is not present in plasma [54]. The D1 and D2 domains comprise most of the 741-amino acid VWFpp. VWFpp is present in platelets, endothelial cells, and plasma, and its intracellular function has been reviewed in detail in Chapter 2. Once the VWFpp is cleaved from pro-VWF by furin intracellularly, the rest of the VWF is referred to as the mature monomer. While VWFpp is present in plasma, no extracellular function has yet been identified for this protein.

The VWF monomer is not detected in plasma; the smallest multimer in plasma is therefore a C-terminal dimer that is dimerized intracellularly through the C-terminus. The higher molecular weight multimers are therefore produced by N-terminal multimerization through cysteines at the C-terminal end of the D3 domain [23,30,34]. The N-terminus of VWF consists of the D' and D3 domains. These two domains contain many intrachain disulfide bonds, and the N-terminus is also the region of VWF that interacts with FVIII. Mutations in this region may cause absent or reduced FVIII binding and result in type 2N VWD [55–57]. This will be discussed later in this chapter in greater detail. The D3 domain is followed by three A domains. The A domains have structural similarities to the I domains of complement proteins and the L domain of Mac-1 [58,59]. The VWF A1 domain has been studied extensively because mutations in this region result in most of the type 2B and type 2M, as well as many of the type 2A, VWD variants [60–62]. While the A2 domain has three-dimensional structural similarity to the A1 and A3 domains, the A2 does not have the long-distance disulfide bond of the A1 and A3 loops [63–66]. However, the A2 domain does contain the ADAMTS13 proteolysis site and the accessory region that is required for this cleavage. Some mutations in this region of VWF increase the proteolytic susceptibility to ADAMTS13 and result in type 2A VWD [67–70]. The A3 domain is structurally similar to the A1, but the major function mapped to this domain is collagen binding [65,66,71]. This will be discussed in greater detail later in this chapter. Proteins, like fibrinogen and VWF that bind to platelet GPIIb/IIIa contain an "RGDS" (Arg-Gly-Asp-Ser) sequence [9,72–74]. This RGDS sequence is located at the C-terminal end of the VWF C1 domain. The extreme C-terminus of VWF contains the cystine knot domain (CK domain) that is critical for the C-terminal interchain disulfide dimerization. The structure/function of these domains will be discussed below.

Biochemistry of VWF

The biosynthesis and organization of VWF has been discussed in Chapter 2 and briefly summarized above. The VWF monomer contains 2050 amino acids that begin with Ser^{764} and end with Lys^{2813}. While reduced SDS gels predict a molecular weight of 220,000 Da for VWF, the actual molecular weight is estimated to be between 255,000 and 260,000, including 225,663 Da from the amino acids and an additional 10–15% from carbohydrate modification [75–77].

Multimers of VWF are exceptionally large, with the largest multimers (>20 million Da) being larger than some viral particles. Electron microscopic imaging of VWF demonstrates globular domains at both the N-terminus and C-terminus of the monomer—both of these regions are rich in cysteines and intrachain disulfide bonding [24,78]. When FVIII imaging has been simultaneously carried out, FVIII associates with the globular domain, presumably on the N-terminus [79]. When unwound, VWF multimers are filamentous strings that are as long as 11,500 angstroms, 25 times the length of fibrinogen. Under native conditions, these long filamentous multimers are compacted in a random coil (ball of string). After vascular injury, Weibel–Palade bodies release VWF that is tethered to endothelial cells by P-selectin or αVβ3 [80–83]. Alternatively, circulating VWF becomes attached to the subendothelial matrix. Under physiologic shear, VWF is unwound to produce the filamentous form. In this extended form, multiple platelet GPIb-binding sites become exposed and participate in the initiation of platelet adhesion. Several groups have demonstrated long strings of VWF with bound platelets appearing as "beads on a string" [81,84–86]. The largest VWF multimers are felt to be most important to this process physiologically. Reduction of multimer size by proteolysis or partial disulfide reduction has a dramatic effect on the platelet agglutinating activity. In type 2A VWF, only the smaller VWF multimers may be present. Smaller multimers have a reduced ability to recruit circulating platelets [64,87]. Small VWF multimers may augment the physiologic adhesive activity through self-association [88–90]. This self-association has the effect of producing a structure similar to the longer, higher molecular weight multimers and involves multiple domains of VWF—even VWF missing A1 or A3 domains. Functional assays of VWF vary in their ability to measure the function of large and small VWF multimers (see Chapter 9), for example assays employing ristocetin primarily measure high molecular weight VWF multimers in contrast to assays using botrocetin, in which even dimeric VWF may have normal activity. Collagen binding activity also reflects primarily high molecular weight VWF.

Interaction of VWF with FVIII

Since the 1970s, VWF has been recognized as the physiologic binding protein for FVIII in plasma [91]. When bound to VWF, FVIII has the same half-life as VWF (approximately 12–15 h), but in the absence of VWF (type 3 VWD), FVIII half-life is less than 2 h [92]. In a patient with type 3 VWD, the FVIII gene is normal but plasma FVIII levels are markedly reduced (3–8% of normal) [93]; this is because the steady-state level of FVIII is reduced in the absence of VWF. When patients with type 3 VWD are treated only with VWF, FVIII survival is prolonged and can reach normal plasma levels over the next 12–24 h if VWF infusions are maintained [92]. Interestingly, in conditions with accelerated clearance of FVIII (antibodies to FVIII or type 2N VWD), survival of VWF appears to be unaffected, but when there is accelerated clearance of VWF, FVIII also has accelerated clearance (antibodies to VWF, type 1C VWD) [94–98].

The light chain of FVIII binds to the N-terminal globular domain of VWF that is represented by the D′ and D3 domains. This is the region that may contain the mutations causing type 2N VWD that will be discussed in Chapter 12. Some of the disulfide bonds in this region have been mapped [99], but this region has not yet been crystallized. When FVIII binding has been studied, there appears to have been 1:1 stoichiometry of FVIII with the monomer of VWF, although this affinity is lower than that seen with multimerized VWF [100–102]. In plasma and in tissue culture expression of VWF with FVIII, there appears to be a 50:1 ratio of VWF with FVIII [103–105]. This may be due to the complex secondary and tertiary structure of VWF. The concentration of VWF in plasma is 10 μg/mL, while the concentration of FVIII is 200 ng/mL. Since these proteins are primarily referred to by their biologic concentration, WHO standardization has established the normal plasma concentration of each as 100 IU/dL for each protein. Thus, 1 IU of VWF is approximately 10 μg and 1 IU of FVIII is 200 ng.

Two sites of interaction between VWF and platelets

The structural interaction between VWF and platelets has been extensively studied, and there are two primary sites of interaction. The A1 domain of VWF interacts with the GPIb complex (GPIbα, GPIbβ, and GPIX) [4,106,107], and the RGDS sequence of the C1 domain interacts with the αIIbβ3 integrin receptor [8,9]. Each of these interactions will be discussed in greater detail.

Much of our early understanding of the interaction of VWF with platelets came from pioneering studies using the antibiotic, ristocetin [108–111]. Ristocetin was developed as an antibiotic but was withdrawn from clinical studies because it caused thrombocytopenia [112]. Studies subsequently demonstrated that ristocetin would aggregate platelets in platelet-rich plasma (PRP) from normal individuals but not from those with type 3 VWD [108,109,111]. Even after formalin fixation of normal platelets, a suspension of fixed platelets agglutinated in response to ristocetin [113]. This approach evolved into the widely used assay for VWF functional interaction with platelets, termed "ristocetin cofactor activity of VWF," or VWF:RCo [114–116].

A1 domain and its interaction with platelet GPIb
When scientists refer to the function of VWF, they are usually referring to its interaction with the GPIb complex on platelets [4,9,117,118]. The site of interaction on the GPIb complex is GPIbα, but GPIbα does not express on the platelet surface unless the other components of the complex are expressed, including GPIbβ and GPIX [118–123]. If a single mutation in GPIbα, GPIbβ, or GPIX prevents surface expression of one of these proteins, the entire complex is not expressed. Absence of this complex results in a hereditary bleeding disorder called Bernard–Soulier syndrome [118,124,125]. Within VWF it is the A1 domain (Figure 3.1) that interacts with GPIbα [9,126,127]. While the GPIb-binding site is within the A1 loop [127], the sites that interact with ristocetin lie just outside of this loop, with one site situated on the N-terminal side of the A1 loop and the other on the C-terminal side [126]. Ristocetin appears to dimerize at the same concentration that induces the binding of VWF to GPIb, and it is this two-site binding of ristocetin that is thought to alter the conformation of the A1 loop to induce its binding to GPIb [128]. While the physiologic stimulus that induces VWF binding to platelet GPIb is shear, ristocetin is used in the clinical laboratory to measure VWF function (see Chapter 9) [109,111,129,130].

There are three types of mutations that affect the binding of VWF to platelet GPIb. These include "gain-of-function" mutations that cause type 2B VWD [131,132], "loss-of-function" mutations that cause type 2M VWD [133–135], and mutations in GPIbα that cause gain-of-function interactions with VWF,

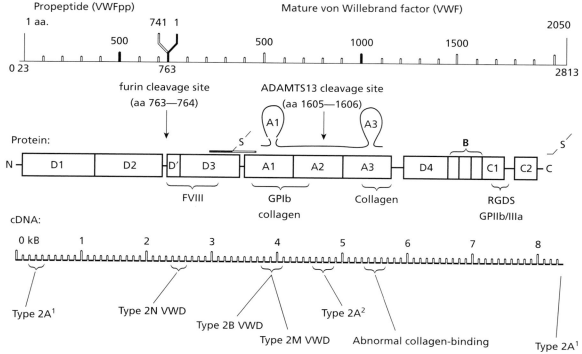

Figure 3.1 This figure provides the structural relationships between the von Willebrand factor (VWF) protein and the cDNA sequence. The mRNA that encodes VWF directs the synthesis of pro-VWF that includes a 22-amino acid signal peptide, a 741-amino acid propeptide (D1-D2), and a 2050-amino acid VWF monomer (D'-CK). In plasma, VWF exists as a large multimeric protein that is the result of N-terminal multimerization (D3 domain) of C-terminal VWF dimers (cystine knot or CK domain). The D'-D3 region includes the FVIII binding site. The A1 domain includes the A1 loop that binds to platelet GPIb. The A2 domain includes the ADAMTS13 cleavage site. The A1 and A3 domains include sites of collagen binding. The C1 domain includes the "RGDS" (Arg-Gly-Asp-Ser) site that binds to platelet GPIIb/IIIa. At the bottom of the illustration are the general regions in which mutations cause potential variants of von Willebrand disease (VWD), including types 2A, 2B, 2M, 2N, and 1C (↑-clearance). The 2A[1] designates mutations causing type 2V VWD by virtue of multimerization defects in contrast to the 2A[2] designation that causes type 2A VWD by virtue of increased sensitivity to ADAMTS13. (Used with permission of RR Montgomery.)

referred to as platelet-type or pseudo-VWD [136,137]. These are discussed in greater detail in Chapters 9 and 12. The crystal structure of the A1 domain has been solved [64,138,139] and has established that type 2B and 2M mutations cluster within the A1 domain [134,140]. Figure 3.2 demonstrates the distribution of these mutations from a recent US VWD study with the localizations based on the crystal structure solved by Emsley and coworkers [64]. *In vivo*, the stimulus for platelet adhesion to VWF is now recognized to be shear. Under shear, VWF is unraveled and exposes repetitive binding sites for platelet GPIb that initiate the immobilization of circulating or flowing platelets [141–143]. This is not a permanent immobilization and other cohesive events must occur in order to irreversibly bind platelets [144–147].

Platelet adhesion as studied with ristocetin does not require metabolically active platelets. In fact, the ristocetin cofactor assay uses formalin-fixed platelets [148]. Recently, studies have been carried out that suggest that the A1 loop of VWF has an active conformational state in which it is easily able to bind to platelet GPIb. A llama-derived antibody fragment binds to the A1 loop of VWF when VWF is in this

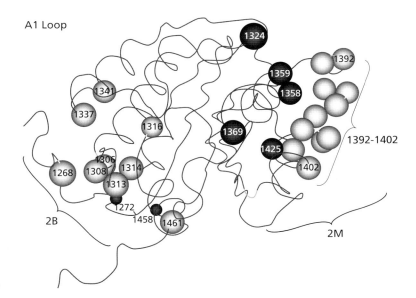

Figure 3.2 The A1 loop of von Willebrand factor (VWF) interacts with platelet GPIb and is formed by the disulfide bond connecting cys1272 and cys1458 (black small spheres). The crystal structure is based on the PDB 1auq structure as solved by Emsley *et al.* [61]. The mutations designated are from the Zimmerman Program Project on von Willebrand disease and include 2B mutations in white and IIm mutations in mid and dark gray. (Used with permission of RR Montgomery.)

active conformation [149–152]. This "activated VWF" is identified in thrombotic thrombocytopenic purpura (TTP) [152], type 2B VWF [152,153], malaria [154,155], HELLP syndrome [156], and antiphospholipid syndrome [151]. It will be important to determine if the state itself confers a thrombotic state or whether a thrombotic state alters VWF so that it interacts in the assay.

Interaction of VWF with platelet GPIIb/IIIa
Following platelet adhesion to VWF, platelets activate and then undergo the aggregation process [157–161]. When studied in a platelet aggregometer, platelets aggregate through the interaction of fibrinogen with the GPIIb/IIIa receptor. This process requires metabolically active platelets and involves intracellular signaling events that alter the conformation of GPIIb/IIIa to an active state. VWF can serve as the ligand for this receptor if the concentration of fibrinogen is low or absent [9,162]. *In vitro*, adenosine diphosphate (ADP) and thrombin induce the binding of VWF to GPIIb/IIIa [163,164]. Monoclonal antibodies to GPIIb/IIIa block this ADP or thrombin-induced VWF from binding to platelets [9,165]. *In vivo*, the local concentration of VWF is increased at sites of vascular injury by the local adsorption of VWF from plasma to the subendothelial matrix and the local release of VWF from platelet α-granules and endothe-

lial cell Weibel–Palade bodies. Studies have demonstrated that the release of VWF by platelets can increase the concentration of VWF to support this platelet–platelet interaction locally [90,166,167]. The GPIIb/IIIa receptors bind ligands containing RGDS. VWF has this RGDS sequence at amino acid positions 1744–1747 in the C1 domain of VWF (see Figure 3.1) [74,168–170]. When subjected to shear, VWF interacts with both the GPIIb/IIIa receptor and the GPIb receptor of platelets [142,171].

Interactions between VWF and collagen

An additional function of VWF is its interaction with collagen. As demonstrated in Figure 3.1, there are two sites on VWF that have been mapped for interaction with collagen. Most work on VWF has focused on the interaction of the A3 domain of VWF, but there are also data to support the interaction of the A1 domain with type VI collagen. The larger VWF multimers have a much higher affinity for collagen. Thus, collagen binding is an indirect measure of multimer size.

A3 domain interaction with collagen
The A3 domain of VWF has been studied extensively for its interaction with type I and III collagen [65,71,172–174]. There have been several reports of

mutations in the A3 domain that affect collagen binding to type I and type III collagen which are associated with clinical bleeding [49,50]. The collagen binding function of VWF (VWF:CB) has not been as extensively studied in patients as the other assays of VWF function [175–177]. A more thorough description of the clinical utility of this assay will be provided in Chapter 9. It is still not clear if collagen binding defects are infrequent or whether the assay simply has not been incorporated into the usual screening tests for VWF function. Figure 3.3 demonstrates the localization of the VWF mutations associated with collagen binding defects mapped on the crystal structure of the A3 domain published by Bienkowska and coworkers [48]. Monoclonal antibodies to the A3 domain have demonstrated inhibition of collagen VWF interactions, but these antibodies have not yet been mapped to specific epitopes within the A3 domain [172].

A1 domain and its interaction with collagen

Studies of type VI collagen have demonstrated its interaction with the A1 domain rather than the A3 domain [178–182]. While some studies suggest that

the A1 domain can substitute for the A3 domain under flow conditions [178], most clinical laboratory assays have looked only at type III and type I collagen [175]. The isolated A1 domain has demonstrated binding to both collagen and GPIb [179].

Proteolysis of VWF

When VWF was first purified and studied, in vitro proteolysis was extensively studied but few of these proteases were subsequently defined in vivo [183,184]. More recently, extensive studies by several groups helped to elucidate a protease that cleaved VWF that, when absent, resulted in TTP [38,185–191]. The enzyme was named ADAMTS13 and was found to be absent in a rare hereditary form of TTP [37] that ultimately led to the identification of the gene for this enzyme [192,193]. Furthermore, the more common acquired forms of TTP were found to be caused by autoantibodies to ADAMTS13 [194–196]. This was an important discovery and will be extensively reviewed in Chapter 4. Recently, leukocyte proteases were also identified that cleaved VWF near to the same site that is cleaved by ADAMTS13 [197]. The

A3 Loop

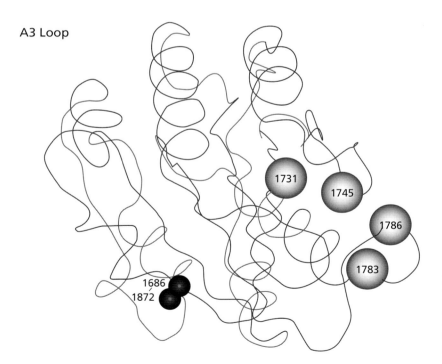

Figure 3.3 The A3 loop of von Willebrand factor (VWF) interacts with types 1 and III collagen. The crystal structure is based on the PDB 1a03 structure as solved by Bienkowska *et al.* [48]. The three mutations that are shown are for mutations that cause collagen binding defects in VWF and are associated with clinical bleeding. These include S1731T as published by Ribba *et al.* [50] and W1745C and S1783 as published by Riddell *et al.* [49]. A fourth mutation, H1786D, was identified by Flood and coworkers in a patient studied in the Zimmerman Program Project on VWD. (Used with permission of RR Montgomery.)

role of these proteases *in vivo* has not yet been well defined, and it is not clear if this protease might be responsible for some of the proteolysis of VWF in myeloproliferative disease [198–202]. Staphylococcal V-8 protease also modifies VWF and may have a role in acute sepsis [203–205].

Studies from a number of laboratories have demonstrated depolymerization of VWF through disulfide exchange with thrombospondin 1 [27,206,207]. This results in a reduction of VWF multimeric size. Some studies have also suggested a role of thrombospondin 1 in the regulation of ADAMTS13 on subendothelial VWF [208].

Carbohydrate modifications of VWF

The majority of carbohydrate modifications are the result of endoplasmic reticulum or Golgi processing steps that were reviewed in Chapter 2. About 15% of VWF by weight is the result of carbohydrate modifications. This carbohydrate is critical to the function and concentration of VWF. While the N-linked sugars are distributed across the VWF molecule, the O-linked sugars are clustered around the A1 domain. Early studies with purified VWF demonstrated that removing the negatively charged sialic acid residues (asialo-VWF) results in VWF that binds spontaneously to platelets without added agonist [209–212]. Modifying sugar moieties also affects VWF clearance. The RIIIS/J mouse is a model of VWD with markedly reduced, but not absent, VWF [213]. Studies on this mouse revealed an interesting mechanism for low VWF, which was an aberrant expression on N-acetylgalactosaminyltransferase [214,215]. In earlier studies, if the sialyl groups were removed, VWF survival changed from 4–5 h to 5 min [216]. The modified VWF bound to the asialoglycoprotein receptor in the liver and was rapidly cleared [217]. Blood group antigens have been recognized on VWF carbohydrate for many years [218,219]. An extensive study on blood group and VWF demonstrated that plasma VWF levels were lower in individuals who were blood type O, presumably because of the carbohydrate differences between blood types [220–223]; the blood group antigen genes are the modifying genes with the greatest effect on the level of plasma VWF [224]. Blood group antigens also affect the sensitivity to proteolysis by ADAMTS13 [225,226]. Studying VWF released by DDAVP, blood type O modifications

of VWF result in accelerated clearance of VWF in blood group O subjects [227]. This mechanism helps to explain the marked effect of blood type on plasma VWF levels [220] and, not surprisingly, results in a higher VWFpp/VWF:Ag ratio, as will be discussed in the next section.

Clearance of VWF

Plasma VWF is predominantly, if not exclusively, derived from endothelial synthesis. It is synthesized, stored, and released on an equimolar basis with its propeptide, VWFpp [92,94,228]. The half-life of VWF is approximately 12–15 h, but the half-life of VWFpp is around 2 h [229]. Modifications that affect VWF clearance will modify the level of plasma VWF but appear not to affect the clearance of the VWFpp. Thus, a number of laboratories have used the VWFpp/VWF:Ag ratio as a measure of VWF clearance [94,95,230–233]. Although VWF and FVIII form a circulating complex, there are differences in their relative clearance. In acquired hemophilia an autoantibody develops against FVIII. While the FVIII clearance is markedly increased, the plasma level of VWF is unaffected [234,235]. In contrast, acquired VWD caused by an autoantibody to VWF results in the clearance of both VWF and FVIII [198,236,237]. Recently, several papers have identified variant forms of type 1 VWD that are caused by accelerated clearance rather than reduced synthesis [94–98,238]. In these individuals the VWFpp/VWF:Ag ratio is markedly elevated and the reduced VWF is paralleled by reduced FVIII. Thus, VWF clearance is usually associated with clearance of FVIII; however, the converse is not usually seen but has been reported after high-dose infusion of FVIII [239]. There have been two recent reviews on VWF clearance [240,241]. These investigators have also established a murine model system in which to study accelerated clearance of VWF [242]. They have identified regions in VWF associated with changes in VWF clearance, including the A1-A3, D′-D3, and D4-CK regions that appear to have an independent importance to the clearance process. When labeled VWF was injected intravenously, most of the protein went to the liver, but some also went to the spleen [242]. To date, the only cell that has been found to take up VWF is the macrophage [243]. Lenting *et al.* have postulated a role for αMβ2 (MAC-1) integrin in this process, but more studies are necessary [240,241]. Understanding VWF clearance is also important for FVIII clearance. In the review by Lenting and coworkers, some recent studies were summarized that have targeted modification of VWF (e.g., PEGylation) in order to prolong the half-life of FVIII. It seems reasonable that if a reduced half-life of VWF results in a reduced half-life of FVIII, the converse will probably be seen with a VWF with long survival. Understanding VWF clearance mechanisms may not just be of biologic interest but might affect therapeutics for both VWD and hemophilia.

Disulfide structure of VWF

The pairing of cysteines, which are abundant in VWF, is critical to the various functions of VWF. Mutations in single cysteines have resulted in functional abnormalities of VWF [244,245]. Sadler and coworkers have mapped the disulfide bonds in two regions of VWF—in the 273-728 tryptic fragment for V8 protease digestion and the cysteine pairings in the cystine knot [99,246]. Other critical pairings include the disulfide bond between cys1272 and cys1458 that constrain the A1 loop and the cys1686–cys1872 disulfide that forms the A3 domain. The C-terminal dimerization of VWF monomers that occurs in the endoplasmic reticulum appears to involve one or more of the three cysteines at 2008, 2010, and/or 2048. In a similar manner, the multimerization of VWF involves cysteines in the D3 domain at positions 1142, 1222, 1225, and/or 1227. When ADAMTS13 cleaves VWF between Y1605 and M1606, proteolysed multimers are created with a truncated C-terminus on one multimer and a truncated N-terminus on the other. One outcome of this proteolysis is the creation of the characteristic triplet structure of VWF multimers (see Chapter 9). If VWF is depolymerized, the multimeric bands remain as singlets [35]. Proteolysis is the primary mechanism of the formation of the characteristic triplet structure of VWF in multimeric analysis [20,40,41].

Effects of shear on VWF

Normally, VWF circulates as a random coil of highly multimerized VWF that has been visualized by electron microscopy [26,247]. When it is unwound, the repeating subunits are visualized. *In vivo*, this transition is achieved by the adhesion of VWF to the exposed subendothelial matrix (e.g., collagen) by the A3 domain. Under shear and the binding of platelets through GPIb to the A1 domain, the A2 domain is stretched [248,249] and undergoes subsequent cleavage by ADAMTS13 [250]. This is a normal regulatory mechanism to limit the formation of platelet thrombi [251,252]. This also focuses the thrombus event at the site of vascular injury and prevents its pathologic propagation downstream. Shear is felt to be the physiologic agonist for the participation of VWF in initiating, propagating, and finally limiting the growing thrombus. Several instruments have been developed to attempt to quantify the effect of shear on VWF function [253–256]. Other than in a research setting, these have not been useful for VWF functional screening.

Structure and function of the VWF propeptide, VWFpp

The primary function of VWFpp as we understand it today is intracellular. This is reviewed in detail in Chapter 2. In the past there were some studies suggesting that VWFpp assisted in the regulation of VWF interaction with collagen; however, this was based on studies using bovine or porcine VWFpp [257–259]. Human VWFpp has not been demonstrated as having this function. Currently, VWFpp serves as a marker of VWF synthesis and its ratio to VWF:Ag can be used to identify clinical states, with accelerated VWF:Ag clearance as discussed above.

Summary

In summary, VWF serves a pivotal role in the functional regulation of hemostasis. VWF binds to collagen through the A3 domain and unravels under shear, enabling platelets to bind through GPIb to the A1 domain of VWF. The interaction of VWF with GPIIb/IIIa helps to stabilize this platelet binding. VWF also serves as a carrier protein for FVIII that binds to VWF through the D′ and D3 domains, but the participation in FVIII delivery to the activated platelet has not been well characterized. Regulation of this process by the effect of ADAMTS13 on the A2 domain helps to limit the propagation of thrombosis. Clearance of VWF is increased in some patients with type 1 VWD or with type 2 variants, but the mechanisms for this are still being defined.

Acknowledgements

The authors acknowledge support from NIH P01 HL081588 (RRM and SLH), R01 HL033721 (RRM and SLH), and P01 HL044612 (RRM).

References

1 Koutts J, Walsh PN, Plow EF, Fenton JW, Bouma BN, Zimmerman TS. Active release of human platelet factor VIII-related antigen by adenosine diphosphate, collagen, and thrombin. *J Clin Invest* 1978; **62**: 1255–63.

2 Nyman D. Interaction of collagen with the factor VIII antigen-activity—von Willebrand factor complex. *Thromb Res* 1977; **11**: 433–8.

3 Koutts J, Walsh PN, Plow EF, Fenton JW, Bouma BN, Zimmerman TS. Active release of human platelet factor VIII-related antigen by adenosine diphosphate, collagen, and thrombin. *J Clin Invest* 1978; **62**: 1255–63.

4 Coller BS, Peerschke EI, Scudder LE, Sullivan CA. Studies with a murine monoclonal antibody that abolishes ristocetin-induced binding of von Willebrand factor to platelets: additional evidence in support of GPIb as a platelet receptor for von Willebrand factor. *Blood* 1983; **61**: 99–110.

5 Goto S, Salomon DR, Ikeda Y, Ruggeri ZM. Characterization of the unique mechanism mediating the shear-dependent binding of soluble von Willebrand factor to platelets. *J Biol Chem* 1995; **270**: 23352–61.

6 Savage B, Saldivar E, Ruggeri ZM. Initiation of platelet adhesion by arrest onto fibrinogen or translocation on von Willebrand factor. *Cell* 1996; **84**: 289–97.

7 Ruggeri ZM, Zimmerman TS. Platelets and von Willebrand disease. *Semin Hematol* 1985; **22**: 203–18.

8 Ruggeri ZM, Bader R, De Marco L. Glanzmann thrombasthenia: deficient binding of von Willebrand factor to thrombin-stimulated platelets. *Proc Natl Acad Sci U S A* 1982; **79**: 6038–41.

9 Ruggeri ZM, De Marco L, Gatti L, Bader R, Montgomery RR. Platelets have more than one binding site for von Willebrand factor. *J Clin Invest* 1983; **72**: 1–12.

10 Fujimoto T, Ohara S, Hawiger J. Thrombin-induced exposure and prostacyclin inhibition of the receptor for factor VIII/von Willebrand factor on human platelets. *J Clin Invest* 1982; **69**: 1212–22.

11 Timmons S, Kloczewiak M, Hawiger J. ADP-dependent common receptor mechanism for binding of von Willebrand factor and fibrinogen to human platelets. *Proc Natl Acad Sci U S A* 1984; **81**: 4935–9.

12 Ginsburg D, Handin RI, Bonthron DT, *et al*. Human von Willebrand factor (vWF): isolation of complementary DNA (cDNA) clones and chromosomal localization. *Science* 1985; **228**: 1401–6.

13 Sadler JE, Shelton-Inloes BB, Sorace JM, Harlan JM, Titani K, Davie EW. Cloning and characterization of two cDNAs coding for human von Willebrand factor. *Proc Natl Acad Sci U S A* 1985; **82**: 6394–8.

14 Verweij CL, de Vries CJ, Distel B, *et al*. Construction of cDNA coding for human von Willebrand factor using antibody probes for colony-screening and mapping of the chromosomal gene. *Nucleic Acids Res* 1985; **13**: 4699–717.

15 Chopek MW, Girma JP, Fujikawa K, Davie EW, Titani K. Human von Willebrand factor: a multivalent protein composed of identical subunits. *Biochemistry* 1986; **25**: 3146–55.

16 Montgomery RR, Zimmerman TS. von Willebrand's disease antigen II. A new plasma and platelet antigen deficient in severe von Willebrand's disease. *J Clin Invest* 1978; **61**: 1498–507.

17 Fay PJ, Kawai Y, Wagner DD, *et al*. Propolypeptide of von Willebrand factor circulates in blood and is identical to von Willebrand antigen II. *Science* 1986; **232**: 995–8.

18 Meyer D, Obert B, Pietu G, Lavergne JM, Zimmerman TS. Multimeric structure of factor VIII/von Willebrand factor in von Willebrand's disease. *J Lab Clin Med* 1980; **95**: 590–602.

19 Ruggeri ZM, Zimmerman TS. Variant von Willebrand's disease: characterization of two subtypes by analysis of multimeric composition of factor VIII/von Willebrand factor in plasma and platelets. *J Clin Invest* 1980; **65**: 1318–25.

20 Ruggeri ZM, Zimmerman TS. The complex multimeric composition of factor VIII/von Willebrand factor. *Blood* 1981; **57**: 1140–3.

21 Wagner DD, Marder VJ. Biosynthesis of von Willebrand protein by human endothelial cells: processing steps and their intracellular localization. *J Cell Biol* 1984; **99**: 2123–30.

22 Wagner DD, Mayadas T, Urban-Pickering M, Lewis BH, Marder VJ. Inhibition of disulfide bonding of von Willebrand protein by monensin results in small, functionally defective multimers. *J Cell Biol* 1985; **101**: 112–20.

23 Wagner DD, Lawrence SO, Ohlsson-Wilhelm BM, Fay PJ, Marder VJ. Topology and order of formation of interchain disulfide bonds in von Willebrand factor. *Blood* 1987; **69**: 27–32.

24 Ohmori K, Fretto LJ, Harrison RL, Switzer ME, Erickson HP, McKee PA. Electron microscopy of human factor VIII/Von Willebrand glycoprotein: effect of reducing reagents on structure and function. *J Cell Biol* 1982; **95**: 632–40.

25 Beck EA, Tranqui-Pouit L, Chapel A, *et al*. Studies on factor VIII-related protein. I. Ultrastructural and

electrophoretic heterogeneity of human factor VIII-related protein. *Biochim Biophys Acta* 1979; **578**: 155–63.

26 Slayter H, Loscalzo J, Bockenstedt P, Handin RI. Native conformation of human von Willebrand protein. Analysis by electron microscopy and quasi-elastic light scattering. *J Biol Chem* 1985; **260**: 8559–63.

27 Pimanda JE, Ganderton T, Maekawa A, *et al.* Role of thrombospondin-1 in control of von Willebrand factor multimer size in mice. *J Biol Chem* 2004; **14**: 21439–48.

28 Furlan M. Von Willebrand factor: molecular size and functional activity. *Ann Hematol* 1996; **72**: 341–8.

29 Gerritsen HE, Turecek PL, Schwarz HP, Lammle B, Furlan M. Assay of von Willebrand factor (vWF)-cleaving protease based on decreased collagen binding affinity of degraded vWF: a tool for the diagnosis of thrombotic thrombocytopenic purpura (TTP). *Thromb Haemost* 1999; **82**:1386–9.

30 Wagner DD, Fay PJ, Sporn LA, Sinha S, Lawrence SO, Marder VJ. Divergent fates of von Willebrand factor and its propolypeptide (von Willebrand antigen II) after secretion from endothelial cells. *Proc Natl Acad Sci U S A* 1987; **84**: 1955–9.

31 Wagner DD. Cell biology of von Willebrand factor. *Annu Rev Cell Biol* 1990; **6**: 217–46.

32 Wagner DD, Marder VJ. Biosynthesis of von Willebrand protein by human endothelial cells. Identification of a large precursor polypeptide chain. *J Biol Chem* 1983; **258**: 2065–7.

33 Handin RI, Wagner DD. Molecular and cellular biology of von Willebrand factor. *Prog Hemost Thromb* 1989; **9**: 233–59.

34 Mayadas T, Wagner DD, Simpson PJ. von Willebrand factor biosynthesis and partitioning between constitutive and regulated pathways of secretion after thrombin stimulation. *Blood* 1989; **73**: 706–11.

35 Turecek PL, Gritsch H, Pichler L, *et al.* In vivo characterization of recombinant von Willebrand factor in dogs with von Willebrand disease. *Blood* 1997; **90**: 3555–67.

36 Schwarz HP, Dorner F, Mitterer A, *et al.* Evaluation of recombinant von Willebrand factor in a canine model of von Willebrand disease. *Haemophilia* 1998; **4** (Suppl. 3): 53–62.

37 Levy GG, Nichols WC, Lian EC, *et al.* Mutations in a member of the ADAMTS gene family cause thrombotic thrombocytopenic purpura. *Nature* 2001; **413**: 488–94.

38 Furlan M, Robles R, Lamie B. Partial purification and characterization of a protease from human plasma cleaving von Willebrand factor to fragments produced by in vivo proteolysis. *Blood* 1996; **87**: 4223–34.

39 Furlan M, Lammle B. von Willebrand factor in thrombotic thrombocytopenic purpura. *Thromb Haemost* 1999; **82**: 592–600.

40 Furlan M, Robles R, Affolter D, Meyer D, Baillod P, Lammle B. Triplet structure of von Willebrand factor reflects proteolytic degradation of high molecular weight multimers. *Proc Natl Acad Sci U S A* 1993; **90**: 7503–7.

41 Fischer BE, Thomas KB, Schlokat U, Dorner F. Triplet structure of human von Willebrand factor. *Biochem J* 1998; **331**: 483–8.

42 Studt JD, Budde U, Schneppenheim R, *et al.* Quantification and facilitated comparison of von Willebrand factor multimer patterns by densitometry. *Am J Clin Pathol* 2001; **116**: 567–74.

43 Budde U, Schneppenheim R, Eikenboom J, *et al.* Detailed von Willebrand factor multimer analysis in patients with von Willebrand disease in the European study, molecular and clinical markers for the diagnosis and management of type 1 von Willebrand disease (MCMDM-1VWD). *J Thromb Haemost* 2008; **6**: 762–71.

44 Scott JP, Montgomery RR. Platelet von Willebrand's antigen II: active release by aggregating agents and a marker of platelet release reaction *in vivo*. *Blood* 1981; **58**: 1075–80.

45 McCarroll DR, Ruggeri ZM, Montgomery RR. The effect of DDAVP on plasma levels of von Willebrand antigen II in normal individuals and patients with von Willebrand's disease. *Blood* 1984; **63**: 532–5.

46 McCarroll DR, Ruggeri ZM, Montgomery RR. Correlation between circulating levels of von Willebrand's antigen II and von Willebrand factor: discrimination between type I and type II von Willebrand's disease. *J Lab Clin Med* 1984; **103**: 704–11.

47 McCarroll DR, Levin EG, Montgomery RR. Endothelial cell synthesis of von Willebrand antigen II, von Willebrand factor, and von Willebrand factor/von Willebrand antigen II complex. *J Clin Invest* 1985; **75**: 1089–95.

48 Bienkowska J, Cruz M, Atiemo A, Handin R, Liddington R. The von Willebrand factor A3 domain does not contain a metal ion-dependent adhesion site motif. *J Biol Chem* 1997; **272**: 25162–7.

49 Riddell AF, Gomez K, Millar CM, *et al.* Characterisation of W1745C and S1783A: two novel mutations causing defective collagen binding in the A3 domain of von Willebrand factor. *Blood* 2009; **114**: 3489–96.

50 Ribba AS, Loisel I, Lavergne JM, *et al.* Ser968Thr mutation within the A3 domain of von Willebrand factor (VWF) in two related patients leads to a defective binding of VWF to collagen. *Thromb Haemost* 2001; **86**: 848–54.

51 Mancuso DJ, Tuley EA, Westfield LA, *et al.* Structure of the gene for human von Willebrand factor. *J Biol Chem* 1989; **264**: 19514–27.

52 Bonthron DT, Handin RI, Kaufman RJ, *et al*. Structure of pre-pro-von Willebrand factor and its expression in heterologous cells. *Nature* 1986; **324**: 270–3.

53 Girma JP, Meyer D, Verweij CL, Pannekoek H, Sixma JJ. Structure–function relationship of human von Willebrand factor. *Blood* 1987; **70**: 605–11.

54 Haberichter SL, Jozwiak MA, Rosenberg JB, Christopherson PA, Montgomery RR. The von Willebrand factor propeptide (VWFpp) traffics an unrelated protein to storage. *Arterioscler Thromb Vasc Biol* 2002; **22**: 921–6.

55 Kroner PA, Friedman KD, Fahs SA, Scott JP, Montgomery RR. Abnormal binding of factor VIII is linked with the substitution of glutamine for arginine 91 in von Willebrand factor in a variant form of von Willebrand disease. *J Biol Chem* 1991; **266**: 19146–9.

56 Kroner PA, Foster PA, Fahs SA, Montgomery RR. The defective interaction between von Willebrand factor and factor VIII in a patient with type 1 von Willebrand disease is caused by substitution of Arg19 and His54 in mature von Willebrand factor. *Blood* 1996; **87**: 1013–21.

57 Cacheris PM, Nichols WC, Ginsburg D. Molecular characterization of a unique von Willebrand disease variant. A novel mutation affecting von Willebrand factor/factor VIII interaction. *J Biol Chem* 1991; **266**: 13499–502.

58 Corbi AL, Kishimoto TK, Miller LJ, Springer TA. The human leukocyte adhesion glycoprotein Mac-1 (complement receptor type 3, CD11b) alpha subunit. Cloning, primary structure, and relation to the integrins, von Willebrand factor and factor B. *J Biol Chem* 1988; **263**: 12403–411.

59 Pytela R. Amino acid sequence of the murine Mac-1 alpha chain reveals homology with the integrin family and an additional domain related to von Willebrand factor. *EMBO J* 1988; **7**: 1371–8.

60 Ginsburg D, Sadler JE. von Willebrand disease: a database of point mutations, insertions, and deletions. For the Consortium on von Willebrand Factor Mutations and Polymorphisms, and the Subcommittee on von Willebrand Factor of the Scientific and Standardization Committee of the International Society on Thrombosis and Haemostasis. *Thromb Haemost* 1993; **69**: 177–84.

61 Sadler JE. A revised classification of von Willebrand disease. For the Subcommittee on von Willebrand Factor of the Scientific and Standardization Committee of the International Society on Thrombosis and Haemostasis. *Thromb Haemost* 1994; **71**: 520–5.

62 Sadler JE, Budde U, Eikenboom JC, *et al*. Update on the pathophysiology and classification of von Willebrand disease: a report of the Subcommittee on von Willebrand Factor. *J Thromb Haemost* 2006; **4**: 2103–14.

63 Emsley J, King SL, Bergelson JM, Liddington RC. Crystal structure of the I domain from integrin alpha-2beta1. *J Biol Chem* 1997; **272**: 28512–17.

64 Emsley J, Cruz M, Handin R, Liddington R. Crystal structure of the von Willebrand Factor A1 domain and implications for the binding of platelet glycoprotein Ib. *J Biol Chem* 1998; **273**: 10396–401.

65 Huizinga EG, Martijn van der Plas R, Kroon J, Sixma JJ, Gros P. Crystal structure of the A3 domain of human von Willebrand factor: implications for collagen binding. *Structure* 1997; **5**: 1147–56.

66 Romijn RA, Bouma B, Wuyster W, Gros P, Kroon J, Sixma JJ, Huizinga EG. Identification of the collagen-binding site of the von Willebrand factor A3-domain. *J Biol Chem* 2001; **276**: 9985–91.

67 Bowen DJ. Increased susceptibility of von Willebrand factor to proteolysis by ADAMTS13: should the multimer profile be normal or type 2A? *Blood* 2004; **103**: 3246.

68 Enayat MS, Guilliatt AM, Surdhar GK, *et al*. Aberrant dimerization of von Willebrand factor as the result of mutations in the carboxy-terminal region: identification of 3 mutations in members of 3 different families with type 2A (phenotype IID) von Willebrand disease. *Blood* 2001; **98**: 674–80.

69 Sutherland JJ, O'Brien LA, Lillicrap D, Weaver DF. Molecular modeling of the von Willebrand factor A2 Domain and the effects of associated type 2A von Willebrand disease mutations. *J Mol Model* 2004; **10**: 259–70.

70 Ginsburg D, Konkle BA, Gill JC, *et al*. Molecular basis of human von Willebrand disease: analysis of platelet von Willebrand factor mRNA. *Proc Natl Acad Sci U S A* 1989; **86**: 3723–7.

71 Lankhof H, van Hoeij M, Schiphorst ME, *et al*. A3 domain is essential for interaction of von Willebrand factor with collagen type III. *Thromb Haemost* 1996; **75**: 950–8.

72 Ruoslahti E, Pierschbacher MD. New perspectives in cell adhesion: RGD and integrins. *Science* 1987; **238**: 491–7.

73 Fressinaud E, Girma JP, Sadler JE, Baumgartner HR, Meyer D. Synthetic RGDS-containing peptides of von Willebrand factor inhibit platelet adhesion to collagen. *Thromb Haemost* 1990; **64**: 589–93.

74 Beacham DA, Wise RJ, Turci SM, Handin RI. Selective inactivation of the Arg-Gly-Asp-Ser (RGDS) binding site in von Willebrand factor by site-directed mutagenesis. *J Biol Chem* 1992; **267**: 3409–15.

75 Wagner DD, Mayadas T, Marder VJ. Initial glycosylation and acidic pH in the Golgi apparatus are required for multimerization of von Willebrand factor. *J Cell Biol* 1986; **102**: 1320–4.

76 Mayadas TN, Wagner DD. In vitro multimerization of von Willebrand factor is triggered by low pH.

Importance of the propolypeptide and free sulfhydryls. *J Biol Chem* 1989; **264**: 13497–503.

77 Vischer UM, Wagner DD. von Willebrand factor proteolytic processing and multimerization precede the formation of Weibel–Palade bodies. *Blood* 1994; **83**: 3536–44.

78 Slayter H, Loscalzo J, Bockenstedt P, Handin RI. Native conformation of human von Willebrand protein. Analysis by electron microscopy and quasi-elastic light scattering. *J Biol Chem* 1985; **260**: 8559–63.

79 Heijnen HF, Koedam JA, Sandberg H, Beeser-Visser NH, Slot JW, Sixma JJ. Characterization of human factor VIII and interaction with von Willebrand factor. An electron microscopic study. *Eur J Biochem* 1990; **194**: 491–8.

80 Padilla A, Moake JL, Bernardo A, *et al.* P-selectin anchors newly released ultra-large von Willebrand factor multimers to the endothelial cell surface. *Blood* 2003; **103**: 2150–6.

81 Lopez JA, Dong JF. Shear stress and the role of high molecular weight von Willebrand factor multimers in thrombus formation. *Blood Coagul Fibrinolysis* 2005; **16** (Suppl. 1): S11–S16.

82 Huang J, Roth R, Heuser JE, Sadler JE. Integrin alpha(v)beta(3) on human endothelial cells binds von Willebrand factor strings under fluid shear stress. *Blood* 2009; **113**: 1589–97.

83 Dole VS, Bergmeier W, Mitchell HA, Eichenberger SC, Wagner DD. Activated platelets induce Weibel–Palade-body secretion and leukocyte rolling *in vivo*: role of P-selectin. *Blood* 2005; **106**: 2334–9.

84 Tao Z, Peng Y, Nolasco L, *et al.* Recombinant CUB-1 domain polypeptide inhibits the cleavage of ULVWF strings by ADAMTS13 under flow conditions. *Blood* 2005; **106**: 4139–45.

85 Arya M, Kolomeisky AB, Romo GM, Cruz MA, Lopez JA, Anvari B. Dynamic force spectroscopy of glycoprotein Ib-IX and von Willebrand factor. *Biophys J* 2005; **88**: 4391–401.

86 Tao Z, Wang Y, Choi H, *et al.* Cleavage of ultralarge multimers of von Willebrand factor by C-terminal-truncated mutants of ADAMTS-13 under flow. *Blood* 2005; **106**: 141–3.

87 O'Brien LA, Sutherland JJ, Hegadorn C, *et al.* A novel type 2A (Group II) von Willebrand disease mutation (L1503Q) associated with loss of the highest molecular weight von Willebrand factor multimers. *J Thromb Haemost* 2004; **2**: 1135–42.

88 Ruggeri ZM. The role of von Willebrand factor in thrombus formation. *Thromb Res* 2007; **120** (Suppl. 1): S5–S9.

89 Ulrichts H, Vanhoorelbeke K, Girma JP, Lenting PJ, Vauterin S, Deckmyn H. The von Willebrand factor self-association is modulated by a multiple domain interaction. *J Thromb Haemost* 2005; **3**: 552–61.

90 Savage B, Sixma JJ, Ruggeri ZM. Functional self-association of von Willebrand factor during platelet adhesion under flow. *Proc Natl Acad Sci U S A* 2002; **99**: 425–30.

91 Zimmerman TS, Edgington TS. Factor VIII coagulant activity and factor VIII-like antigen: independent molecular entities. *J Exp Med* 1973; **138**: 1015–20.

92 Menache D, Aronson DL, Darr F, *et al.* Pharmacokinetics of von Willebrand factor and factor VIIIC in patients with severe von Willebrand disease (type 3 VWD): estimation of the rate of factor VIIIC synthesis. Cooperative Study Groups. *Br J Haematol* 1996; **94**: 740–5.

93 Nichols WL, Hultin MB, James AH, *et al.* von Willebrand disease (VWD): evidence-based diagnosis and management guidelines, the National Heart, Lung, and Blood Institute (NHLBI) Expert Panel report (USA). *Haemophilia* 2008; **14**: 171–232.

94 Haberichter SL, Balistreri M, Christopherson P, *et al.* Assay of the von Willebrand factor (VWF) propeptide to identify patients with type 1 von Willebrand disease with decreased VWF survival. *Blood* 2006; **108**: 3344–51.

95 Haberichter SL, Castaman G, Budde U, *et al.* Identification of type 1 von Willebrand disease patients with reduced von Willebrand factor survival by assay of the VWF propeptide in the European study: molecular and clinical markers for the diagnosis and management of type 1 VWD (MCMDM-1VWD). *Blood* 2008; **111**: 4979–85.

96 Casonato A, Pontara E, Sartorello F, *et al.* Reduced von Willebrand factor survival in type Vicenza von Willebrand disease. *Blood* 2002; **99**: 180–4.

97 Castaman G, Federici AB, Bernardi M, Moroni B, Bertoncello K, Rodeghiero F. Factor VIII and von Willebrand factor changes after desmopressin and during pregnancy in type 2M von Willebrand disease Vicenza: a prospective study comparing patients with single (R1205H) and double (R1205H-M740I) defect. *J Thromb Haemost* 2006; **4**: 357–60.

98 Sztukowska M, Gallinaro L, Cattini MG, *et al.* Von Willebrand factor propeptide makes it easy to identify the shorter Von Willebrand factor survival in patients with type 1 and type Vicenza von Willebrand disease. *Br J Haematol* 2008; **143**: 107–14.

99 Dong Z, Thoma RS, Crimmins DL, McCourt DW, Tuley EA, Sadler JE. Disulfide bonds required to assemble functional von Willebrand factor multimers. *J Biol Chem* 1994; **269**: 6753–8.

100 Zimmerman TS. Purification of factor VIII by monoclonal antibody affinity chromatography. *Semin Hematol* 1988; **25**: 25–6.

101 Weinstein RE. Immunoaffinity purification of factor VIII. *Ann Clin Lab Sci* 1989; **19**: 84–91.

102 Leyte A, Verbeet MP, Brodniewicz-Proba T, Van Mourik JA, Mertens K. The interaction between human

blood-coagulation factor VIII and von Willebrand factor. Characterization of a high-affinity binding site on factor VIII. *Biochem J* 1989; **257**: 679–83.

103 Kaufman RJ, Wasley LC, Dorner AJ. Synthesis, processing, and secretion of recombinant human factor VIII expressed in mammalian cells. *J Biol Chem* 1988; **263**: 6352–62.

104 Kaufman RJ, Wasley LC, Davies MV, Wise RJ, Israel DI, Dorner AJ. Effect of von Willebrand factor coexpression on the synthesis and secretion of factor VIII in Chinese hamster ovary cells. *Mol Cell Biol* 1989; **9**: 1233–42.

105 Kaufman RJ, Pipe SW. Regulation of factor VIII expression and activity by von Willebrand factor. *Thromb Haemost* 1999; **82**: 201–8.

106 Ruggeri ZM, Pareti FI, Mannucci PM, Ciavarella N, Zimmerman TS. Heightened interaction between platelets and factor VIII/von Willebrand factor in a new subtype of von Willebrand's disease. *N Engl J Med* 1980; **302**: 1047–51.

107 Miller JL, Kupinski JM, Castella A, Ruggeri ZM. von Willebrand factor binds to platelets and induces aggregation in platelet-type but not type IIB von Willebrand disease. *J Clin Invest* 1983; **72**: 1532–42.

108 Howard MA, Firkin BG. Ristocetin–a new tool in the investigation of platelet aggregation. *Thromb Diath Haemorrh* 1971; **26**: 362–9.

109 Howard MA, Sawers RJ, Firkin BG. Ristocetin: a means of differentiating von Willebrand's disease into two groups. *Blood* 1973; **41**: 687–90.

110 Weiss HJ, Hoyer IW. Von Willebrand factor: dissociation from antihemophilic factor procoagulant activity. *Science* 1973; **182**: 1149–51.

111 Weiss HJ, Hoyer LW, Rickles FR, Varma A, Rogers J. Quantitative assay of a plasma factor deficient in von Willebrand's disease that is necessary for platelet aggregation. Relationship to factor VIII procoagulant activity and antigen content. *J Clin Invest* 1973; **52**: 2708–16.

112 Gangarosa EJ, Johnson TR, Ramos HS. Ristocetin-induced thrombocytopenia: site and mechanism of action. *Arch Intern Med* 1960; **105**: 83–9.

113 Allain JP, Cooper HA, Wagner RH, Brinkhous KM. Platelets fixed with paraformaldehyde: a new reagent for assay of von Willebrand factor and platelet aggregating factor. *J Lab Clin Med* 1975; **85**: 318–28.

114 Zuzel M, Nilsson IM, Aberg M. A method for measuring plasma ristocetin cofactor activity. Normal distribution and stability during storage. *Thromb Res* 1978; **12**: 745–54.

115 Blatt PM, Brinkhous KM, Culp HR, Krauss JS, Roberts HR. Antihemophilic factor concentrate therapy in von Willebrand disease. Dissociation of bleeding-time factor and ristocetin-cofactor activities. *JAMA* 1976; **236**: 2770–2.

116 Rodeghiero F, Castaman G. Calibration of lyophilized standards for ristocetin cofactor activity of von Willebrand Factor (vWF) requires vWF-deficient plasma as diluent for dose-response curves. *Thromb Haemost* 1987; **58**: 978–81.

117 Coller BS, Gralnick HR. Studies on the mechanism of ristocetin-induced platelet agglutination. Effects of structural modification of ristocetin and vancomycin. *J Clin Invest* 1977; **60**: 302–12.

118 Montgomery RR, Kunicki TJ, Taves C, Pidard D, Corcoran M. Diagnosis of Bernard–Soulier syndrome and Glanzmann's thrombasthenia with a monoclonal assay on whole blood. *J Clin Invest* 1983; **71**: 385–9.

119 Nurden AT, Didry D, Rosa JP. Molecular defects of platelets in Bernard–Soulier syndrome. *Blood Cells* 1983; **9**: 333–58.

120 Ware J, Russell SR, Vicente V, *et al*. Nonsense mutation in the glycoprotein Ib alpha coding sequence associated with Bernard–Soulier syndrome. *Proc Natl Acad Sci U S A* 1990; **87**: 2026–30.

121 Ware J, Russell SR, Marchese P, *et al*. Point mutation in a leucine-rich repeat of platelet glycoprotein Ib alpha resulting in the Bernard–Soulier syndrome. *J Clin Invest* 1993; **92**: 1213–20.

122 Kenny D, Morateck PA, Gill JC, Montgomery RR. The critical interaction of glycoprotein (GP) IBbeta with GPIX-a genetic cause of Bernard–Soulier syndrome. *Blood* 1999; **93**: 2968–75.

123 Kenny D, Morateck PA, Montgomery RR. The cysteine knot of platelet glycoprotein Ib beta (GPIb beta) is critical for the interaction of GPIb beta with GPIX. *Blood* 2002; **99**: 4428–33.

124 Kenny D, Newman PJ, Morateck PA, Montgomery RR. A dinucleotide deletion results in defective membrane anchoring and circulating soluble glycoprotein Ib alpha in a novel form of Bernard–Soulier syndrome. *Blood* 1997; **90**: 2626–33.

125 Moran N, Morateck PA, Deering A, *et al*. Surface expression of glycoprotein ib alpha is dependent on glycoprotein ib beta: evidence from a novel mutation causing Bernard–Soulier syndrome. *Blood* 2000; **96**: 532–9.

126 Mohri H, Fujimura Y, Shima M, *et al*. Structure of the von Willebrand factor domain interacting with glycoprotein Ib. *J Biol Chem* 1988; **263**: 17901–4.

127 Berndt MC, Ward CM, Booth WJ, Castaldi PA, Mazurov AV, Andrews RK. Identification of aspartic acid 514 through glutamic acid 542 as a glycoprotein Ib-IX complex receptor recognition sequence in von Willebrand factor. Mechanism of modulation of von Willebrand factor by ristocetin and botrocetin. *Biochemistry* 1992; **31**: 11144–51.

128 Scott JP, Montgomery RR, Retzinger GS. Dimeric ristocetin flocculates proteins, binds to platelets, and

mediates von Willebrand factor-dependent agglutination of platelets. *J Biol Chem* 1991; **266**: 8149–55.

129 Meyer D, Jenkins CS, Dreyfus MD, Fressinaud E, Larrieu MJ. Willebrand factor and ristocetin. II. Relationship between Willebrand factor, Willebrand antigen and factor VIII activity. *Br J Haematol* 1974; **28**: 579–99.

130 Brinkhous KM, Graham JE, Cooper HA, Allain JP, Wagner RH. Assay of von Willebrand factor in von Willebrand's disease and hemophilia: use of a macroscopic platelet aggregation test. *Thromb Res* 1975; **6**: 267–72.

131 Kroner PA, Kluessendorf ML, Scott JP, Montgomery RR. Expressed full-length von Willebrand factor containing missense mutations linked to type IIB von Willebrand disease shows enhanced binding to platelets. *Blood* 1992; **79**: 2048–55.

132 Cooney KA, Nichols WC, Bruck ME, *et al*. The molecular defect in type IIB von Willebrand disease. Identification of four potential missense mutations within the putative GpIb binding domain. *J Clin Invest* 1991; **87**: 1227–33.

133 Mancuso DJ, Kroner PA, Christopherson PA, Vokac EA, Gill JC, Montgomery RR. Type 2M:Milwaukee-1 von Willebrand disease: an in-frame deletion in the Cys509-Cys695 loop of the von Willebrand factor A1 domain causes deficient binding of von Willebrand factor to platelets. *Blood* 1996; **88**: 2559–68.

134 Hillery CA, Mancuso DJ, Evan SJ, *et al*. Type 2M von Willebrand disease: F606I and I662F mutations in the glycoprotein Ib binding domain selectively impair ristocetin- but not botrocetin-mediated binding of von Willebrand factor to platelets. *Blood* 1998; **91**: 1572–81.

135 Rabinowitz I, Tuley EA, Mancuso DJ, *et al*. von Willebrand disease type B: a missense mutation selectively abolishes ristocetin-induced von Willebrand factor binding to platelet glycoprotein Ib. *Proc Natl Acad Sci U S A* 1992; **89**: 9846–9.

136 Miller JL, Castella A. Platelet-type von Willebrand's disease: characterization of a new bleeding disorder. *Blood* 1982; **60**: 790–4.

137 Weiss HJ, Meyer D, Rabinowitz R, *et al*. Pseudo-von Willebrand's disease. An intrinsic platelet defect with aggregation by unmodified human factor VIII/von Willebrand factor and enhanced adsorption of its high-molecular-weight multimers. *N Engl J Med* 1982; **306**: 326–33.

138 Celikel R, Varughese KI, Madhusudan, Yoshioka A, Ware J, Ruggeri ZM. Crystal structure of the von Willebrand factor A1 domain in complex with the function blocking NMC-4 Fab. *Nat Struct Biol* 1998; **5**: 189–94.

139 Huizinga EG, Tsuji S, Romijn RA, *et al*. Structures of glycoprotein Ibalpha and its complex with von Willebrand factor A1 domain. *Science* 2002; **297**: 1176–9.

140 Cruz MA, Diacovo TG, Emsley J, Liddington R, Handin RI. Mapping the glycoprotein Ib-binding site in the von willebrand factor A1 domain. *J Biol Chem* 2000; **275**: 19098–105.

141 Moake JL, Turner NA, Stathopoulos NA, Nolasco L, Hellums JD. Shear-induced platelet aggregation can be mediated by vWF released from platelets, as well as by exogenous large or unusually large vWF multimers, requires adenosine diphosphate, and is resistant to aspirin. *Blood* 1988; **71**: 1366–74.

142 Ikeda Y, Handa M, Kawano K, *et al*. The role of von Willebrand factor and fibrinogen in platelet aggregation under varying shear stress. *J Clin Invest* 1991; **87**: 1234–40.

143 Kroll MH, Hellums JD, McIntire LV, Schafer AI, Moake JL. Platelets and shear stress. *Blood* 1996; **88**: 1525–41.

144 Ruggeri ZM, Ruggeri ZM. Platelet and von Willebrand factor interactions at the vessel wall. *Hamostaseologie* 2004; **24**: 1–11.

145 Bergmeier W, Piffath CL, Goerge T, *et al*. The role of platelet adhesion receptor GPIbalpha far exceeds that of its main ligand, von Willebrand factor, in arterial thrombosis. *Proc Natl Acad Sci U S A* 2006; **103**: 16900–5.

146 Reininger AJ, Heijnen HF, Schumann H, Specht HM, Schramm W, Ruggeri ZM. Mechanism of platelet adhesion to von Willebrand factor and microparticle formation under high shear stress. *Blood* 2006; **107**: 3537–45.

147 Ruggeri ZM, Orje JN, Habermann R, Federici AB, Reininger AJ. Activation-independent platelet adhesion and aggregation under elevated shear stress. *Blood* 2006; **108**: 1903–10.

148 Ramsey R, Evatt BL. Rapid assay for von Willebrand factor activity using formalin-fixed platelets and microtitration technic. *Am J Clin Pathol* 1979; **72**: 996–9.

149 Groot E, Fijnheer R, Sebastian SA, de Groot PG, Lenting PJ. The active conformation of von Willebrand factor in patients with thrombotic thrombocytopenic purpura in remission. *J Thromb Haemost* 2009; **7**: 962–9.

150 Groot E, de Groot PG, Fijnheer R, Lenting PJ. The presence of active von Willebrand factor under various pathological conditions. *Curr Opin Hematol* 2007; **14**: 284–9.

151 Hulstein JJ, Lenting PJ, de Laat B, Derksen RH, Fijnheer R, de Groot PG. beta2-Glycoprotein I inhibits von Willebrand factor dependent platelet adhesion and aggregation. *Blood* 2007; **110**: 1483–91.

152 Hulstein JJ, de Groot PG, Silence K, Veyradier A, Fijnheer R, Lenting PJ. A novel nanobody that detects the gain-of-function phenotype of von Willebrand factor in ADAMTS13 deficiency and von Willebrand disease type 2B. *Blood* 2005; **106**: 3035–42.

153 Stakiw J, Bowman M, Hegadorn C, *et al.* The effect of exercise on von Willebrand factor and ADAMTS-13 in individuals with type 1 and type 2B von Willebrand disease. *J Thromb Haemost* 2007; **6**: 90–6.

154 de MQ, Groot E, Asih PB, Syafruddin D, Oosting M, Sebastian S, Ferwerda B, Netea MG, de Groot PG, van d, V, Fijnheer R. ADAMTS13 deficiency with elevated levels of ultra-large and active von Willebrand factor in P. falciparum and P. vivax malaria. *Am J Trop Med Hyg* 2009; **80**: 492–498.

155 de Mast Q, Groot E, Lenting PJ, *et al.* Thrombocytopenia and release of activated von Willebrand Factor during early Plasmodium falciparum malaria. *J Infect Dis* 2007; **196**: 622–8.

156 Hulstein JJ, van Runnard Heimel PJ, Franx A, *et al.* Acute activation of the endothelium results in increased levels of active von Willebrand factor in hemolysis, elevated liver enzymes and low platelets (HELLP) syndrome. *J Thromb Haemost* 2006; **4**: 2569–75.

157 Ruggeri ZM, De Marco L, Gatti L, Bader R, Montgomery RR. Platelets have more than one binding site for von Willebrand factor. *J Clin Invest* 1983; **72**: 1–12.

158 Phillips DR, Fitzgerald LA, Charo IF, Parise LV. The platelet membrane glycoprotein IIb/IIIa complex. Structure, function, and relationship to adhesive protein receptors in nucleated cells. *Ann N Y Acad Sci* 1987; **509**: 177–87.

159 De Marco L, Girolami A, Zimmerman TS, Ruggeri ZM. Interaction of purified type IIB von Willebrand factor with the platelet membrane glycoprotein Ib induces fibrinogen binding to the glycoprotein IIb/IIIa complex and initiates aggregation. *Proc Natl Acad Sci U S A* 1985; **82**: 7424–8.

160 Grainick HR, Williams SB, Coller BS. Asialo von Willebrand factor interactions with platelets. Interdependence of glycoproteins Ib and IIb/IIIa for binding and aggregation. *J Clin Invest* 1985; **75**: 19–25.

161 Lombardo VT, Hodson E, Roberts JR, Kunicki TJ, Zimmerman TS, Ruggeri ZM. Independent modulation of von Willebrand factor and fibrinogen binding to the platelet membrane glycoprotein IIb/IIIa complex as demonstrated by monoclonal antibody. *J Clin Invest* 1985; **76**: 1950–8.

162 Schullek J, Jordan J, Montgomery RR. Interaction of von Willebrand factor with human platelets in the plasma milieu. *J Clin Invest* 1984; **73**: 421–8.

163 Fujimoto T, Ohara S, Hawiger J. Thrombin-induced exposure and prostacyclin inhibition of the receptor for factor VIII/von Willebrand factor on human platelets. *J Clin Invest* 1982; **69**: 1212–22.

164 Fujimoto T, Hawiger J. Adenosine diphosphate induces binding of von Willebrand factor to human platelets. *Nature* 1982; **297**: 154–6.

165 Schullek J, Jordan J, Montgomery RR. Interaction of von Willebrand factor with human platelets in the plasma milieu. *J Clin Invest* 1984; **73**: 421–8.

166 Ruggeri ZM. Role of von Willebrand factor in platelet thrombus formation. *Ann Med* 2000; **32** (Suppl. 1): 2–9.

167 Ruggeri ZM, Dent JA, Saldivar E. Contribution of distinct adhesive interactions to platelet aggregation in flowing blood. *Blood* 1999; **94**: 172–8.

168 Saelman EU, Hese KM, Nieuwenhuis HK, *et al.* Aggregate formation is more strongly inhibited at high shear rates by dRGDW, a synthetic RGD-containing peptide. *Arterioscler Thromb* 1993; **13**: 1164–70.

169 Litjens PE, Van WG, Weeterings C, *et al.* A tripeptide mimetic of von Willebrand factor residues 981–983 enhances platelet adhesion to fibrinogen by signaling through integrin alpha(IIb)beta3. *J Thromb Haemost* 2005; **3**: 1274–83.

170 Jumilly AL, Veyradier A, Ribba AS, Meyer D, Girma JP. Selective inactivation of Von Willebrand factor binding to glycoprotein IIb/IIIa and to inhibitor monoclonal antibody 9 by site-directed mutagenesis. *Hematol J* 2001; **2**: 180–7.

171 O'Brien JR, Salmon GP. Shear stress activation of platelet glycoprotein IIb/IIIa plus von Willebrand factor causes aggregation: filter blockage and the long bleeding time in von Willebrand's disease. *Blood* 1987; **70**: 1354–61.

172 Zhao Y, Dong N, Shen F, *et al.* Two novel monoclonal antibodies to VWFA3 inhibit VWF-collagen and VWF–platelet interactions. *J Thromb Haemost* 2007; **5**: 1963–70.

173 Nishida N, Sumikawa H, Sakakura M, *et al.* Collagen-binding mode of vWF-A3 domain determined by a transferred cross-saturation experiment. *Nat Struct Biol* 2003; **10**: 53–8.

174 Romijn RA, Westein E, Bouma B, *et al.* Mapping the collagen-binding site in the von Willebrand factor A3-domain. *J Biol Chem* 2003; **278**: 15035–9.

175 Favaloro EJ. Toward a new paradigm for the identification and functional characterization of von Willebrand disease. *Semin Thromb Hemost* 2009; **35**: 60–75.

176 Favaloro EJ. An update on the von Willebrand factor collagen binding assay: 21 years of age and beyond adolescence but not yet a mature adult. *Semin Thromb Hemost* 2007; **33**: 727–44.

177 Favaloro EJ, Henniker A, Facey D, Hertzberg M. Discrimination of von Willebrands disease (VWD) subtypes: direct comparison of von Willebrand factor:collagen binding assay (VWF:CBA) with monoclonal antibody (MAB) based VWF-capture systems. *Thromb Haemost* 2000; **84**: 541–7.

178 Bonnefoy A, Romijn RA, Vandervoort PA, Van Rompaey I, Vermylen J, Hoylaerts MF. von Willebrand

factor A1 domain can adequately substitute for A3 domain in recruitment of flowing platelets to collagen. *J Thromb Haemost* 2006; **4**: 2151–61.

179 Morales LD, Martin C, Cruz MA. The interaction of von Willebrand factor-A1 domain with collagen: mutation G1324S (type 2M von Willebrand disease) impairs the conformational change in A1 domain induced by collagen. *J Thromb Haemost* 2006; **4**: 417–25.

180 Rand JH, Wu XX, Potter BJ, Uson RR, Gordon RE. Co-localization of von Willebrand factor and type VI collagen in human vascular subendothelium. *Am J Pathol* 1993; **142**: 843–50.

181 Rand JH, Patel ND, Schwartz E, Zhou SL, Potter BJ. 150-kD von Willebrand factor binding protein extracted from human vascular subendothelium is type VI collagen. *J Clin Invest* 1991; **88**: 253–9.

182 Rand JH, Glanville RW, Wu XX, *et al.* The significance of subendothelial von Willebrand factor. *Thromb Haemost* 1997; **78**: 445–50.

183 Bonnefoy A, Legrand C. Proteolysis of subendothelial adhesive glycoproteins (fibronectin, thrombospondin, and von Willebrand factor) by plasmin, leukocyte cathepsin G, and elastase. *Thromb Res* 2000; **98**: 323–32.

184 Kunicki TJ, Montgomery RR, Schullek J. Cleavage of human von Willebrand factor by platelet calcium-activated protease. *Blood* 1985; **65**: 352–6.

185 Moake JL, Byrnes JJ. Thrombotic microangiopathies associated with drugs and bone marrow transplantation. *Hematol Oncol Clin North Am* 1996; **10**: 485–97.

186 Moake JL. Thrombotic thrombocytopenic purpura. *Thromb Haemost* 1995; **74**: 240–5.

187 Moake JL. The role of von Willebrand factor (vWF) in thrombotic thrombocytopenic purpura (TTP) and the hemolytic-uremic syndrome (HUS). *Prog Clin Biol Res* 1990; **337**: 135–40.

188 Furlan M, Lammle B. Assays of von Willebrand factor-cleaving protease: a test for diagnosis of familial and acquired thrombotic thrombocytopenic purpura. *Semin Thromb Hemost* 2002; **28**: 167–72.

189 Furlan M, Robles R, Solenthaler M, Lammle B. Acquired deficiency of von Willebrand factor-cleaving protease in a patient with thrombotic thrombocytopenic purpura. *Blood* 1998; **91**: 2839–46.

190 Tsai HM. Physiologic cleavage of von Willebrand factor by a plasma protease is dependent on its conformation and requires calcium ion. *Blood* 1996; **87**: 4235–44.

191 Tsai HM, Sussman II, Nagel RL. Shear stress enhances the proteolysis of von Willebrand factor in normal plasma. *Blood* 1994; **83**: 2171–9.

192 Zheng X, Chung D, Takayama TK, Majerus EM, Sadler JE, Fujikawa K. Structure of von Willebrand factor-cleaving protease (ADAMTS13), a metalloprotease involved in thrombotic thrombocytopenic purpura. *J Biol Chem* 2001; **276**: 41059–63.

193 Zheng X, Majerus EM, Sadler JE. ADAMTS13 and TTP. *Curr Opin Hematol* 2002; **9**: 389–94.

194 Rieger M, Mannucci PM, Kremer Hovinga JA, *et al.* ADAMTS13 autoantibodies in patients with thrombotic microangiopathies and other immunomediated diseases. *Blood* 2005; **106**: 1262–7.

195 Pham PT, Danovitch GM, Wilkinson AH, *et al.* Inhibitors of ADAMTS13: a potential factor in the cause of thrombotic microangiopathy in a renal allograft recipient. *Transplantation* 2002; **74**: 1077–80.

196 Tsai HM. Deficiency of ADAMTS13 and thrombotic thrombocytopenic purpura. *Transfusion* 2002; **42**: 1523–4.

197 Raife TJ, Cao W, Atkinson BS, *et al.* Leukocyte proteases cleave von Willebrand factor at or near the ADAMTS13 cleavage site. *Blood* 2009; **114**: 1666–74.

198 Federici AB. Acquired von Willebrand syndrome: is it an extremely rare disorder or do we see only the tip of the iceberg? *J Thromb Haemost* 2008; **6**: 565–8.

199 Federici AB. Acquired von Willebrand syndrome: an underdiagnosed and misdiagnosed bleeding complication in patients with lymphoproliferative and myeloproliferative disorders. *Semin Hematol* 2006; **43**: S48–S58.

200 Federici AB, Rand JH, Mannucci PM. Acquired von Willebrand syndrome: an important bleeding complication to be considered in patients with lymphoproliferative and myeloproliferative disorders. *Hematol J* 2001; **2**: 358–62.

201 Landolfi R. Bleeding and thrombosis in myeloproliferative disorders. *Curr Opin Hematol* 1998; **5**: 327–31.

202 Kessler CM. Propensity for hemorrhage and thrombosis in chronic myeloproliferative disorders. *Semin Hematol* 2004; **41**: 10–14.

203 Kroh HK, Panizzi P, Bock PE. Von Willebrand factor-binding protein is a hysteretic conformational activator of prothrombin. *Proc Natl Acad Sci U S A* 2009; **106**: 7786–91.

204 Herrmann M, Hartleib J, Kehrel B, Montgomery RR, Sixma JJ, Peters G. Interaction of von Willebrand factor with *Staphylococcus aureus*. *J Infect Dis* 1997; **176**: 984–91.

205 Mascari LM, Ross JM. Quantification of staphylococcal-collagen binding interactions in whole blood by use of a confocal microscopy shear-adhesion assay. *J Infect Dis* 2003; **188**: 98–107.

206 Xie L, Chesterman CN, Hogg PJ. Control of von Willebrand factor multimer size by thrombospondin-1. *J Exp Med* 2001; **193**: 1341–9.

207 Bonnefoy A, Moura R, Hoylaerts MF. The evolving role of thrombospondin-1 in hemostasis and vascular biology. *Cell Mol Life Sci* 2008; **65**: 713–27.

208 Bonnefoy A, Daenens K, Feys HB, *et al.* Thrombospondin-1 controls vascular platelet recruit-

ment and thrombus adherence in mice by protecting (sub)endothelial VWF from cleavage by ADAMTS13. *Blood* 2006; **107**: 955–64.

209 Grainick HR, Williams SB, Coller BS. Asialo von Willebrand factor interactions with platelets. Interdependence of glycoproteins Ib and IIb/IIIa for binding and aggregation. *J Clin Invest* 1985; **75**: 19–25.

210 De Marco L, Shapiro SS. Properties of human asialo-factor VIII. A ristocetin-independent platelet-aggregating agent. *J Clin Invest* 1981; **68**: 321–8.

211 Sodetz JM, Paulson JC, Pizzo SV, McKee PA. Carbohydrate on human factor VIII/von Willebrand factor. Impairment of function by removal of specific galactose residues. *J Biol Chem* 1978; **253**: 7202–6.

212 Miller JL, Ruggeri ZM, Lyle VA. Unique interactions of asialo von Willebrand factor with platelets in platelet-type von Willebrand disease. *Blood* 1987; **70**: 1804–9.

213 Sweeney JD, Novak EK, Reddington M, Takeuchi KH, Swank RT. The RIIIS/J inbred mouse strain as a model for von Willebrand disease. *Blood* 1990; **76**: 2258–65.

214 Johnsen JM, Levy GG, Westrick RJ, Tucker PK, Ginsburg D. The endothelial-specific regulatory mutation, Mvwf1, is a common mouse founder allele. *Mamm Genome* 2008; **19**: 32–40.

215 Nichols WC, Cooney KA, Mohlke KL, *et al.* von Willebrand disease in the RIIIS/J mouse is caused by a defect outside of the von Willebrand factor gene. *Blood* 1994; **83**: 3225–31.

216 Sodetz JM, Pizzo SV, McKee PA. Relationship of sialic acid to function and *in vivo* survival of human factor VIII/von Willebrand factor protein. *J Biol Chem* 1977; **252**: 5538–46.

217 Sorensen AL, Rumjantseva V, Nayeb-Hashemi S, *et al.* Role of sialic acid for platelet lifespan: exposure of {beta}galactose results in the rapid clearance of platelets from the circulation by asialoglycoprotein receptor-expressing liver macrophages and hepatocytes. *Blood* 2009; **114**: 1645–54.

218 Sodetz JM, Paulson JC, McKee PA. Carbohydrate composition and identification of blood group A, B, and H oligosaccharide structures on human Factor VIII/von Willebrand factor. *J Biol Chem* 1979; **254**: 10754–60.

219 Kao KJ, Pizzo SV, McKee PA. Factor VIII/von Willebrand protein. Modification of its carbohydrate causes reduced binding to platelets. *J Biol Chem* 1980; **255**: 10134–9.

220 Gill JC, Endres-Brooks J, Bauer PJ, Marks WJ, Jr., Montgomery RR. The effect of ABO blood group on the diagnosis of von Willebrand disease. *Blood* 1987; **69**: 1691–5.

221 Jenkins PV, O'Donnell JS. ABO blood group determines plasma von Willebrand factor levels: a biologic function after all? *Transfusion* 2006; **46**: 1836–44.

222 Tirado I, Mateo J, Soria JM, *et al.* The ABO blood group genotype and factor VIII levels as independent risk factors for venous thromboembolism. *Thromb Haemost* 2005; **93**: 468–74.

223 Castaman G, Eikenboom JC. ABO blood group also influences the von Willebrand factor (VWF) antigen level in heterozygous carriers of VWF null alleles, type 2N mutation Arg854Gln, and the missense mutation Cys2362Phe. *Blood* 2002; **100**: 1927–8.

224 Levy G, Ginsburg D. Getting at the variable expressivity of von Willebrand disease. *Thromb Haemost* 2001; **86**: 144–8.

225 O'Donnell J, McKinnon TA, Crawley JT, Lane DA, Laffan MA. Bombay phenotype is associated with reduced plasma-VWF levels and an increased susceptibility to ADAMTS13 proteolysis. *Blood* 2005; **106**: 1988–91.

226 Bowen DJ. An influence of ABO blood group on the rate of proteolysis of von Willebrand factor by ADAMTS13. *J Thromb Haemost* 2003; **1**: 33–40.

227 Gallinaro L, Cattini MG, Sztukowska M, *et al.* A shorter von Willebrand factor survival in O blood group subjects explains how ABO determinants influence plasma von Willebrand factor. *Blood* 2008; **111**: 3540–5.

228 Van Mourik JA, Boertjes R, Huisveld IA, *et al.* von Willebrand factor propeptide in vascular disorders: A tool to distinguish between acute and chronic endothelial cell perturbation. *Blood* 1999; **94**: 179–85.

229 Haberichter SL, Merricks EP, Fahs SA, Christopherson PA, Nichols TC, Montgomery RR. Re-establishment of VWF-dependent Weibel–Palade bodies in VWD endothelial cells. *Blood* 2005; **105**: 145–52.

230 Vischer UM, Emeis JJ, Bilo HJ, *et al.* von Willebrand factor (vWf) as a plasma marker of endothelial activation in diabetes: improved reliability with parallel determination of the vWf propeptide (vWf:AgII). *Thromb Haemost* 1998; **80**: 1002–7.

231 Vischer UM, Ingerslev J, Wollheim CB, *et al.* Acute von Willebrand factor secretion from the endothelium *in vivo*: assessment through plasma propeptide (vWf:AgII) levels. *Thromb Haemost* 1997; **77**: 387–93.

232 Hollestelle MJ, Donkor C, Mantey EA, *et al.* von Willebrand factor propeptide in malaria: evidence of acute endothelial cell activation. *Br J Haematol* 2006; **133**: 562–9.

233 Nossent AY, Van Marion V, Van Tilburg NH, *et al.* von Willebrand factor and its propeptide: the influence of secretion and clearance on protein levels and the risk of venous thrombosis. *J Thromb Haemost* 2006; **4**: 2556–62.

234 Zakarija A, Green D. Acquired hemophilia: diagnosis and management. *Curr Hematol Rep* 2002; **1**: 27–33.

235 Boggio LN, Green D. Acquired hemophilia. *Rev Clin Exp Hematol* 2001; **5**: 389–404.

236 Collins P, Budde U, Rand JH, Federici AB, Kessler CM. Epidemiology and general guidelines of the management of acquired haemophilia and von Willebrand syndrome. *Haemophilia* 2008; **14** (Suppl. 3): 49–55.

237 Federici AB, Budde U, Rand JH. Acquired von Willebrand syndrome 2004: International Registry–diagnosis and management from online to bedside. *Hamostaseologie* 2004; **24**: 50–5.

238 Gadisseur A, Berneman Z, Schroyens W, Michiels JJ. Laboratory diagnosis of von Willebrand disease type 1/2E (2A subtype IIE), type 1 Vicenza and mild type 1 caused by mutations in the D3, D4, B1-B3 and C1-C2 domains of the von Willebrand factor gene. Role of von Willebrand factor multimers and the von Willebrand factor propeptide/antigen ratio. *Acta Haematol* 2009; **121**: 128–38.

239 Rock G, Adamkiewicz T, Blanchette V, Poon A, Sparling C. Acquired von Willebrand factor deficiency during high-dose infusion of recombinant factor VIII. *Br J Haematol* 1996; **93**: 684–7.

240 Denis CV, Christophe OD, Oortwijn BD, Lenting PJ. Clearance of von Willebrand factor. *Thromb Haemost* 2008; **99**: 271–8.

241 Lenting PJ, Van Schooten CJ, Denis CV. Clearance mechanisms of von Willebrand factor and factor VIII. *J Thromb Haemost* 2007; **5**: 1353–60.

242 Lenting PJ, Westein E, Terraube V, *et al.* An experimental model to study the in vivo survival of von Willebrand factor. Basic aspects and application to the R1205H mutation. *J Biol Chem* 2004; **279**: 12102–9.

243 Van Schooten CJ, Shahbazi S, Groot E, *et al.* Macrophages contribute to the cellular uptake of von Willebrand factor and factor VIII in vivo. *Blood* 2008; **112**: 1704–12.

244 Schooten CJ, Tjernberg P, Westein E, *et al.* Cysteine-mutations in von Willebrand factor associated with increased clearance. *J Thromb Haemost* 2005; **3**: 2228–37.

245 Tjernberg P, Vos HL, Castaman G, Bertina RM, Eikenboom JC. Dimerization and multimerization defects of von Willebrand factor due to mutated cysteine residues. *J Thromb Haemost* 2004; **2**: 257–65.

246 Katsumi A, Tuley EA, Bodo I, Sadler JE. Localization of disulfide bonds in the cystine knot domain of human von Willebrand factor. *J Biol Chem* 2000; **275**: 25585–94.

247 Ohmori K, Fretto LJ, Harrison RL, Switzer ME, Erickson HP, McKee PA. Electron microscopy of human factor VIII/Von Willebrand glycoprotein: effect of reducing reagents on structure and function. *J Cell Biol* 1982; **95**: 632–40.

248 Zhang X, Halvorsen K, Zhang CZ, Wong WP, Springer TA. Mechanoenzymatic cleavage of the ultralarge vascular protein von Willebrand factor. *Science* 2009; **324**: 1330–4.

249 Zhang Q, Zhou YF, Zhang CZ, Zhang X, Lu C, Springer TA. Structural specializations of A2, a force-sensing domain in the ultralarge vascular protein von Willebrand factor. *Proc Natl Acad Sci U S A* 2009; **106**: 9226–31.

250 Shim K, Anderson PJ, Tuley EA, Wiswall E, Sadler JE. Platelet-VWF complexes are preferred substrates of ADAMTS13 under fluid shear stress. *Blood* 2007; **111**: 651–7.

251 Turner NA, Nolasco L, Ruggeri ZM, Moake JL. Endothelial cell ADAMTS-13 and VWF: production, release and VWF string cleavage. *Blood* 2009; **114**: 5102–11.

252 Donadelli R, Orje JN, Capoferri C, Remuzzi G, Ruggeri ZM. Size regulation of von Willebrand factor-mediated platelet thrombi by ADAMTS13 in flowing blood. *Blood* 2006; **107**: 1943–50.

253 Favaloro EJ. Clinical utility of the PFA-100. *Semin Thromb Hemost* 2008; **34**: 709–33.

254 Quiroga T, Goycoolea M, Munoz B, *et al.* Template bleeding time and PFA-100 have low sensitivity to screen patients with hereditary mucocutaneous hemorrhages: comparative study in 148 patients. *J Thromb Haemost* 2004; **2**: 892–8.

255 Shenkman B, Savion N, Dardik R, Tamarin I, Varon D. Testing of platelet deposition on polystyrene surface under flow conditions by the cone and plate(let) analyzer: role of platelet activation, fibrinogen and von Willebrand factor. *Thromb Res* 2000; **99**: 353–61.

256 Ikeda Y, Murata M, Goto S. Von Willebrand factor-dependent shear-induced platelet aggregation: basic mechanisms and clinical implications. *Ann N Y Acad Sci* 1997; **811**: 325–36.

257 Royo T, Vidal M, Badimon L. Porcine platelet von Willebrand antigen II (vW AgII): inhibitory effect on collagen-induced aggregation and comparative distribution with human platelets. *Thromb Haemost* 1998; **80**: 677–85.

258 Fujisawa T, Takagi J, Sekiya F, Goto A, Miake F, Saito Y. Monoclonal antibodies that inhibit binding of propolypeptide of von Willebrand factor to collagen. Localization of epitopes. *Eur J Biochem* 1991; **196**: 673–7.

259 Takagi J, Kasahara K, Sekiya F, Inada Y, Saito Y. A collagen-binding glycoprotein from bovine platelets is identical to propolypeptide of von Willebrand factor. *J Biol Chem* 1989; **264**: 10425–30.

Modulation of von Willebrand factor by ADAMTS13

Jennifer Barr[1] *and David Motto*[2]

[1]Department of Anatomy and Cell Biology, University of Iowa Carver College of Medicine, Iowa City, IA, USA

[2]Departments of Internal Medicine and Pediatrics, University of Iowa Carver College of Medicine, Iowa City, IA, USA

Pathogenesis of TTP and discovery of ADAMTS13

First described in 1925, thrombotic thrombocytic purpura (TTP) is a systemic hematologic disorder characterized by the inappropriate deposition of platelet- and von Willebrand factor (VWF)-rich thrombi throughout the microvasculature [1]. The clinical findings of TTP are diverse and reflect the systemic nature of the disease. Severe thrombocytopenia (<20,000/µL) is common and likely results secondary to widespread platelet deposition in the microvasculature [2]. Intravascular hemolysis is thought to result from high fluid shear stress through partially occluded vessels, and schistocytes and red blood cell fragments are prevalent in the peripheral blood smear [2]. The presence of thrombi throughout the microvasculature can result in ischemia of the heart, brain, kidneys, and other organs, with accompanying cardiac, neurologic, renal, and other symptoms [3]. Untreated, TTP typically progresses rapidly and results in death in over 80% of cases [4,5]. Prompt initiation of therapeutic plasma is the current standard of care, which has decreased the TTP mortality rate to approximately 20% [4,5].

Investigators of TTP pathogenesis had for some time focused on the roles played by endothelial cell and platelet dysfunction [6,7]; however, more recently, the role of abnormal VWF homeostasis has become the most widely supported hypothesis regarding TTP pathogenesis. VWF is a large and abundant plasma glycoprotein that provides the initial adhesive link between circulating blood platelets and sites of vascular injury. Additionally, VWF serves as a carrier for, and significantly prolongs the half-life of, coagulation factor VIII (FVIII) [8–13].

The importance of VWF in maintaining hemostasis is illustrated clinically in patients with von Willebrand disease (VWD). While type 1 VWD is associated with modestly decreased levels of circulating VWF with mild clinical bleeding, type 3 VWD (severe VWF deficiency) can clinically mimic hemophilia A. VWF is synthesized in endothelial cells and megakaryocytes where it is processed from an initial propeptide monomer into considerably larger multimeric forms (Figure 4.1). Endothelial cell VWF is synthesized and released in both a constitutive and regulated manner. VWF that is not released constitutively is transported to, and subsequently stored in, specialized organelles called Weibel–Palade bodies. Upon endothelial cell stimulation, Weibel–Palade body VWF is released into the circulation in a form termed ultralarge VWF (UL-VWF), which is thought to represent the most thrombogenic form of this molecule [14,15]. Soon after release into the circulation, UL-VWF is processed into smaller and less thrombogenic multimers, and is therefore not typically detected upon multimer analysis of normal healthy human plasma.

Identification of the crucial link between VWF metabolism and TTP pathogenesis was made in 1982 when Moake and colleagues [16] demonstrated the presence of UL-VWF in the plasma of patients with

Von Willebrand Disease, 1st edition. Edited by Augusto B. Federici, Christine A. Lee, Erik E. Berntorp, David Lillicrap, Robert R. Montgomery. © 2011 Blackwell Publishing Ltd.

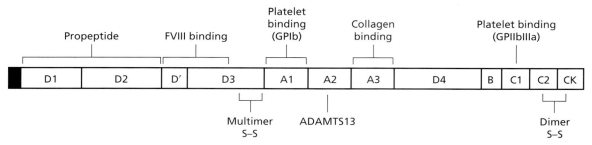

Figure 4.1 Structure of von Willebrand factor. Binding regions are indicated for FVIII, platelet glycoprotein Ib alpha (GPIb), collagen, and platelet glycoprotein αIIb/βIII (GPIIb/IIIa). The cleavage site for ADAMTS13 (Tyr[1605]–Met[1606]) is located within the A2 domain. The locations of intersubunit disulfide bonds (S–S) are shown.

a congenital form of TTP. These investigators prophetically hypothesized that deficiency of a VWF "depolymerase" was the underlying cause of TTP, and that UL-VWF played an important role in the formation of the platelet- and VWF-rich clots characteristic of this disease. Later also referred to as the "VWF-cleaving protease" [17,18], in 2001 this molecule was ultimately identified as the metalloprotease ADAMTS13 [19,20]. As discussed further below, deficiency of ADAMTS13 can either be genetic (the rare Upshaw–Schulman syndrome) or, more commonly, acquired in the form of inhibitory anti-ADAMTS13 autoantibodies [21–28].

Overall, the annual incidence of TTP in the USA is estimated to be one in 250,000 and appears to be increasing [29,30]. As with many diseases with an autoimmune component, females are at a greater risk, with a female-to-male ratio of at least 3:2 [31–35]. While patients with familial TTP can be successfully treated with plasma infusions to replace ADAMTS13, the mainstay of treatment for acquired TTP is plasma exchange, which is additionally thought to remove the inhibitory autoantibodies. Although this therapy carries considerable morbidity including exposure to blood products from multiple donors, plasma exchange has reduced the mortality of acquired TTP from 90% to approximately 20% [4,36–38]. Unfortunately, about 30% of acquired TTP cases become chronic, and significant morbidity remains a clinical challenge [39,40].

It is becoming increasingly clear that ADAMTS13 deficiency does not underlie all cases that carry the diagnosis of TTP. Averaging the clinical studies reported to date demonstrates that approximately 75% of patients diagnosed with acquired TTP exhibit severe ADAMTS13 deficiency, with the range spanning from 33% to 100% [21,22,41–44]. This large variability most certainly reflects many underlying causes, including differences in diagnostic and selection criteria, differences in ADAMTS13 assays, and potentially other etiologies of disease pathogenesis. However, this distinction is likely clinically relevant as those with severe ADAMTS13 deficiency are much more likely to exhibit high-titer anti-ADAMTS13 antibodies, are more prone to relapse [45–47], and may respond differentially to plasma exchange [48]. Nevertheless, without additional prospective studies investigating the efficacy of plasma exchange (and newer therapies such as rituximab) in patients with and without severe ADAMTS13 deficiency, plasma exchange should remain the standard of care for all patients diagnosed with acquired TTP, as well as those with whom there is a reasonable degree of clinical suspicion [49–52].

Regarding familial TTP, there is a striking age-dependent clustering of the first acute TTP episode. Approximately half of these patients suffer an initial TTP episode before the age of 5 years, while in the other half of patients an initial episode of TTP is delayed until adulthood [53]. It is unclear why some patients experience TTP episodes early in life while others survive for decades with no apparent symptoms. Clearly, in addition to ADAMTS13 deficiency, additional genetic and/or environmental factors are required for the pathogenesis of both familial and acquired TTP [53]. Pregnancy-associated TTP deserves special consideration, as pregnancy has long been recognized as a prothrombotic state that seems to be a particular risk factor for triggering episodes of both familial TTP and acquired TTP [54–59].

ADAMTS13 structure, synthesis, and secretion

Once sequenced, the VWF-cleaving protease was recognized as a member of the ADAMTS protease family and was subsequently named ADAMTS13 [20]. The ADAMTS family comprises 19 members that share several common motifs including a hydrophobic signal sequence, a propeptide sequence, a metalloprotease domain, thrombospondin type 1 (TSP-1) motif, a disintegrin-like domain, a cysteine-rich domain, and a spacer domain [19,20]. ADAMTS13 also contains seven additional TSP-1 motifs following the spacer domain and two C-terminal CUB domains (Figure 4.2). Among the ADAMTS family members, the CUB domains are unique to ADAMTS13 and are named after motifs first identified in complement components C1r, C1s, the sea urchin protein UEGF, and bone morphogenetic protein [60]. The *ADAMTS13* gene is located on chromosome 9q34, spans 37 kb in length, and comprises 29 exons. Several possible alternatively spliced variants have been identified; however, their significance remains unknown [19,20].

The peptide sequence of human ADAMTS13 comprises 1427 amino acid residues with a calculated molecular weight of 145 kDa [19,20]. The difference between this calculated weight and its actual migration of ~190 kDa by sodium dodecyl sulfate polyacrylamide gel electrophoresis (SDS-PAGE) is attributed to glycosylation and other post-translational modifications [61].

Northern blot analysis, as well as semiquantitative polymerase chain reaction (PCR), has shown high levels of ADAMTS13 expression in the liver [17,19, 20,62]. *In situ* hybridization, immunohistochemistry, and real-time (RT)-PCR analysis revealed that hepatic stellate cells, rather than hepatocytes, are the cells responsible for synthesizing ADAMTS13 in the liver [63,64]. Patients with liver cirrhosis or with significant activation and proliferation of hepatic stellate cells display variable levels of plasma ADAMTS13 activity [54]. Expression of ADAMTS13 has also been observed by endothelial cells [65,66] and platelets [67], although transcript levels appear to be much lower than liver expression. It remains unclear what relative contributions to circulating plasma ADAMTS13 are made by hepatic stellate cells and endothelial cells and what physiologic role is played by platelet ADAMTS13.

The mechanism by which ADAMTS13 synthesized in endothelial cells becomes targeted to the apical (luminal) membrane has been investigated in cell culture. ADAMTS13 expressed in polarized Madin-Darby canine kidney (MDCK) cells is preferentially delivered to the apical membrane [65]. Disruption or deletion of the ADAMTS13 CUB domains abolishes this preferential targeting, which appears to occur through interaction of the CUB domains themselves with lipid rafts on the cell membrane [65].

ADAMTS13 gene mutations

Well over 50 mutations in the *ADAMTS13* gene have been identified in patients with familial TTP (Figure 4.3) [19,68–81]. These mutations are located within both introns and exons and there does not appear to be any mutation clustering or "hot spots" throughout the gene, implying structural and functional importance of many of the domains. The majority of reported mutations are missense, followed by splice site, nonsense, and frameshift [82,83]. Heterozygous mutations are more commonly observed; however, homozygous mutations have been found in some families [19,68–76,84].

Studies in cell culture have demonstrated that the mechanism by which most missense mutations result in decreased ADAMTS13 plasma activity likely occurs through impairment of secretion of this molecule, although some also abrogate proteolytic activity [72,76,83]. Additionally, over 10 ADAMTS13

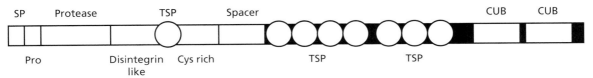

Figure 4.2 Schematic diagram of ADAMTS13. SP, signal peptide; pro, propeptide; protease, metalloprotease; disintegrin like, disintegrin-like domain; cys-rich, cysteine-rich domain; TSP, thrombospondin type-1 motif; CUB, CUB domain.

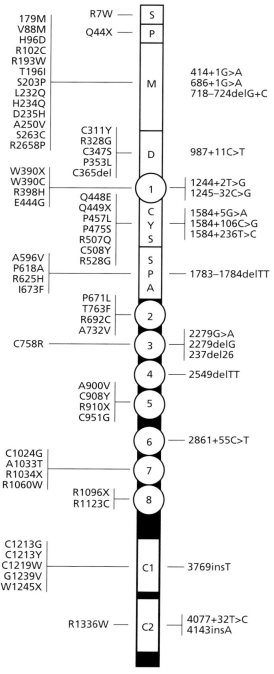

Figure 4.3 Localization of ADAMTS13 mutations. Mutations found in patients with congenital thrombotic thrombocytopenic purpura are indicated. Point mutations resulting in single amino acid substitutions and premature stop codons (X) are shown to the left of the structure of ADAMTS13. Mutations resulting in alternative splicing of *ADAMTS13* mRNA or frameshifts are listed to the right of the structure of ADAMTS13. S, signal peptide; P, propeptide; M, metalloprotease; D, disintegrin domain; 1, the first thrombospondin type 1 (TSP-1) repeat; CYS, cysteine-rich domain; SPA, spacer domain; 2 through 8, the second to eighth TSP repeats; C1 and C2, the CUB domains 1 and 2.

missense mutations involving cysteine residues have been reported, likely indicating that proper disulfide bond formation is important for the function of the protease [82,83].

Not surprisingly, *ADAMTS13* gene mutations that cause protein truncations have also been shown to impair secretion and reduce ADAMTS13 activity. For example, the frameshift mutation 4143–4144insA dysregulates apical secretion of ADAMTS13 from MDCK cells [65,68]. This familial TTP mutation truncates ADAMTS13 within the second CUB domain, demonstrating the importance of this CUB domain both *in vitro* and *in vivo* [65]. In another example, the truncating nonsense mutation Q449X was also shown to be correctly secreted in cell culture but shows greatly decreased proteolytic activity, demonstrating the necessity of the spacer domain and distal sequences for ADAMTS13 activity [69,85,86]. Finally, several splice site mutations have been found in *ADAMTS13* [19,72].

Multiple single nucleotide polymorphisms (SNPs) have been reported in the *ADAMTS13* gene that do not show a clear association with TTP [19,69, 83]. However, when expressed in cell culture, the presence of several SNPs in combination has been shown to modulate secretion and specific activity of ADAMTS13 [87]. This finding raises the interesting possibility that inheritance of a combination of *ADAMTS13* SNPs on a single allele might, in some instances, be equivalent to a disease-causing familial TTP mutation.

Autoantibodies against ADAMTS13

Deficiency of ADAMTS13 associated with acquired TTP is caused by anti-ADAMTS13 autoantibodies, which, in most cases, inhibit enzymatic activity (in the presence of a detectable ADAMTS13 antigen) but in some instances may increase ADAMTS13 clearance, resulting in low ADAMTS13 antigen levels [88]. Besides improving our ability to detect anti-ADAMTS13 antibodies in patient plasma, the development of enzyme-linked immunosorbant assays (ELISAs) has also demonstrated the existence of non-inhibitory anti-ADAMTS13 antibodies [89–91]. Recent use of these assays has demonstrated that among patients with acquired TTP and severe ADAMTS13 deficiency, anti-ADAMTS13 IgG anti-

bodies can be detected in as high as 97% of individuals, with IgM antibodies also present in approximately 10% [88,89,92]. To our knowledge, anti-ADAMTS13 antibodies typically do not develop in patients with familial TTP secondary to repeated plasma infusion therapy.

Epitope mapping of anti-ADAMTS13 antibodies has demonstrated that most patients with acquired TTP and severe ADAMTS13 deficiency seem to have developed a polyclonal response to the molecule [82,86,93]. Although the individual domains of ADAMTS13 that are targeted vary across individuals, all patients reported to date possess antibodies against the cysteine-rich/spacer region of the protein, demonstrating that this region likely harbors the critical epitope(s) needed to develop severe ADAMTS13 deficiency [82,86,93]. Indeed, mutagenesis studies involving the generation of chimeric ADAMTS13 peptide fragments in which regions of the protein were exchanged for homologous regions of the ADAMTS1 sequence indicated that amino acid residues Thr^{572}-Asn^{579} and Val^{657}-Gly^{666} comprise a core region in the spacer domain that is recognized by ADAMTS13 antibodies from patients with acquired TTP [94].

ADAMTS13 activity and regulation

Regarding the regulation of ADAMTS13 activity, an important factor to consider is that, to date, the only known substrate for ADAMTS13 is VWF. Additionally, unlike most plasma proteases, ADAMTS13 appears to be fully active upon secretion into the circulation. Many proteases of the metzincin superfamily (to which ADAMTS13 belongs) possess amino-terminal propeptides, that upon cleavage trigger enzyme activation [95]. Although the ADAMTS13 propeptide indeed contains a typical propeptide cleavage site, RQRR, ADAMTS13 appears to be active even before cleavage of the propeptide [61]. Consistent with this finding is the absence of a cysteine residue in a "cysteine-switch" sequence context in the human ADAMTS13 propeptide, as well as in ADAMTS13 from other species [61]. However, despite the fact that ADAMTS13 in circulation is constitutively active, plasma VWF does not become proteolyzed down to monomeric form. Thus, regulation of VWF cleavage by ADAMTS13 must occur via another mechanism.

Interestingly, the first clues into understanding this mechanism came from studies of type 2A VWD, which, as described in detail elsewhere in this volume, is characterized by clinical bleeding secondary to a qualitative defect of VWF comprising loss of large- and intermediate-sized multimers in the plasma. In 1986 Zimmerman and colleagues [96] described how plasma from several patients with type 2A VWD also contained increased concentrations of 176 kDa and 140 kDa cleavage fragments of VWF, which were found only in trace amounts in normal plasma. Subsequently, the origin of these fragments was determined to be cleavage of VWF between Tyr^{1605} and Met^{1606} within the A2 domain [97]. These investigators therefore hypothesized that type 2A VWF mutations likely induce structural changes within the VWF A2 domain that expose a cryptic bond to the action of a specific, but unknown, protease.

These observations naturally led to questions centering on the mechanism by which the putative cryptic cleavage site within the A2 domain becomes exposed in wild-type VWF under physiologic conditions. Insight into these questions came through the initial characterization of the VWF-cleaving protease that was deficient in TTP. Importantly, this protease was found to cleave between Tyr^{1605} and Met^{1606} within the VWF A2 domain (Figure 4.1). Additionally, it was demonstrated that both fluid shear stress [98] and exposure of VWF to mild chemical denaturants, such as urea or guanidine, greatly enhances proteolysis of VWF by the protease, with only trace cleavage occurring under nondenaturing static conditions [18,99].

These observations proved pivotal in understanding VWF physiology as they established that the protease deficient in TTP appeared to be the same protease whose activity was responsible for many instances of type 2A VWD and that, under normal conditions, the Tyr^{1605}–Met^{1606} bond within the wild-type VWF A2 domain was indeed cryptic and nonaccessible to the protease but could be exposed in vitro under denaturing conditions, possibly through partial unfolding of the A2 domain. Furthermore, these observations suggested that, in vivo, the protease (eventually identified as ADAMTS13) could gain access to the Tyr^{1605}–Met^{1606} bond secondary to unfolding of the A2 domain concomitant to VWF exposure to fluid shear stress in the circulation.

Recently, elucidation of the crystal structure of the VWF A2 domain and sophisticated studies with laser tweezers have demonstrated the structural basis for the cryptic nature of the Tyr^{1605}–Met^{1606} bond and established the mechanism by which the A2 domain becomes unfolded in response to external force [100,101]. Based on crystal structure solved by Zhang and colleagues [100], the Tyr^{1605} and Met^{1606} residues are buried at the center of a β-sheet in the hydrophobic core of the A2 domain, demonstrating that in order to be cleaved by ADAMTS13, this domain would have to become unfolded at least up to its β4 strand. Additionally, using laser tweezers to grab and manipulate the ends of single A2 domain molecules, this same group demonstrated that forces applied within the range experienced by VWF in circulation indeed result in unfolding of the A2 domain, allowing its subsequent cleavage by ADAMTS13 [101]. The A2 domain crystal structure further demonstrates that these forces are likely transmitted from the A1 and A3 domains through O-glycosylated linkers to the N- and C-termini of the A2 domain, and that unfolding then probably proceeds from its C-terminal side [100]. Thus, these studies demonstrated definitively that unfolding of the A2 domain is required for ADAMTS13 cleavage, and strongly suggested that the force required for this phenomenon derives from the fluid shear stress to which VWF is subjected in the circulation.

The involvement of the A1 and A3 domains in VWF cleavage by ADAMTS13 has been investigated through the use of recombinant VWF constructs containing the A2 domain with and without the adjacent A1 and A3 domains [102]. Interestingly, the presence of the adjacent A1 domain (but not the A3 domain) resulted in a decreased rate of cleavage, suggesting that the A1 domain can function to stabilize the native folded conformation of the A2 domain or prevent binding of ADAMTS13 [102]. Furthermore, the presence of recombinant GPIbα substantially enhanced cleavage of the A1A2A3 construct (even allowing for cleavage in the absence of urea), suggesting that binding of GPIbα to the A1 domain may facilitate unfolding of the A2 domain and subsequent cleavage by ADAMTS13 [102].

In addition to recombinant GPIbα, platelets bound to VWF via the GPIbα/VWF A1 domain interaction also significantly enhance ADAMTS13 cleavage of multimeric VWF under flowing conditions *in vitro* [103], possibly by amplifying the force on VWF exerted by fluid shear stress. Similarly, binding of coagulation factor VIII to VWF also significantly enhances cleavage of multimeric VWF by ADAMTS13 under flowing conditions *in vitro* through an unknown mechanism [104].

Other factors may also influence ADAMTS13 regulation and activity. The inflammatory cytokine interleukin 6 has been shown to inhibit ADAMTS13 cleavage of VWF–platelet complexes under flowing conditions *in vitro* [105], and free hemoglobin also has an inhibitory affect on ADAMTS13 activity *in vitro* [106]. Finally, thrombin, coagulation factor Xa, and plasmin have all been shown to cleave and inactivate ADAMTS13 *in vitro*, suggesting one or more of these enzymes may be involved in downregulation of ADAMTS13 activity during different phases of thrombus formation and dissolution [107].

Thus, although ADAMTS13 in plasma is constitutively active, from the above studies (and many others) it is now clear that its activity in effect is regulated principally through access to its substrate, the Tyr^{1605}–Met^{1606} bond, within the A2 domain of VWF. This interesting arrangement in which the substrate is regulated rather than the enzyme perhaps makes it less likely that additional substrates exist for ADAMTS13 other than VWF.

ADAMTS13 interaction with VWF

The specific domains of VWF required for ADAMTS13 binding and cleavage have not yet been entirely elucidated. The minimal fragment of VWF that can be cleaved efficiently by ADAMTS13 is VWF73, a fragment derived from the central A2 domain of VWF (Asp^{1596} to Arg^{1668}), indicating that at least one ADAMTS13 binding site exists within this sequence [108]. Indeed, several additional studies have demonstrated the presence of a high-affinity binding site within the A2 domain that interacts with the spacer domain of ADAMTS13 with possible contributions from the disintegrin, first TSP-1, and cysteine-rich domains [109–113].

As discussed above, the Y^{1605}–M^{1606} bond of VWF only becomes accessible to ADAMTS13 in its unfolded conformation. Indeed, the crystal structure of the A2 domain demonstrates that VWF73 corresponds to the A2 domain unfolded from the C-terminus up to the α3-β4 loop [100]. However, the observation that the VWF-cleaving protease could be copurified with VWF from plasma [114] strongly suggests that ADAMTS13 can also bind to VWF in its native conformation, likely at a site apart from the A2 domain. Additionally, several recent studies demonstrate that there likely exists a second VWF-binding region in ADAMTS13 as well [110,115,116].

Using surface plasmon resonance under flowing conditions, ADAMTS13 mutants lacking the CUB domains show a fivefold reduction in binding affinity (compared with full-length ADAMTS13) for VWF, and ADAMTS13 truncated after the spacer domain almost completely abolishes binding of ADAMTS13 to VWF under flow [110]. Adding the distal TSP-1 repeats back to the CUB domains restores binding for VWF, and constructs comprising the distal TSP-1 repeats and CUB domains inhibit ADAMTS13 cleavage of VWF [110]. Additionally, a peptide derived from the first CUB domain of ADAMTS13 has been shown to inhibit cleavage of VWF under flowing, but not static, conditions [117]. Finally, several strains of laboratory mice express a form of ADAMTS13 truncated after the sixth TSP-1 motif, which also demonstrates greatly decreased cleavage of multimeric VWF [118]. Together, these data suggest a cooperative activity between the distal TSP-1 repeats and CUB domains of ADAMTS13 that aid in recognition and/or binding to multimeric VWF under flowing conditions.

Building on these observations, a second site of interaction between ADAMTS13 and VWF has recently been identified in both proteins [119]. Using plate binding assays and surface plasmon resonance, the C-terminal domains of ADAMTS13 were shown to interact with a portion of VWF that contained the D4 domain and spanning residues 1874–2813 (Figure 4.1) [119]. This interaction occurs under static conditions when the A2 domain presumably is not accessible to ADAMTS13 and, interestingly, an antibody directed against the VWF D4 domain inhibits ADAMTS13 cleavage of VWF under flowing conditions [119]. These investigators therefore proposed a multistep model for ADAMTS13 cleavage of VWF, whereby ADAMTS13 is first constitutively associated with VWF via an interaction between the distal TSP-1 and CUB domains of ADAMTS13 and the C-terminal sequences of VWF. Subsequently, as VWF traverses the circulation and encounters shear stress, the ADAMTS13 spacer domain (and possibly other nearby sequences) are able to interact with the newly unfolded A2 domain, allowing for ensuing cleavage of the Tyr^{1605}–Met^{1606} bond.

ADAMTS13 and VWD

As discussed above and elsewhere in this volume, type 2A VWD is characterized by clinical bleeding secondary to a qualitative defect of VWF comprising loss of large- and intermediate-sized multimers in the plasma. Unlike other VWD subtypes, the etiology of type 2A VWD is heterogeneous in nature, as deficiency of large and intermediate-sized multimers may result from either aberrant synthesis and secretion of VWF, increased susceptibility to ADAMTS13-mediated cleavage in the plasma, or to a combination of both of these factors [97,120–124].

Thus, at least for a subset of type 2A VWD, it appears that ADAMTS13 activity is required for expression of the disease phenotype. Although this hypothesis has not formerly been addressed experimentally, many recombinant type IIA VWF mutants indeed exhibit greatly increased susceptibility to ADAMTS13 cleavage *in vitro* [122–127]. Additionally, the increased presence of the 176 kDa and 140 kDa cleavage fragments of VWF (which result from cleavage of VWF at Tyr^{1605}–Met^{1606}) in plasma from patients with type 2A VWD also strongly argues for a requirement for ADAMTS13 activity in the pathogenesis of type 2A VWD, as ADAMTS13 is the only enzyme known to cleave VWF at this site.

It has also been hypothesized that ADAMTS13 plays a role in some cases of type 1 VWD [128,129]. In support of this notion, among the different human ABO blood groups, VWF isolated from individuals with blood type O exhibits the highest susceptibility to cleavage by ADAMTS13, followed by types B, A, and AB [130–133]. This difference in cleavage susceptibility is presumably due to differences in VWF glycosylation among individuals with differing ABO blood groups. As individuals with blood type O also have the lowest VWF antigen levels [132], increased susceptibility to cleavage by ADAMTS13 might further decrease the efficacy of VWF function at a site of vascular injury [130,134].

Additionally, several VWF polymorphisms also demonstrate increased susceptibility to ADAMTS13 cleavage *in vitro* [129,135]. This finding, coupled with the recent observation that many individuals diagnosed with type 1 VWD actually have subtle qualitative multimer abnormalities consistent with type 2 VWD [136], suggests that in some instances the clinical phenotype of type 1 VWD might also result from increased VWF susceptibility to ADAMTS13 cleavage. Although investigation of these arguably fine points of disease pathogenesis will not immediately impact the treatment of patients with type 1 VWD, elucidation of these processes will undoubtedly contribute to our better understanding of the physiology and pathophysiology of hemostasis and thrombosis. Finally, although it is possible that mutations in ADAMTS13 that increase its ability to cleave VWF could also result in a VWD-like phenotype, to our knowledge this has never been reported.

Conclusions

The VWF-cleaving protease implicated in TTP pathogenesis was identified as ADAMTS13 in 2001. Since that time, considerable progress has been made into understanding the pathophysiology of TTP, including the roles played by both ADAMTS13 and VWF. Much of this work has contributed greatly to our understanding of how these molecules function in "normal" physiology and hemostasis. Continued investigation should therefore lead not only to more refined knowledge of, and therapy for, TTP and similar disorders, but also to a globally improved understanding of VWF physiology, VWD, hemostasis, and thrombosis.

References

1 Moschcowitz E. Hyaline thrombosis of the terminal arterioles and capillaries: a hitherto undescribed disease. *Proc N Y Pathol Soc* 1924; **24**: 21–4.

2 Sadler JE, Moake JL, Miyata T, George JN. Recent advances in thrombotic thrombocytopenic purpura. *Hematology Am Soc Hematol Educ Program* 2004; 407–23.

3 Tsai HM. The molecular biology of thrombotic micro-angiopathy. *Kidney Int* 2006 ; **70**: 16–23.

4 George JN. How I treat patients with thrombotic thrombocytopenic purpura-hemolytic uremic syndrome. *Blood* 2000; **96**: 1223–9.

5 Rock GA, Shumak KH, Buskard NA, *et al.* Comparison of plasma exchange with plasma infusion in the treatment of thrombotic thrombocytopenic purpura. Canadian Apheresis Study Group. *N Engl J Med* 1991; **325**: 393–7.

6 Burns ER, Zucker-Franklin D. Pathologic effects of plasma from patients with thrombotic thrombocytopenic purpura on platelets and cultured vascular endothelial cells. *Blood* 1982; **60**: 1030–7.

7 Sims PJ, Boswell EB. Elevated platelet-bound IgG associated with an episode of thrombotic thrombocytopenic purpura. *Blood* 1981; **58**: 682–4.

8 Vlot AJ, Koppelman SJ, Bouma BN, Sixma JJ. Factor VIII and von Willebrand factor. *Thromb Haemost* 1998; **79**: 456–65.

9 Weiss HJ, Sussman, II, Hoyer LW. Stabilization of factor VIII in plasma by the von Willebrand factor. Studies on posttransfusion and dissociated factor VIII and in patients with von Willebrand's disease. *J Clin Invest* 1977; **60**: 390–404.

10 Over J, Sixma JJ, Bouma BN, Bolhuis PA, Vlooswijk RA, Beeser-Visser NH. Survival of iodine-125-labeled factor VIII in patients with von Willebrand's disease. *J Lab Clin Med* 1981; **97**: 332–44.

11 Koedam JA, Meijers JC, Sixma JJ, Bouma BN. Inactivation of human factor VIII by activated protein C. Cofactor activity of protein S and protective effect of von Willebrand factor. *J Clin Invest* 1988; **82**: 1236–43.

12 Koedam JA, Hamer RJ, Beeser-Visser NH, Bouma BN, Sixma JJ. The effect of von Willebrand factor on activation of factor VIII by factor Xa. *Eur J Biochem* 1990; **189**: 229–34.

13 Tuddenham EG, Lane RS, Rotblat F, *et al.* Response to infusions of polyelectrolyte fractionated human factor VIII concentrate in human haemophilia A and von Willebrand's disease. *Br J Haematol* 1982; **52**: 259–67.

14 Furlan M. Von Willebrand factor: molecular size and functional activity. *Ann Hematol* 1996; **72**: 341–8.

15 Arya M, Anvari B, Romo GM, *et al.* Ultralarge multimers of von Willebrand factor form spontaneous high-strength bonds with the platelet glycoprotein Ib–IX complex: studies using optical tweezers. *Blood* 2002; **99**: 3971–7.

16 Moake JL, Rudy CK, Troll JH, *et al.* Unusually large plasma factor VIII: von Willebrand factor multimers in chronic relapsing thrombotic thrombocytopenic purpura. *N Engl J Med* 1982; **307**: 1432–5.

17 Soejima K, Mimura N, Hirashima M, *et al.* A novel human metalloprotease synthesized in the liver and secreted into the blood: possibly, the von Willebrand factor-cleaving protease? *J Biochem* 2001; **130**: 475–80.

18 Furlan M, Robles R, Lamie B. Partial purification and characterization of a protease from human plasma cleaving von Willebrand factor to fragments produced by in vivo proteolysis. *Blood* 1996; **87**: 4223–34.

19 Levy GG, Nichols WC, Lian EC, *et al.* Mutations in a member of the ADAMTS gene family cause thrombotic thrombocytopenic purpura. *Nature* 2001; **413**: 488–94.

20 Zheng X, Chung D, Takayama TK, Majerus EM, Sadler JE, Fujikawa K. Structure of von Willebrand factor-cleaving protease (ADAMTS13), a metalloprotease involved in thrombotic thrombocytopenic purpura. *J Biol Chem* 2001; **276**: 41059–63.

21 Furlan M, Robles R, Solenthaler M, Lammle B. Acquired deficiency of von Willebrand factor-cleaving protease in a patient with thrombotic thrombocytopenic purpura. *Blood* 1998; **91**: 2839–46.

22 Tsai HM, Lian EC. Antibodies to von Willebrand factor-cleaving protease in acute thrombotic thrombocytopenic purpura. *N Engl J Med* 1998; **339**: 1585–94.

23 Furlan M, Robles R, Solenthaler M, Wassmer M, Sandoz P, Lammle B. Deficient activity of von Willebrand factor-cleaving protease in chronic relapsing thrombotic thrombocytopenic purpura. *Blood* 1997; **89**: 3097–103.

24 Furlan M, Lammle B. Deficiency of von Willebrand factor-cleaving protease in familial and acquired thrombotic thrombocytopenic purpura. *Bailliteres Clin Haematol* 1998; **11**: 509–14.

25 Furlan M, Robles R, Galbusera M, *et al.* von Willebrand factor-cleaving protease in thrombotic thrombocytopenic purpura and the hemolytic-uremic syndrome. *N Engl J Med* 1998; **339**: 1578–84.

26 Furlan M, Robles R, Morselli B, Sandoz P, Lammle B. Recovery and half-life of von Willebrand factor-cleaving protease after plasma therapy in patients with thrombotic thrombocytopenic purpura. *Thromb Haemost* 1999; **81**: 8–13.

27 Schulman I, Pierce M, Lukens A, Currimbhoy Z. Studies on thrombopoiesis. I. A factor in normal human plasma required for platelet production; chronic thrombocytopenia due to its deficiency. *Blood* 1960; **16**: 943–57.

28 Upshaw JD, Jr. Congenital deficiency of a factor in normal plasma that reverses microangiopathic hemolysis and thrombocytopenia. *N Engl J Med* 1978; **298**: 1350–2.

29 Terrell DR, Williams LA, Vesely SK, Lammle B, Hovinga JA, George JN. The incidence of thrombotic thrombocytopenic purpura-hemolytic uremic syndrome:

all patients, idiopathic patients, and patients with severe ADAMTS-13 deficiency. *J Thromb Haemost* 2005; **3**: 1432–6.

30 Frederiksen H, Schmidt K. The incidence of idiopathic thrombocytopenic purpura in adults increases with age. *Blood* 1999; **94**: 909–13.

31 Ruggenenti P, Remuzzi G. Thrombotic thrombocytopenic purpura and related disorders. *Hematol Oncol Clin North Am* 1990; **4**: 219–41.

32 Ridolfi RL, Bell WR. Thrombotic thrombocytopenic purpura. Report of 25 cases and review of the literature. *Medicine (Baltimore)* 1981; **60**: 413–28.

33 Cuttner J. Thrombotic thrombocytopenic purpura: a ten-year experience. *Blood* 1980; **56**: 302–6.

34 Pettitt AR, Clark RE. Thrombotic microangiopathy following bone marrow transplantation. *Bone Marrow Transplant* 1994; **14**: 495–504.

35 George JN, el-Harake MA, Raskob GE. Chronic idiopathic thrombocytopenic purpura. *N Engl J Med* 1994; **331**: 1207–11.

36 Allford SL, Hunt BJ, Rose P, Machin SJ. Guidelines on the diagnosis and management of the thrombotic microangiopathic haemolytic anaemias. *Br J Haematol* 2003; **120**: 556–73.

37 Kwaan HC, Soff GA. Management of thrombotic thrombocytopenic purpura and hemolytic uremic syndrome. *Semin Hematol* 1997; **34**: 159–66.

38 Lankford KV, Hillyer CD. Thrombotic thrombocytopenic purpura: new insights in disease pathogenesis and therapy. *Transfus Med Rev* 2000; **14**: 244–57.

39 McMillan R, Durette C. Long-term outcomes in adults with chronic ITP after splenectomy failure. *Blood* 2004; **104**: 956–60.

40 Bourgeois E, Caulier MT, Delarozee C, Brouillard M, Bauters F, Fenaux P. Long-term follow-up of chronic autoimmune thrombocytopenic purpura refractory to splenectomy: a prospective analysis. *Br J Haematol* 2003; **120**: 1079–88.

41 Vesely SK, George JN, Lammle B, *et al*. ADAMTS13 activity in thrombotic thrombocytopenic purpura-hemolytic uremic syndrome: relation to presenting features and clinical outcomes in a prospective cohort of 142 patients. *Blood* 2003; **102**: 60–8.

42 Veyradier A, Obert B, Houllier A, Meyer D, Girma JP. Specific von Willebrand factor-cleaving protease in thrombotic microangiopathies: a study of 111 cases. *Blood* 2001; **98**: 1765–72.

43 Mori Y, Wada H, Gabazza EC, *et al*. Predicting response to plasma exchange in patients with thrombotic thrombocytopenic purpura with measurement of vWF-cleaving protease activity. *Transfusion* 2002; **42**: 572–80.

44 Studt JD, Kremer Hovinga JA, Alberio L, Bianchi V, Lammle B. Von Willebrand factor-cleaving protease

(ADAMTS-13) activity in thrombotic microangiopathies: diagnostic experience 2001/2002 of a single research laboratory. *Swiss Med Wkly* 2003; **133**: 325–32.

45 Ferrari S, Mudde GC, Rieger M, Veyradier A, Kremer Hovinga JA, Scheiflinger F. IgG-subclass distribution of anti-ADAMTS13 antibodies in patients with acquired thrombotic thrombocytopenic purpura. *J Thromb Haemost* 2009; **7**: 1703–10.

46 Bresin E, Gastoldi S, Daina E, *et al*. Rituximab as pre-emptive treatment in patients with thrombotic thrombocytopenic purpura and evidence of anti-ADAMTS13 autoantibodies. *Thromb Haemost* 2009; **101**: 233–8.

47 Zheng XL, Kaufman RM, Goodnough LT, Sadler JE. Effect of plasma exchange on plasma ADAMTS13 metalloprotease activity, inhibitor level, and clinical outcome in patients with idiopathic and nonidiopathic thrombotic thrombocytopenic purpura. *Blood* 2004; **103**: 4043–9.

48 Scaramucci L, Niscola P, Palumbo R, *et al*. Rapid response and sustained remission by rituximab in four cases of plasma-exchange-failed acute thrombotic thrombocytopenic purpura. *Int J Hematol* 2009; **89**: 398–9.

49 Coppo P, Bussel A, Charrier S, *et al*. High-dose plasma infusion versus plasma exchange as early treatment of thrombotic thrombocytopenic purpura/hemolytic-uremic syndrome. *Medicine (Baltimore)* 2003; **82**: 27–38.

50 Brunskill SJ, Tusold A, Benjamin S, Stanworth SJ, Murphy MF. A systematic review of randomized controlled trials for plasma exchange in the treatment of thrombotic thrombocytopenic purpura. *Transfus Med* 2007; **17**: 17–35.

51 Zheng X, Pallera AM, Goodnough LT, Sadler JE, Blinder MA. Remission of chronic thrombotic thrombocytopenic purpura after treatment with cyclophosphamide and rituximab. *Ann Intern Med* 2003; **138**: 105–8.

52 Tsai HM. High titers of inhibitors of von Willebrand factor-cleaving metalloproteinase in a fatal case of acute thrombotic thrombocytopenic purpura. *Am J Hematol* 2000; **65**: 251–5.

53 Furlan M, Lammle B. Aetiology and pathogenesis of thrombotic thrombocytopenic purpura and haemolytic uraemic syndrome: the role of von Willebrand factor-cleaving protease. *Best Pract Res Clin Haematol* 2001; **14**: 437–54.

54 Mannucci PM, Canciani MT, Forza I, Lussana F, Lattuada A, Rossi E. Changes in health and disease of the metalloprotease that cleaves von Willebrand factor. *Blood* 2001; **98**: 2730–5.

55 McCrae KR, Cines DB. Thrombotic microangiopathy during pregnancy. *Semin Hematol* 1997; **34**: 148–58.

56 Esplin MS, Branch DW. Diagnosis and management of thrombotic microangiopathies during pregnancy. *Clin Obstet Gynecol* 1999; **42**: 360–7.

57 George JN. The association of pregnancy with thrombotic thrombocytopenic purpura-hemolytic uremic syndrome. *Curr Opin Hematol* 2003; **10**: 339–44.

58 Gerth J, Schleussner E, Kentouche K, Busch M, Seifert M, Wolf G. Pregnancy-associated thrombotic thrombocytopenic purpura. *Thromb Haemost* 2009; **101**: 248–51.

59 Ehsanipoor RM, Rajan P, Holcombe RF, Wing DA. Limitations of ADAMTS-13 activity level in diagnosing thrombotic thrombocytopenic purpura in pregnancy. *Clin Appl Thromb Hemost* 2008; **15**: 585–7.

60 Bork P, Beckmann G. The CUB domain. A widespread module in developmentally regulated proteins. *J Mol Biol* 1993; **231**: 539–45.

61 Majerus EM, Zheng X, Tuley EA, Sadler JE. Cleavage of the ADAMTS13 propeptide is not required for protease activity. *J Biol Chem* 2003; **278**: 46643–8.

62 Plaimauer B, Zimmermann K, Volkel D, *et al.* Cloning, expression, and functional characterization of the von Willebrand factor-cleaving protease (ADAMTS13). *Blood* 2002; **100**: 3626–32.

63 Zhou W, Inada M, Lee TP, *et al.* ADAMTS13 is expressed in hepatic stellate cells. *Lab Invest* 2005; **85**: 780–8.

64 Uemura M, Tatsumi K, Matsumoto M, *et al.* Localization of ADAMTS13 to the stellate cells of human liver. *Blood* 2005; **106**: 922–4.

65 Shang D, Zheng XW, Niiya M, Zheng XL. Apical sorting of ADAMTS13 in vascular endothelial cells and Madin-Darby canine kidney cells depends on the CUB domains and their association with lipid rafts. *Blood* 2006; **108**: 2207–15.

66 Turner N, Nolasco L, Tao Z, Dong JF, Moake J. Human endothelial cells synthesize and release ADAMTS-13. *J Thromb Haemost* 2006; **4**: 1396–404.

67 Liu L, Choi H, Bernardo A, *et al.* Platelet-derived VWF-cleaving metalloprotease ADAMTS-13. *J Thromb Haemost* 2005; **3**: 2536–44.

68 Pimanda JE, Maekawa A, Wind T, Paxton J, Chesterman CN, Hogg PJ. Congenital thrombotic thrombocytopenic purpura in association with a mutation in the second CUB domain of ADAMTS13. *Blood* 2004; **103**: 627–9.

69 Kokame K, Matsumoto M, Soejima K, *et al.* Mutations and common polymorphisms in ADAMTS13 gene responsible for von Willebrand factor-cleaving protease activity. *Proc Natl Acad Sci U S A* 2002; **99**: 11902–7.

70 Antoine G, Zimmermann K, Plaimauer B, *et al.* ADAMTS13 gene defects in two brothers with constitutional thrombotic thrombocytopenic purpura and normalization of von Willebrand factor-cleaving protease activity by recombinant human ADAMTS13. *Br J Haematol* 2003; **120**: 821–4.

71 Assink K, Schiphorst R, Allford S, *et al.* Mutation analysis and clinical implications of von Willebrand factor-cleaving protease deficiency. *Kidney Int* 2003; **63**: 1995–9.

72 Matsumoto M, Kokame K, Soejima K, *et al.* Molecular characterization of ADAMTS13 gene mutations in Japanese patients with Upshaw-Schulman syndrome. *Blood* 2004; **103**: 1305–10.

73 Savasan S, Lee SK, Ginsburg D, Tsai HM. ADAMTS13 gene mutation in congenital thrombotic thrombocytopenic purpura with previously reported normal VWF cleaving protease activity. *Blood* 2003; **101**: 4449–51.

74 Schneppenheim R, Budde U, Oyen F, *et al.* von Willebrand factor cleaving protease and ADAMTS13 mutations in childhood TTP. *Blood* 2003; **101**: 1845–50.

75 Licht C, Stapenhorst L, Simon T, Budde U, Schneppenheim R, Hoppe B. Two novel ADAMTS13 gene mutations in thrombotic thrombocytopenic purpura/hemolytic-uremic syndrome (TTP/HUS). *Kidney Int* 2004; **66**: 955–8.

76 Uchida T, Wada H, Mizutani M, *et al.* Identification of novel mutations in ADAMTS13 in an adult patient with congenital thrombotic thrombocytopenic purpura. *Blood* 2004; **104**: 2081–3.

77 Donadelli R, Banterla F, Galbusera M, *et al.* In-vitro and in-vivo consequences of mutations in the von Willebrand factor cleaving protease ADAMTS13 in thrombotic thrombocytopenic purpura. *Thromb Haemost* 2006; **96**: 454–64.

78 Tao Z, Anthony K, Peng Y, *et al.* Novel ADAMTS-13 mutations in an adult with delayed onset thrombotic thrombocytopenic purpura. *J Thromb Haemost* 2006; **4**: 1931–5.

79 Shibagaki Y, Matsumoto M, Kokame K, *et al.* Novel compound heterozygote mutations (H234Q/R1206X) of the ADAMTS13 gene in an adult patient with Upshaw–Schulman syndrome showing predominant episodes of repeated acute renal failure. *Nephrol Dial Transplant* 2006; **21**: 1289–92.

80 Schneppenheim R, Kremer Hovinga JA, Becker T, *et al.* A common origin of the 4143insA ADAMTS13 mutation. *Thromb Haemost* 2006; **96**: 3–6.

81 Veyradier A, Lavergne JM, Ribba AS, *et al.* Ten candidate ADAMTS13 mutations in six French families with congenital thrombotic thrombocytopenic purpura (Upshaw-Schulman syndrome). *J Thromb Haemost* 2004; **2**: 424–9.

82 Zheng XL, Sadler JE. Pathogenesis of thrombotic microangiopathies. *Annu Rev Pathol* 2008; **3**: 249–77.

83 Kokame K, Miyata T. Genetic defects leading to hereditary thrombotic thrombocytopenic purpura. *Semin Hematol* 2004; **41**: 34–40.

84 Palla R, Lavoretano S, Lombardi R, *et al*. The first deletion mutation in the TSP1–6 repeat domain of ADAMTS13 in a family with inherited thrombotic thrombocytopenic purpura. *Haematologica* 2009; **94**: 289–93.

85 Zheng X, Nishio K, Majerus EM, Sadler JE. Cleavage of von Willebrand factor requires the spacer domain of the metalloprotease ADAMTS13. *J Biol Chem* 2003; **278**: 30136–41.

86 Soejima K, Matsumoto M, Kokame K, *et al*. ADAMTS-13 cysteine-rich/spacer domains are functionally essential for von Willebrand factor cleavage. *Blood* 2003; **102**: 3232–7.

87 Plaimauer B, Fuhrmann J, Mohr G, *et al*. Modulation of ADAMTS13 secretion and specific activity by a combination of common amino acid polymorphisms and a missense mutation. *Blood* 2006; **107**: 118–25.

88 Scheiflinger F, Knobl P, Trattner B, *et al*. Nonneutralizing IgM and IgG antibodies to von Willebrand factor-cleaving protease (ADAMTS-13) in a patient with thrombotic thrombocytopenic purpura. *Blood* 2003; **102**: 3241–3.

89 Rieger M, Mannucci PM, Kremer Hovinga JA, *et al*. ADAMTS13 autoantibodies in patients with thrombotic microangiopathies and other immunomediated diseases. *Blood* 2005; **106**: 1262–7.

90 Whitelock JL, Nolasco L, Bernardo A, Moake J, Dong JF, Cruz MA. ADAMTS-13 activity in plasma is rapidly measured by a new ELISA method that uses recombinant VWF-A2 domain as substrate. *J Thromb Haemost* 2004; **2**: 485–91.

91 Zhou W, Tsai HM. An enzyme immunoassay of ADAMTS13 distinguishes patients with thrombotic thrombocytopenic purpura from normal individuals and carriers of ADAMTS13 mutations. *Thromb Haemost* 2004; **91**: 806–11.

92 Dong L, Chandrasekaran V, Zhou W, Tsai HM. Evolution of ADAMTS13 antibodies in a fatal case of thrombotic thrombocytopenic purpura. *Am J Hematol* 2008; **83**: 815–17.

93 Klaus C, Plaimauer B, Studt JD, *et al*. Epitope mapping of ADAMTS13 autoantibodies in acquired thrombotic thrombocytopenic purpura. *Blood* 2004; **103**: 4514–19.

94 Luken BM, Turenhout EA, Kaijen PH, *et al*. Amino acid regions 572–579 and 657–666 of the spacer domain of ADAMTS13 provide a common antigenic core required for binding of antibodies in patients with acquired TTP. *Thromb Haemost* 2006; **96**: 295–301.

95 Stocker W, Grams F, Baumann U, *et al*. The metzincins—topological and sequential relations between the astacins, adamalysins, serralysins, and matrixins (collagenases) define a superfamily of zinc-peptidases. *Protein Sci* 1995; **4**: 823–40.

96 Zimmerman TS, Dent JA, Ruggeri ZM, Nannini LH. Subunit composition of plasma von Willebrand factor. Cleavage is present in normal individuals, increased in IIA and IIB von Willebrand disease, but minimal in variants with aberrant structure of individual oligomers (types IIC, IID, and IIE). *J Clin Invest* 1986; **77**: 947–51.

97 Dent JA, Berkowitz SD, Ware J, Kasper CK, Ruggeri ZM. Identification of a cleavage site directing the immunochemical detection of molecular abnormalities in type IIA von Willebrand factor. *Proc Natl Acad Sci U S A* 1990; **87**: 6306–10.

98 Tsai HM, Sussman, II, Nagel RL. Shear stress enhances the proteolysis of von Willebrand factor in normal plasma. *Blood* 1994; **83**: 2171–9.

99 Tsai HM. Physiologic cleavage of von Willebrand factor by a plasma protease is dependent on its conformation and requires calcium ion. *Blood* 1996; **87**: 4235–44.

100 Zhang Q, Zhou YF, Zhang CZ, Zhang X, Lu C, Springer TA. Structural specializations of A2, a force-sensing domain in the ultralarge vascular protein von Willebrand factor. *Proc Natl Acad Sci U S A* 2009; **106**: 9226–31.

101 Zhang X, Halvorsen K, Zhang CZ, Wong WP, Springer TA. Mechanoenzymatic cleavage of the ultralarge vascular protein von Willebrand factor. *Science* 2009; **324**: 1330–4.

102 Nishio K, Anderson PJ, Zheng XL, Sadler JE. Binding of platelet glycoprotein Ibalpha to von Willebrand factor domain A1 stimulates the cleavage of the adjacent domain A2 by ADAMTS13. *Proc Natl Acad Sci U S A* 2004; **101**: 10578–83.

103 Shim K, Anderson PJ, Tuley EA, Wiswall E, Sadler JE. Platelet–VWF complexes are preferred substrates of ADAMTS13 under fluid shear stress. *Blood* 2008; **111**: 651–7.

104 Cao W, Krishnaswamy S, Camire RM, Lenting PJ, Zheng XL. Factor VIII accelerates proteolytic cleavage of von Willebrand factor by ADAMTS13. *Proc Natl Acad Sci U S A* 2008; **105**: 7416–21.

105 Bernardo A, Ball C, Nolasco L, Moake JF, Dong JF. Effects of inflammatory cytokines on the release and cleavage of the endothelial cell-derived ultralarge von Willebrand factor multimers under flow. *Blood* 2004; **104**: 100–6.

106 Studt JD, Hovinga JA, Antoine G, *et al*. Fatal congenital thrombotic thrombocytopenic purpura with

apparent ADAMTS13 inhibitor: in vitro inhibition of ADAMTS13 activity by hemoglobin. *Blood* 2005; **105**: 542–4.

107 Crawley JT, Lam JK, Rance JB, Mollica LR, O'Donnell JS, Lane DA. Proteolytic inactivation of ADAMTS13 by thrombin and plasmin. *Blood* 2005; **105**: 1085–93.

108 Kokame K, Matsumoto M, Fujimura Y, Miyata T. VWF73, a region from D1596 to R1668 of von Willebrand factor, provides a minimal substrate for ADAMTS-13. *Blood* 2004; **103**: 607–12.

109 Majerus EM, Anderson PJ, Sadler JE. Binding of ADAMTS13 to von Willebrand factor. *J Biol Chem* 2005; **280**: 21773–8.

110 Zhang P, Pan W, Rux AH, Sachais BS, Zheng XL. The cooperative activity between the carboxyl-terminal TSP1 repeats and the CUB domains of ADAMTS13 is crucial for recognition of von Willebrand factor under flow. *Blood* 2007; **110**: 1887–94.

111 Zanardelli S, Crawley JT, Chion CK, Lam JK, Preston RJ, Lane DA. ADAMTS13 substrate recognition of von Willebrand factor A2 domain. *J Biol Chem* 2006; **281**: 1555–63.

112 Gao W, Anderson PJ, Majerus EM, Tuley EA, Sadler JE. Exosite interactions contribute to tension-induced cleavage of von Willebrand factor by the antithrombotic ADAMTS13 metalloprotease. *Proc Natl Acad Sci U S A* 2006; **103**: 19099–104.

113 Wu JJ, Fujikawa K, McMullen BA, Chung DW. Characterization of a core binding site for ADAMTS-13 in the A2 domain of von Willebrand factor. *Proc Natl Acad Sci U S A* 2006; **103**: 18470–4.

114 Fujikawa K, Suzuki H, McMullen B, Chung D. Purification of human von Willebrand factor-cleaving protease and its identification as a new member of the metalloproteinase family. *Blood* 2001; **98**: 1662–6.

115 Ai J, Smith P, Wang S, Zhang P, Zheng XL. The proximal carboxyl-terminal domains of ADAMTS13 determine substrate specificity and are all required for cleavage of von Willebrand factor. *J Biol Chem* 2005; **280**: 29428–34.

116 Akiyama M, Takeda S, Kokame K, Takagi J, Miyata T. Production, crystallization and preliminary crystallographic analysis of an exosite-containing fragment of human von Willebrand factor-cleaving proteinase ADAMTS13. *Acta Crystallogr Sect F Struct Biol Cryst Commun* 2009; **65**: 739–42.

117 Tao Z, Peng Y, Nolasco L, *et al*. Recombinant CUB-1 domain polypeptide inhibits the cleavage of ULVWF strings by ADAMTS13 under flow conditions. *Blood* 2005; **106**: 4139–45.

118 Zhou W, Bouhassira EE, Tsai HM. An IAP retrotransposon in the mouse ADAMTS13 gene creates ADAMTS13 variant proteins that are less effective in cleaving von Willebrand factor multimers. *Blood* 2007; **110**: 886–93.

119 Zanardelli S, Chion AC, Groot E, *et al*. A novel binding site for ADAMTS13 constitutively exposed on the surface of globular VWF. *Blood* 2009; **114**: 2819–28.

120 Sadler JE. New concepts in von Willebrand disease. *Annu Rev Med* 2005; **56**: 173–91.

121 Lyons SE, Bruck ME, Bowie EJ, Ginsburg D. Impaired intracellular transport produced by a subset of type IIA von Willebrand disease mutations. *J Biol Chem* 1992; **267**: 4424–30.

122 Dent JA, Galbusera M, Ruggeri ZM. Heterogeneity of plasma von Willebrand factor multimers resulting from proteolysis of the constituent subunit. *J Clin Invest* 1991; **88**: 774–82.

123 Gralnick HR, Williams SB, McKeown LP, *et al*. In vitro correction of the abnormal multimeric structure of von Willebrand factor in type IIa von Willebrand's disease. *Proc Natl Acad Sci U S A* 1985; **82**: 5968–72.

124 Kunicki TJ, Montgomery RR, Schullek J. Cleavage of human von Willebrand factor by platelet calcium-activated protease. *Blood* 1985; **65**: 352–6.

125 Hassenpflug WA, Budde U, Obser T, *et al*. Impact of mutations in the von Willebrand factor A2 domain on ADAMTS13-dependent proteolysis. *Blood* 2006; **107**: 2339–45.

126 Tsai HM, Sussman, II, Ginsburg D, Lankhof H, Sixma JJ, Nagel RL. Proteolytic cleavage of recombinant type 2A von Willebrand factor mutants R834W and R834Q: inhibition by doxycycline and by monoclonal antibody VP-1. *Blood* 1997; **89**: 1954–62.

127 Michiels JJ, Gadisseur A, Vangenegten I, Schroyens W, Berneman Z. Recessive von Willebrand disease type 2 Normandy: variable expression of mild hemophilia and VWD type 1. *Acta Haematol* 2009; **121**: 119–27.

128 Brown SA, Eldridge A, Collins PW, Bowen DJ. Increased clearance of von Willebrand factor antigen post-DDAVP in Type 1 von Willebrand disease: is it a potential pathogenic process? *J Thromb Haemost* 2003; **1**: 1714–7.

129 Bowen DJ, Collins PW. An amino acid polymorphism in von Willebrand factor correlates with increased susceptibility to proteolysis by ADAMTS13. *Blood* 2004; **103**: 941–7.

130 Bowen DJ. An influence of ABO blood group on the rate of proteolysis of von Willebrand factor by ADAMTS13. *J Thromb Haemost* 2003; **1**: 33–40.

131 Ginsburg D. Molecular genetics of von Willebrand disease. *Thromb Haemost* 1999; **82**: 585–91.

132 Gill JC, Endres-Brooks J, Bauer PJ, Marks WJ, Jr., Montgomery RR. The effect of ABO blood group on the diagnosis of von Willebrand disease. *Blood* 1987; **69**: 1691–5.

133 Zuberi L, Yerasuri D, Kuriakose P. Effect of blood group on idiopathic thrombotic thrombocytopenic purpura. *J Clin Apher* 2009; **24**: 131–3.

134 Staropoli JF, Stowell CP, Tuncer HH, Marques MB. An inquiry into the relationship between ABO blood group and thrombotic thrombocytopenic purpura. *Vox Sang* 2009; **96**: 344–8

135 Pruss CM, Notley CR, Hegadorn CA, O'Brien LA, Lillicrap D. ADAMTS13 cleavage efficiency is altered by mutagenic and, to a lesser extent, polymorphic sequence changes in the A1 and A2 domains of von Willebrand factor. *Br J Haematol* 2008; **143**: 552–8.

136 Goodeve A, Eikenboom J, Castaman G, *et al*. Phenotype and genotype of a cohort of families historically diagnosed with type 1 von Willebrand disease in the European study, molecular and clinical markers for the diagnosis and management of type 1 von Willebrand Disease (MCMDM-1VWD). *Blood* 2007; **109**: 112–21.

5 Animal models in von Willebrand disease

Cécile V. Denis, Olivier D. Christophe and Peter J. Lenting

INSERM U770, Université Paris-sud, Le Kremlin-Bicêtre, France

von Willebrand disease (VWD), caused by quantitative or qualitative abnormalities in von Willebrand factor (VWF), is considered the most common inherited bleeding disorder in humans. Interestingly, this hemorrhagic syndrome has not spared animals and over the years several animal species have also been described as suffering from VWD [1]. Although some of these animal models have been genetically engineered, others arose from spontaneous mutations not only in the *VWF* gene itself (pigs, dogs) but also in some modifier genes affecting VWF (mice). Independent of the underlying mechanisms leading to the onset of the disease, these different models that reproduce the various types of VWD have greatly contributed to improving our knowledge about VWF biology and functions and have also been very useful for testing new therapies.

Genetic and phenotypic characterization of the different VWD animal models

Porcine VWD

In 1941, a hemophilia-like disorder affecting swine was described by Hogan *et al.* [2] These pigs were initially reported to display an extremely prolonged ear bleeding time but it was 20 years later that other similarities with human severe (type 3) VWD were recognized, such as reduced levels of factor VIII (FVIII), an overresponse of FVIII to transfusion of plasma, and reduced retention of platelets in glass beads columns (Table 5.1) [1]. As such, the pigs with VWD represent the oldest known animal model of a human bleeding diathesis. A complete survey of hemostatic parameters was conducted in 1973 in order to compare values found in normal pigs with pigs with VWD [3]. Platelet counts and platelet aggregation in the presence of the ADP nucleotide were not different between pigs with VWD and normal pigs; however, FVIII levels were reduced to 30% of normal pig levels. This value is much higher than FVIII levels in human patients with type 3 VWD where residual FVIII levels are below 10%. However, it should be noted that although hemostasis in pigs is not very different from in humans, notable differences do exist, mostly in coagulation factor activities. Indeed, the activities of factors V, VIII, IX, XI, and XII are much higher than in humans, with levels between 450% and 1000% when expressed in terms of a normal human standard [1]. As a consequence, pigs with VWD can bleed while still expressing FVIII levels, which would be supranormal in humans. This hemorrhagic phenotype leads to an increased number of postnatal deaths and a reduction in litter size of affected pigs [16].

Transmission of the disease is autosomal recessive [1]. The bleeder swine are homozygous for the defect while carriers are heterozygous [16]. These carriers are asymptomatic with normal bleeding times and normal FVIII levels, although VWF:Ag and VWF:RCo are reduced to 30–40% of normal [17].

Von Willebrand Disease, 1st edition. Edited by Augusto B. Federici, Christine A. Lee, Erik E. Berntorp, David Lillicrap, Robert R. Montgomery. © 2011 Blackwell Publishing Ltd.

Table 5.1 Animal models of von Willebrand disease.

Type	Species	Breed/strain	Genetic defect	VWF:Ag (%)	FVIII (% of wild-type)	Reference
I	Dog	Various breeds	G7437A, splice junction mutation resulting in instable mRNA	Variably decreased	Variably decreased	4, 5
	Mouse	C57Bl/6 or any breed	Heterozygous state of the genetically induced model	50	50	7
	Mouse	RIIIS/J	Post-translational modifications due to a mutation in a glycosyltransferase, resulting in rapid clearance of von Willebrand factor	30–50	30–50	8
II	Dog	German shorthair pointers	Unknown	12–27	Reduced	9
		German wirehair pointers	Unknown	4–6	19–25	10
III	Pig		Reduced transcription Post-transcriptional defects	Traces	30	2, 3, 6
	Dog	Scottish terrier	Single base deletion at position 255 in exon 4 induces a stop codon downstream	Undetectable	15–50	11, 12
	Dog	Chesapeake Bay retriever	Unknown	Undetectable	18–30	13
	Dog	Dutch kooiker	G→A mutation in donor splice site of intron 16 induces downstream stop codon	Traces	30–50	14, 15
	Dog	Shetland sheepdog	Single base deletion at position 735 induces a stop codon downstream	Undetectable	73–77	5
	Mouse	C57Bl/6 or any breed	Genetically induced	Undetectable	15–20	7

The molecular basis of porcine VWD is not precisely known but the defect appears to be linked to the *VWF* locus [6]. Southern blot experiments revealed that the porcine *VWF* gene is grossly normal in affected pigs, indicating that the defect does not result from a deletion or a major rearrangement of the gene but more likely from a small insertion/deletion within it [6]. It is also important to note that pigs with VWD are not completely deficient in VWF. Low amounts of VWF:Ag can be detected both in platelets and in endothelial cells from the pulmonary artery and from the inferior vena cava [18]. Analysis of the mRNA revealed a two-third decrease in VWF message levels compared with wild-type levels [19]. However, mRNA levels in pigs with VWD are still significant and do not correlate with the very low amounts of VWF:Ag, suggesting that post-transcriptional defects are involved, for example defects in translation or instability of the transcripts [19].

Canine VWD

The first incidence of VWD in dogs was reported almost 40 years ago in German shepherds [20]. This breed of German shepherds was characterized by a mild-to-severe bleeding diathesis, and laboratory analysis revealed similarities to the defects of human VWD. Since then, many other dog breeds have been identified that also carry the disease, and VWD is now considered the most common bleeding disorder in dogs. Clinical manifestations in canine VWD are associated with a broad phenotypic heterogeneity [21,22]. An intriguing aspect is that platelet VWF, which represents approximately 10–20% of total VWF in humans, is markedly reduced in canine platelets, which contain ~2% of total circulating VWF [1]. This amount may vary between breeds since no VWF could be detected in canine platelets from Scottish terriers [23]. VWF deficiency in dogs is associated with moderately reduced FVIII levels, varying between 20% and 50% in type 3 VWF-deficient dogs. It should be noted that FVIII plasma levels are threefold higher in dogs than in humans.

Various types of VWD can be distinguished in dogs (Table 5.1). The most common is type 1 VWD, which affects a large number of breeds including golden retrievers, German shepherds, and Doberman pinschers. In Doberman pinschers, up to 70% of the dogs may be carriers of the disease. The disease was found to be transmitted as an autosomal dominant trait with variable penetrance [24]. Reduced VWF levels in this breed originate from a reduced constitutive release of VWF from endothelial cells combined with a decrease in VWF mRNA [25]. The genetic defect has been identified recently. A mutation at nucleotide 7437 (G–A) at the end of exon 43 changes the consensus splice junction sequence. Consequently, the splice junction is used less frequently, with the resulting mRNA being less stable. A similar mutation has also been found in other breeds, such as Bernese mountain dogs, Manchester terrier, poodles, and Pembroke Welsh corgis [4].

Type 2 VWD is rarely found in dogs. One report related to German shorthair pointers, which were characterized by bleeding episodes and absence of high molecular weight multimers [9]. VWF from dogs with type 2 VWD is also characterized by impaired collagen binding because of the lack of high multimers. Also, a colony of German wirehair pointers has been reported to carry type 2 VWD. These dogs lack high molecular weight multimers and have reduced VWF-dependent platelet aggregation activity [10]. At present, the genetic defects that cause the type 2 phenotype in dogs are unknown.

Type 3 VWD is present in a number of breeds, including Scottish terriers, Shetland sheepdogs, Chesapeake Bay retrievers and Dutch kooikers. The VWF antigen and activity is virtually absent, resulting in severe bleeding tendencies in homozygous dogs [26–28]. Heterozygous dogs are usually clinically asymptomatic, although heterozygous Shetland sheepdogs can present some clinical bleeding problems [29]. Different genetic defects have been found— for Dutch kooiker dogs, a point mutation has been identified. This mutation (G–A) transition at the first position of the donor splice site sequence of intron 16 introduces a stop codon at amino acid residue 729 in the propolypeptide of VWF [14,15]. VWF deficiency in Scottish terriers is caused by a single base deletion at position 255 in exon 4, and this frameshift mutation leads to a new stop codon 103 base pairs downstream [11,12]. A third variant causing type 3 VWD in dogs has been found in Shetland sheepdogs. Here, deletion of a single base pair at position 735 introduces a stop codon 244 base pairs downstream [5].

Murine VWD

Although much more recently described that porcine and canine VWD, murine models of VWD have quickly become the models of choice in research. The most commonly used is the VWF-deficient mouse engineered through homologous recombination. However, there are also a number of various murine models in which VWF is affected owing to the presence of gene modifiers with or without a direct link to the *VWF* gene (Table 5.1).

Genetically Induced Model. Mice deficient in VWF were engineered via classic gene targeting techniques with insertion of the neomycin resistance gene in the murine *VWF* locus [7]. No trace of VWF protein is detectable in any of the compartments where VWF is normally present. FVIII levels are reduced to 15–20% of that found in wild-type mice. Homozygous knock-out mice do not suffer any major bleeding complications, although a small percentage of pups suffer from lethal abdominal bleeding shortly after birth. However, in the tail clip assay bleeding time of VWF-deficient mice is infinite. These mice represent a good model for human type 3 VWD. Heterozygous mice display antigen levels down to 50% and FVIII levels between 50% and 60% of wild-type mice, mimicking human type 1 VWD [7].

Gene Modifiers and Murine Models of VWD. Plasma VWF levels among inbred mouse strains are highly variable. Ginsburg [8] has taken advantage of this observation to identify candidate VWF modifier genes. Random testing of bleeding times in common mouse strains first led to the identification of the RIIIS/J strain, which is characterized by a prolonged bleeding time (>15 min) and plasma VWF:Ag levels 50–75% lower than in normal mouse plasma [8]. FVIII was similarly reduced and the activated partial thromboplastin time (aPTT) was prolonged 2.5-fold. In contrast to the reduced plasma level, platelet VWF was normal [30]. The multimeric profile showed presence of all multimers, although reduced in concentration—a hallmark of type 1 VWD. Extensive genetic analysis of this strain led to the discovery of the first gene modifier of VWF in mice, named *Mvwf1* for modifier of VWF 1 [8]. *Mvwf1* is a mutation that causes a tissue-specific switch in the expression of an N-acetylgalactosaminyltransferase, B4GALNT2, from intestinal epithelium to vascular endothelium. This switch leads to the B4GALNT2-mediated transfer of N-acetylgalactosamine onto VWF, and this aberrantly modified VWF gets cleared rapidly from the circulation by the asialoglycoprotein receptor (ASPGR), explaining the low plasma antigen levels. A recent study reported that *Mvwf1* and low VWF phenotype is not restricted to the RIIIS/J strain exclusively but can also be found in 13 other inbred strains, including five wild-derived strains [31].

Since the first description of *Mvwf1*, other gene modifiers have been identified. Indeed, in the CASA/RkJ mouse strain, very high VWF plasma levels were reported. Comparison with the A/J strain revealed levels that were increased eightfold [32]. The CASA/RkJ strain appears to carry a single nucleotide polymorphism associated to an amino acid change (R2657Q) in the *VWF* gene. This modification, named *Mvwf2*, accounts for a significant proportion of the increased VWF levels in CASA/RkJ compared with the A/J strain, an effect mediated through increased VWF biosynthesis/secretion [32]. Additional genetic analysis led to the identification of two other regions on the mouse genome that also co-segregate with VWF level variation between the CASA/RkJ and A/J strains [33]. One region on chromosome 4 was named *Mvwf3* and a second region on chromosome 13 was named *Mvwf4*. These two candidate loci are independent of the *VWF* gene, which is localized on mouse chromosome 6. Neither the specific genes underlying *Mvwf3* and *Mvwf4*, nor the mechanisms by which they influence VWF levels, have been identified so far [33].

Another group of *VWF* gene modifiers have also been discovered following gene targeting of other genes independently of VWF. For example, deficiency in the ST3Gal-IV sialyltransferase induces a dominant 50% reduction in VWF plasma levels accompanied by a similar decrease in FVIII and a prolonged tail bleeding time [34]. By masking galactose linkages on VWF, ST3Gal-IV normally prevents accelerated clearance of VWF by the ASPGR. Conversely, gene targeting of the Ashwell receptor (Asgr-1) leads to a 1.5-fold increase in VWF and FVIII plasma levels as well as a reduction in tail bleeding time, suggesting that this hepatocyte ASPGR contributes to VWF homeostasis [35]. Interestingly, combined deficiency of ST3Gal-IV and Asgr-1 resulted in normalization of VWF plasma levels and of bleeding time in mice [35].

The presence of such modifier genes probably also contribute to the wide variability in VWF levels observed in humans, and the results obtained in the mouse model will certainly help to identify candidate genetic loci that could potentially regulate hemostasis/thrombosis in humans.

Contribution of VWD animal models in improving VWD therapy

Even before their usefulness to investigate VWF role in various experimental settings, VWD animal models are extremely precious as models of the human pathology in order to test new therapies. As the first existing model, the VWD pigs were used to assess the efficacy of VWF transfusion to treat the hemostatic defect. From the different studies that were performed, it appeared that although correction of VWF:Ag and FVIII levels was easily obtained, it did not translate into a significant reduction of the bleeding time, whether porcine cryoprecipitate or human recombinant VWF were transfused [1]. The canine severe VWD model was also used to test the therapeutic efficacy of a recombinant VWF preparation [36]. A reduction of bleeding intensity and successful treatment of bleeding episodes were observed without cuticle bleeding time correction. These results were very much predictive of the situations in humans where, despite an overall improvement of their hemostatic status, patients with severe VWD rarely see a correction of their bleeding time upon VWF infusion whereas inconsistent results were obtained in moderate and variants types of VWD [37,38].

In all animal models as well as in humans with VWD, infusion of VWF normalizes the survival of FVIII and keeps its level elevated for 8–12 h. This phenomenon was studied using pigs with VWD where it was shown to be independent of FVIII mRNA induction in the liver [39].

The efficacy of interleukin 11 to raise VWF plasma levels was first demonstrated in murine and canine models with type 1 VWD [40,41] and these studies provided the basis for the clinical trials that are currently under way in human patients with type 1 VWD [42].

Dogs deficient in VWF have also been used in the initial testing of recombinant factor VIIa [43]. In contrast to the correction observed in FVIII- and FIX-deficient dogs, no correction of bleeding time was detected in VWF-deficient dogs. Since bleeding time may not be the right parameter to judge efficacy of VWF-treatment, it is not surprising that application of recombinant factor VIIa was finally found to be successful in human patients with type 3 VWD [44].

The feasibility of a gene therapy approach to treat VWF has also recently been tested using VWF-deficient mice. Considering the large size of the VWF cDNA as well as its complex post-translational processing, such a task appeared very difficult. However, hydrodynamic gene transfer of murine VWF cDNA resulted in expression of fully functional VWF by liver hepatocytes and correction of bleeding time in VWF-deficient mice [45,46]. Additionally, endothelial cells isolated from VWF-deficient dogs have been used for similar purposes. Blood-outgrowth endothelial cells were isolated and transduced with lentiviral vectors encoding VWF [47]. This approach resulted in endothelial cells producing fully multimerized VWF.

Altogether, these data underscore the utility of VWD animal models in providing an experimental basis for further clinical testing.

Contribution of VWD animal models in improving knowledge of VWF functions

The role of VWF in atherosclerosis

Animal models of VWD have helped to uncover a number of unsuspected functions of VWF besides its classic involvement in hemostasis/thrombosis (Figure 5.1). The first insight in these uncharted areas

- Gene therapy
- Thrombosis
- TTP

VWD models

- Bone marrow transplantation
- Atherosclerosis
- Thrombosis
- TTP

- Gene therapy
- Thrombosis
- Atherosclerosis
- Endocarditis
- TTP
- Metastasis
- Encephalomyelitis
- Ischemic stroke
- Intimal hyperplasia
- Sepsis
- Inflammation
- Clearance

Figure 5.1 Presentation of the various animal models of von Willebrand disease and the research areas in which they have been used. Illustration provided by Servier Medical Art. TTP, thrombotic thrombocytopenic purpura. Illustration provided by Servier Medical Art.

came from a report published in 1978, describing a protection against atherosclerosis development in pigs with VWD both spontaneously or after diet [48]. However, later studies did not confirm the direct link between the absence of VWF and decreased atherosclerosis, attributing the observed differences to higher diet-induced hypercholesterolemia in normal pigs [1] and/or to the presence of a polymorphism at the apolipoprotein B100 locus [1]. Although these results appeared in agreement with ultrasonography studies in patients with type 3 VWD [49] showing presence of atherosclerosis lesions, they also highlighted the difficulty of working with animal models that do not possess a homogenous genetic background. To clarify this issue, further studies were performed in VWF-deficient mice backcrossed to atherosclerosis-sensitive strains, low-density lipoprotein receptor-deficient mice, or apolipoprotein E-deficient mice. In the absence of VWF, the formation of atherosclerotic lesions was significantly delayed. Interestingly, this protective effect was observed mainly in regions of disturbed flow at branch points on the aorta [50]. Thus, the role of VWF in lesion development is apparent only in the syngenic murine model, suggesting that murine and human atherogenesis have different molecular bases or that role of VWF is too subtle to be detectable in humans where many other genes also have significant involvement.

The role of VWF in platelet adhesion and thrombus formation

Besides atherosclerosis, the porcine model also paved the way for improving our understanding of the role of VWF in platelet adhesion and thrombus formation. In particular, shear rate-dependent VWF involvement in mediating platelet–vessel wall interactions was first studied in the porcine model. Platelet deposition on pig thoracic aortas was reduced in the absence of plasma VWF, mostly at high shear rate [1]. At low shear rate in damaged coronary arteries, although no difference in platelet deposition was observed, platelet activation was reduced in the absence of VWF [51]. In a completely different experimental setting, that is the laser-injury thrombosis model in mesenteric vessels of VWF-deficient mice, this role in platelet activation was not confirmed [52].

Platelet plug formation in the absence of VWF was also first monitored in pigs with VWD by microscopic examination of the structure of the hemostatic plug after ear incision [53]. Although large platelet aggregates could form in pigs with VWD, they were largely ineffective in stopping bleeding. Indeed, they did not cover the ends of transected vessels and were penetrated by channels, allowing bleeding to continue. Similar findings were reported in VWF-deficient mice where ferric chloride-induced injury not only led to delayed thrombus formation but also resulted in non-occlusive thrombus with persistent high-shear channels [54]. Arterial thrombosis was also evaluated in one of the very few research studies performed with the canine model. It was shown that dogs with VWD do not develop occlusive thrombosis following stenosis and injury of carotid arteries [55].

Although very different vessel injury methods were used, all models—porcine, canine, and murine—thus confirmed a critical role for VWF in thrombus formation. In dogs and pigs, thrombosis was mostly evaluated at its endpoint by looking at isolated vessels with a microscope. Only in mice can thrombus formation be monitored in real-time using fluorescently labeled platelets and intravital microscopy [56]. It is interesting to note that the biggest disparities concerning the role of VWF have not been observed in comparing the different animal models but rather between the existing murine thrombosis models. Indeed, VWF absence does not significantly affect thrombus growth in the laser-induced injury model [46] but it plays a major role both in mesenteric arterioles and venules after ferric chloride-induced injury [56]. The laser injury model is dominated by tissue factor-mediated thrombin generation and it is therefore possible that thrombin has the capacity to overcome the thrombosis defect associated with VWF deficiency. Further insight in the molecular basis of the role of VWF in thrombus formation was recently gained from VWF-deficient mice transiently expressing VWF mutants in plasma. Those transient models were obtained by hydrodynamic injection of murine VWF cDNAs carrying mutations in VWF binding domains to fibrillar collagen, glycoprotein Ibα, or glycoprotein IIb/IIIa. With this new approach, the relative importance of VWF interactions with its ligands was evaluated in the ferric chloride-induced thrombosis model. Results showed that all three interactions are critical for optimal thrombus formation and that the VWF-glycoprotein IIb/IIIa binding step is essential for thrombus stability [46].

A distinct role for VWF in platelet adhesion independently of vessel wall injury was also uncovered using VWF-deficient mice. Intravital microscopy observations showed that release of VWF from Weibel–Palade bodies following endothelial stimulation leads to immediate and transient platelet interaction with the endothelium, a process that allows rapid recruitment of platelets to sites of inflammation [57].

In all above-mentioned studies, thrombosis was investigated in healthy vessels, which does not reflect the pathologic situations where thrombosis occurs following plaque rupture. A more clinically relevant experiment was carried out in VWD and normal pigs fed a high-cholesterol diet. Although both groups displayed coronary atherosclerosis at the end of the diet period, a stenosis/injury protocol did not induce occlusive thrombosis in pigs with VWD as opposed to normal pigs [58].

Other VWF functions

Owing to its significant involvement in platelet adhesion and thrombus formation, VWF is likely to play a role in diseases in which these two processes are involved. The availability of animal VWD models has allowed such working hypotheses to be tested *in vivo*. For example, based on the evidence that platelets are important in the pathogenesis of experimental infectious endocarditis, both normal pigs and pigs with VWD were submitted to a protocol involving trauma to the aortic valve and endocardium followed by injection of group C streptococci. Endocarditis was present in all control animals but failed to develop in pigs with VWD, suggesting that platelet–vessel wall interactions are crucial in the pathogenesis of this disease [59].

Although the murine VWD model has been increasingly used in the past decade, the porcine model can still provide very useful information. A recent study provided initial evidence that VWF deficiency associated with inflammation modulation leads to prolonged pulmonary xenograft survival in experiments where porcine lungs were transplanted in baboons [60].

The role of VWF in the thrombotic syndrome known as thrombotic thrombocytopenic purpura (TTP) was assessed in canine, porcine, and murine models. First, induction of experimental TTP by injection of the snake venom botrocetin revealed a complete protection against TTP onset in the absence of VWF in dogs and pigs [23]. Later, a similar protection was observed in a murine model of congenital TTP, that is mice deficient for the VWF-cleaving protease ADAMTS13 after shigatoxin challenge [61]. Altogether, these results emphasize the crucial role of VWF in the pathogenesis of TTP.

As mentioned, the murine model has now become the most common model to test hypotheses concerning the role of VWF in various pathologies, and several studies in this regard have been published in the past few years. Experimental metastases experiments performed with the murine melanoma cell line B16-BL6 resulted in the surprising observation that VWF-deficient mice exhibit a significant increase in pulmonary nodules compared with their wild-type litter mates—a phenotype that could be corrected by restoring VWF plasma levels in the mice with VWD [62].

Other functions for VWF revealed with the murine models include a protective role in experimental allergic encephalomyelitis and blood–brain barrier permeability [63]—an important role in modulation of infarct volume after ischemic stroke induced by middle cerebral artery occlusion [64] and a potential implication in smooth muscle cell proliferation and intimal hyperplasia [65]. In sepsis, according to the experimental model used, different results have been obtained. Indeed, VWF deficiency does not affect mortality in LPS-induced endotoxemia [61], but it significantly improves survival in a cecum ligature and puncture model known to reproduce human sepsis more accurately than lipopolysaccharide (LPS)-injection [66]. Finally, the VWF-deficient mice also displayed reduced leukocyte rolling in mesenteric venules and a decrease in leukocyte recruitment in a cytokine-induced meningitis model, as well as in early skin wounds [67]. This particular study highlighted for the first time the critical importance of VWF in endothelial cell biology since the impaired inflammatory response was mostly an indirect consequence of VWF deficiency. Indeed, absence of VWF led to a secondary absence of Weibel–Palade bodies, which in turn resulted in a defective P-selectin expression at the surface of inflamed vessels. Similar indirect mechanisms may also underlie the encephalomyelitis study [63].

69

Contribution of VWD animal models to improving knowledge of VWF biology

Weibel–Palade body formation

Weibel–Palade bodies (WPBs) are unique to vascular endothelial cells of vertebrates. They have a single membrane and a dense interior composed of closely packed VWF multimers, resulting in a fibrillar appearance. No such structures could be detected in the vessels of pigs with VWD by transmission electron microscopy [68]. Endothelial cells obtained from the mice with VWF confirmed this absence of WPBs [67]. In dogs with type 3 VWF, biogenesis of these organelles could be restored upon expression of VWF [11].

The absence of VWF and of WBPs may have some unexpected consequences. Indeed, there are many other proteins localized in WPBs: P-selectin, CD63, interleukin 8, osteoprotegerin, and angiopoietin 2, to name a few [69]. As mentioned in the previous paragraph, defective leukocyte recruitment was observed in the murine VWD model as a consequence of P-selectin mislocalization. In the absence of WPBs, P-selectin was detected partially in lysosomes and partially in small round, unidentified organelles that undergo inefficient secretion upon activation [67]. The potential pathologic consequences of other WPB protein mislocalization have not yet been addressed.

Compartmentalization

Usually, VWF is present in plasma, endothelial cells, subendothelium, and platelets. To address the issue of the relative importance of the different VWF compartments, bone marrow transplantation experiments were performed in pigs. Transplantation of a normal bone marrow in a pig with VWD resulted in a chimera with VWF-positive platelets and VWF-negative endothelium [70]. The plasmatic compartment was only minimally replenished by platelet VWF, suggesting that most plasma VWF is endothelial-derived. Platelet VWF was able to improve only partially the hemostatic status in type 3 VWD. Infusion of VWF concentrate in these transplanted pigs resulted in a normalization of thrombus formation [1], suggesting that both platelet and plasma VWF are needed for optimal function. In the opposite setting, that is transplantation of a normal pig with bone marrow from a pig with VWD, bleeding time remained normal, suggesting that plasma and subendothelial VWF are the main determinants of bleeding time [1]. In the canine and murine models, plasma VWF appears to be sufficient to fully correct bleeding time [45,71].

The inherent differences of the various species such as the quasi-absence of VWF in canine platelets in addition with the very different experimental settings such as infusion of VWF versus high expression of VWF after gene therapy in the mouse make it very difficult to draw any definitive conclusion about this aspect of VWF biology.

Clearance

An important aspect of VWF biology that was recently investigated using the VWF-deficient mice is how the protein is removed from the circulation. Injection of VWF into these mice revealed that the bulk of exogenously administered VWF is directed toward the liver and, more precisely, in liver macrophages, toward the Kupffer cells [72]. *In vivo* depletion of Kupffer cells in mice by injection of gadolinium chloride led to a significantly increased half-life of infused VWF in VWF-deficient mice (mean residence time of 2.7 h in saline-treated mice compared with 4.5 h in gadolinium-treated mice) and doubling of endogenous VWF levels in wild-type mice. Whether Kupffer cells take up VWF through a receptor-mediated or receptor-independent process is not known. However, the sheer physical dimensions of VWF seem to preclude endocytosis through classic pathways involving clathrin-coated pits or caveolae.

Whether abnormal clearance can lead to VWD was also investigated in the mouse system. Indeed, no simple cellular systems can identify mutants that are synthesized and secreted normally but whose elimination is defective. Recently, the causative effect on accelerated clearance of four different mutations (R1205H, C1130F, C1149R, and C2671T) was confirmed in the VWF-deficient mouse [72].

Other murine models, such as the RIIIS/J mouse and mice deficient in ST3Gal-IV sialyltransferase and Ashwell receptor, have also contributed to improve our knowledge about VWF clearance, particularly concerning the importance of glycosylation and sialylation in this process [8,34].

Concluding remarks

The different available animal models of VWD have already proven very useful in characterizing this disease and uncovering some new functions of VWF. No doubt they will continue to be an important asset for testing and developing new treatments, in particular gene therapy approaches. The direction of future research will probably rely on developing new murine models expressing VWF variants through knock-in technologies, allowing a subtle approach of VWF structure–function relationships.

References

1 Denis CV, Wagner DD. Insights from von Willebrand disease animal models. *Cell Mol Life Sci* 1999; **56**: 977–90.

2 Hogan AG, Muhrer ME, Bogart R. A hemophilia-like disease in swine. *Proc Soc Exptl Biol Med* 1941; **48**: 217–19.

3 Bowie EJW, Owen CAJ, Zollman PE, Thompson JHJ, Fass DN. Test of hemostasis in swine: normal values and values in pigs affected with von Willebrand's disease. *Am J Vet Res* 1973; **34**: 1405–7.

4 Whitely M. Composition and methods for detection of von Willebrand's disease. 2003. U.S. patent number 2003/0207272.

5 Venta PJ, Brewer GJ, Yuzbasiyan-Gurkan V, Schall WD. DNA encoding canine von Willebrand factor and methods of use. 2004. U.S. patent number US 6,767,707.

6 Bahou WF, Bowie EJW, Fass DN, Ginsburg D. Molecular genetic analysis of porcine von Willebrand disease: tight linkage to the von Willebrand factor locus. *Blood* 1988; **72**: 308–13.

7 Denis C, Methia N, Frenette PS, *et al*. A mouse model of severe von Willebrand disease: defects in hemostasis and thrombosis. *Proc Natl Acad Sci USA* 1998; **95**: 9524–9.

8 Ginsburg D. Identifying novel genetic determinants of hemostatic balance. *J Thromb Haemost* 2005; **3**: 1561–8.

9 Johnson GS, Turrentine MA, Dodds WJ. Type II von Willebrand's disease in German shorthair pointers. *Vet Clin Pathol* 1987; **16**: 7.

10 van Dongen AM, van Leeuwen M, Slappendel RJ. Canine von Willebrand's disease type 2 in German wire-hair pointers in the Netherlands. *The Veterinary record* 2001; **148**: 80–2.

11 Haberichter SL, Merricks EP, Fahs SA, Christopherson PA, Nichols TC, Montgomery RR. Re-establishment of VWF-dependent Weibel–Palade bodies in VWD endothelial cells. *Blood* 2005; **105**: 145–52.

12 Venta PJ, Li J, Yuzbasiyan-Gurkan V, Brewer GJ, Schall WD. Mutation causing von Willebrand's disease in Scottish terriers. *J Vet Intern Med* 2000; **14**: 10–19.

13 Johnson GS, Lees GE, Rosborough TK, Dodds WJ. A bleeding disorder (von Willebrand's disease) in a Chesapeake Bay retriever. *J Am Vet Med Assoc* 1980; **176**: 1261–3.

14 Rieger M, Schwarz HP, Turecek PL, Dorner F, van Mourik JA, Mannhalter C. Identification of mutations in the canine von Willebrand factor gene associated with type III von Willebrand disease. *Thromb Haemost* 1998; **80**: 332–7.

15 van Oost BA, Versteeg SA, Slappendel RJ. DNA testing for type III von Willebrand disease in Dutch kooiker dogs. *J Vet Intern Med* 2004; **18**: 282–8.

16 Fass DN, Bowie EJW, Owen CAJ, Zollman PE. Inheritance of porcine von Willebrand's disease: study of a kindred of over 700 pigs. *Blood* 1979; **53**: 712–19.

17 Fass DN, Brockway WJ, Owen CAJ, Bowie EJW. Factor VIII (Willebrand) antigen and ristocetin-Willebrand factor in pigs with von Willebrand's disease. *Thromb Res* 1976; **8**: 319–27.

18 Wu QY, Drouet L, Carrier JL, *et al*. Differential distribution of von Willebrand factor in endothelial cells. Comparison between normal pigs and pigs with von Willebrand disease. *Arteriosclerosis* 1987; **7**: 47–54.

19 Wu QY, Bahnak BR, Coulombel L, *et al*. Analysis of von Willebrand factor mRNA from the lungs of pigs with severe von Willebrand disease by using a human cDNA probe. *Blood* 1988; **71**: 1341–6.

20 Dodds WJ. Canine von Willebrand's disease. *J Lab Clin Med* 1970; **76**: 713–21.

21 Brooks MB, Erb HN, Foureman PA, Ray K. von Willebrand disease phenotype and von Willebrand factor marker genotype in Doberman pinschers. *Am J Vet Res* 2001; **62**: 364–9.

22 Dodds WJ. Further studies of canine von Willebrand's disease. *Blood* 1975; **45**: 221–30.

23 Sanders WE, Jr., Reddick RL, Nichols TC, Brinkhous KM, Read MS. Thrombotic thrombocytopenia induced in dogs and pigs. The role of plasma and platelet vWF in animal models of thrombotic thrombocytopenic purpura. *Arterioscler Thromb Vasc Biol* 1995; **15**: 793–800.

24 Riehl J, Okura M, Mignot E, Nishino S. Inheritance of von Willebrand's disease in a colony of Doberman pinschers. *Am J Vet Res* 2000; **61**: 115–20.

25 Meinkoth JH, Meyers KM. Measurement of von Willebrand factor-specific mRNA and release and storage of von Willebrand factor from endothelial cells of dogs with type-I von Willebrand's disease. *Am J Vet Res* 1995; **56**: 1577–85.

26 Benson RE, Johnson GS, Dodds WJ. Binding of low-molecular-weight canine factor VIII coagulant from von Willebrand plasma to canine factor VIII-related antigen. *Brit J Haematol* 1981; **49**: 541–50.

27 Brinkhous KM, Read MS, Reddick RL, Griggs TR. Pathophysiology of platelet-aggregating von Willebrand factor: applications of the venom coagglutinin vWF assay. *Ann Ny Acad Sci* 1981; **370**: 191–204.

28 Pathak EJ. Type 3 von Willebrand's disease in a Shetland sheepdog. *Can Vet J* 2004; **45**: 685–7.

29 Raymond SL, Jones DW, Brooks MB, Dodds WJ. Clinical and laboratory features of a severe form of von Willebrand disease in Shetland sheepdogs. *J Am Vet Med Assoc* 1990; **10**: 1342–6.

30 Sweeney JD, Novak EK, Reddington M, Takeuchi KH, Swank RT. The RIIIS/J inbred mouse strain as a model for von Willebrand disease. *Blood* 1990; **76**: 2258–65.

31 Johnsen JM, Levy GG, Westrick RJ, Tucker PK, Ginsburg D. The endothelial-specific regulatory mutation, Mvwf1, is a common mouse founder allele. *Mamm Genome* 2008; **19**: 32–40.

32 Lemmerhirt HL, Shavit JA, Levy GG, Cole SM, Long JC, Ginsburg D. Enhanced VWF biosynthesis and elevated plasma VWF due to a natural variant in the murine Vwf gene. *Blood* 2006; **108**: 3061–7.

33 Lemmerhirt HL, Broman KW, Shavit JA, Ginsburg D. Genetic regulation of plasma von Willebrand factor levels: quantitative trait loci analysis in a mouse model. *J Thromb Haemost* 2007; **5**: 329–35.

34 Ellies LG, Ditto D, Levy GG, *et al.* Sialyltransferase ST3Gal-IV operates as a dominant modifier of hemostasis by concealing asialoglycoprotein receptor ligands. *Proc Natl Acad Sci U S A* 2002; **99**: 10042–7.

35 Grewal PK, Uchiyama S, Ditto D, *et al.* The Ashwell receptor mitigates the lethal coagulopathy of sepsis. *Nat Med* 2008; **14**: 648–55.

36 Schwarz HP, Schlokat U, Mitterer A, *et al.* Recombinant von Willebrand factor—insight into structure and function through infusion studies in animals with severe von Willebrand disease. *Semin Thromb Hemost* 2002; **28**: 215–26.

37 Fressinaud E, Veyradier A, Sigaud M, Boyer-Neumann C, Le Boterff C, Meyer D. Therapeutic monitoring of von Willebrand disease: interest and limits of a platelet function analyser at high shear rates. *Brit J Haematol* 1999; **106**: 777–83.

38 Perkins HA. Correction of the hemostatic defects in von Willebrand's disease. *Blood* 1967; **30**: 375–80.

39 Kaufman RJ, Dorner AJ, Fass DN. von Willebrand factor elevates plasma factor VIII without induction of factor VIII messenger RNA in the liver. *Blood* 1999; **93**: 193–7.

40 Denis CV, Kwack K, Saffaripour S, *et al.* Interleukin 11 significantly increases plasma von Willebrand factor and factor VIII in wild type and von Willebrand disease mouse models. *Blood* 2001; **97**: 465–72.

41 Olsen EH, McCain AS, Merricks EP, *et al.* Comparative response of plasma VWF in dogs to up-regulation of VWF mRNA by interleukin-11 versus Weibel–Palade body release by desmopressin (DDAVP). *Blood* 2003; **102**: 436–41.

42 Ragni MV, Jankowitz RC, Chapman HL, *et al.* A phase II prospective open-label escalating dose trial of recombinant interleukin-11 in mild von Willebrand disease. *Haemophilia* 2008; **14**: 968–77.

43 Brinkhous KM, Hedner U, Garris JB, Diness V, Read MS. Effect of recombinant factor VIIa on the hemostatic defect in dogs with hemophilia A, hemophilia B, and von Willebrand disease. *Proc Natl Acad Sci U S A* 1989; **86**: 1382–6.

44 Franchini M, Veneri D, Lippi G. The use of recombinant activated factor VII in congenital and acquired von Willebrand disease. *Blood Coagul Fibrinolysis* 2006; **17**: 615–19.

45 De Meyer SF, Vandeputte N, Pareyn I, *et al.* Restoration of plasma von Willebrand factor deficiency is sufficient to correct thrombus formation after gene therapy for severe von Willebrand disease. *Arterioscler Thromb Vasc Biol* 2008; **28**: 1621–6.

46 Marx I, Christophe OD, Lenting PJ, *et al.* Altered thrombus formation in von Willebrand factor-deficient mice expressing von Willebrand factor variants with defective binding to collagen or GPIIbIIIa. *Blood* 2008; **112**: 603–9.

47 De Meyer SF, Vanhoorelbeke K, Chuah MK, *et al.* Phenotypic correction of von Willebrand disease type 3 blood-derived endothelial cells with lentiviral vectors expressing von Willebrand factor. *Blood* 2006; **107**: 4728–36.

48 Fuster V, Bowie EJW, Lewis JC, Fass DN, Owen CAJ. Resistance to atherosclerosis in pigs with von Willebrand's disease. Spontaneous and high cholesterol diet-induced arteriosclerosis. *J Clin Invest* 1978; **61**: 722–30.

49 Sramek A, Bucciarelli P, Federici AB, *et al.* Patients with type 3 severe von Willebrand disease are not protected against atherosclerosis: results from a multicenter study in 47 patients. *Circulation* 2004; **109**: 740–4.

50 Methia N, Andre P, Denis CV, Economopoulos M, Wagner DD. Localized reduction of atherosclerosis in von Willebrand factor-deficient mice. *Blood* 2001; **98**: 1424–8.

51 Reddick RL, Griggs TR, Lamb MA, Brinkhous KM. Platelet adhesion to damaged coronary arteries: comparison in normal and von Willebrand disease swine. *Proc Natl Acad Sci U S A* 1982; **79**: 5076–9.

52 Dubois C, Panicot-Dubois L, Gainor JF, Furie BC, Furie B. Thrombin-initiated platelet activation *in vivo* is vWF

independent during thrombus formation in a laser injury model. *J Clin Invest* 2007; **117**: 953–60.

53 Sawada Y, Fass DN, Katzman JA, Bahn RC, Bowie EJW. Hemostatic plug formation in normal and von Willebrand pigs: the effect of administration of cryoprecipitate and a monoclonal antibody to von Willebrand factor. *Blood* 1986; **67**: 1229–39.

54 Ni H, Denis CV, Subbarao S, *et al.* Persistence of platelet thrombus formation in arterioles of mice lacking both von Willebrand factor and fibrinogen. *J Clin Invest* 2000; **106**: 385–92.

55 Nichols TC, Bellinger DA, Reddick RL, *et al.* The roles of von Willebrand factor and factor VIII in arterial thrombosis: studies in canine von Willebrand disease and hemophilia. *Blood* 1993; **81**: 2644–51.

56 Denis CV, Wagner DD. Platelet adhesion receptors and their ligands in mouse models of thrombosis. *Arterioscler Thromb Vasc Biol* 2007; **27**: 728–39.

57 Andre P, Denis CV, Ware J, *et al.* Platelets adhere to and translocate on von Willebrand factor presented by endothelium in stimulated veins. *Blood* 2000; **96**: 3322–8.

58 Nichols TC, Bellinger DA, Tate DA, *et al.* von Willebrand factor and occlusive arterial thrombosis. A study in normal and von Willebrand's disease pigs with diet-induced hypercholesterolemia and atherosclerosis. *Arteriosclerosis* 1990; **10**: 449–61.

59 Johnson CM, Bowie EJ. Pigs with von Willebrand disease may be resistant to experimental infective endocarditis. *J Lab Clin Med* 1992; **120**: 553–8.

60 Cantu E, Balsara KR, Li B, *et al.* Prolonged function of macrophage, von Willebrand factor-deficient porcine pulmonary xenografts. *Am J Transplant* 2007; **7**: 66–75.

61 Chauhan AK, Walsh MT, Zhu G, Ginsburg D, Wagner DD, Motto DG. The combined roles of ADAMTS13 and VWF in murine models of TTP, endotoxemia, and thrombosis. *Blood* 2008; **111**: 3452–7.

62 Terraube V, Pendu R, Baruch D, *et al.* Increased metastatic potential of tumor cells in von Willebrand factor-deficient mice. *J Thromb Haemost* 2006; **4**: 519–26.

63 Noubade R, del Rio R, McElvany B, *et al.* von-Willebrand factor influences blood brain barrier permeability and brain inflammation in experimental allergic encephalomyelitis. *Am J Pathol* 2008; **173**: 892–900.

64 Zhao BQ, Chauhan AK, Canault M, *et al.* von Willebrand factor-cleaving protease ADAMTS13 reduces ischemic brain injury in experimental stroke. *Blood* 2009; **114**: 3329–34.

65 Qin F, Impeduglia T, Schaffer P, Dardik H. Overexpression of von Willebrand factor is an independent risk factor for pathogenesis of intimal hyperplasia: preliminary studies. *J Vasc Surg* 2003; **37**: 433–9.

66 Lerolle N, Dunois-Larde C, Badirou I, *et al.* von Willebrand factor is a major determinant of ADAMTS-13 decrease during mouse sepsis induced by cecum ligation and puncture. *J Thromb Haemost* 2009; **7**: 843–50.

67 Denis CV, Andre P, Saffaripour S, Wagner DD. Defect in regulated secretion of P-selectin affects leukocyte recruitment in von Willebrand factor-deficient mice. *Proc Natl Acad Sci U S A* 2001; **98**: 4072–7.

68 Gebrane-Younes J, Drouet L, Caen JP, Orcel L. Heterogeneous distribution of Weibel–Palade bodies and von Willebrand factor along the porcine vascular tree. *Am J Pathol* 1991; **139**: 1471–84.

69 Rondaij MG, Bierings R, Kragt A, van Mourik JA, Voorberg J. Dynamics and plasticity of Weibel–Palade bodies in endothelial cells. *Arterioscler Thromb Vasc Biol* 2006; **26**: 1002–7.

70 Bowie EJW, Solberg LAJ, Fass DN, *et al.* Transplantation of normal bone marrow into a pig with severe von Willebrand's disease. *J Clin Invest* 1986; **78**: 26–30.

71 Stokol T, Parry B. Efficacy of fresh-frozen plasma and cryoprecipitate in dogs with von Willebrand's disease or hemophilia A. *J Vet Intern Med* 1998; **12**: 84–92.

72 Denis CV, Christophe OD, Oortwijn BD, Lenting PJ. Clearance of von Willebrand factor. *Thromb Haemost* 2008; **99**: 271–8.

6

Classification of von Willebrand disease

Javier Batlle[1,2], Almudena Pérez-Rodríguez[1] and María Fernanda López-Fernández[1]

[1]Servicio de Hematología y Hemoterapia, Complexo Hospitalario Universitario de A Coruña, A Coruña, Spain

[2]Department of Medicine, School of Medicine, University of Santiago de Compostela, Spain

von Willebrand disease (VWD) is a genetic bleeding disorder transmitted by autosomal genetic factors and related to quantitative and/or qualitative abnormalities of the von Willebrand factor (VWF). Many different types have been described based on phenotypic characteristics of the protein. VWD is heterogeneous in its clinical and laboratory manifestations and underlying pathogenetic mechanisms. Moreover, genetic analysis has identified additional heterogeneity within types with similar phenotypical characteristics. Acquired disorders that mimic VWD are referred to as acquired von Willebrand syndrome (aVWS) and are discussed in Chapter 20. The present chapter focuses exclusively on the classification of inherited VWD.

The old nomenclature of VWD: some historical steps

After the first description of the disease, made by Erik Adolf von Willebrand in 1926, a very elegant immunologic distinction between hemophilia A and VWD was accomplished by Zimmerman *et al.* in 1971 [1]. He used the Laurell technique employing a polyclonal antibody against FVIII/VWF, which precipitates the VWF (Figure 6.1). Hemophilia showed normal antigen levels whereas patients with VWD had decreased levels of VWF, initially called VIII:RAg (currently VWF:Ag), because VWF and FVIII were not yet considered to be different molecular entities. The first step in categorization of VWD in 1972 was provided by Holmberg and Nilsson [2], who demonstrated that some patients with VWD had normal plasma concentrations of the VWF antigen. Using crossed immunoelectrophoresis (CIE), the VWF antigen in these patients was shown to have a rapid mobility consistent with a structural abnormality (Figure 6.1) [3,4].

Subsequent electrophoretic separation of VWF multimers, which replaced the CIE method because of its greater electrophoretic resolution (Figure 6.1), showed that high-molecular-weight multimers (HMWMs) of VWF were lower in plasma from patients with abnormal CIE patterns (Figure 6.1) [5]. This led to the conventional distinction of using roman numerals to identify type I and type II VWD. Type I was characterized by a normal distribution of multimers, whereas type II VWD was characterized by an absence of HMWMs. The particularly severe recessive form of the disease, characterized by the virtual absence of any VWF in plasma or platelets, came to be referred to as type III VWD [6].

In 1980, Ruggeri differentiated between two major variants of type II VWD: IIA, with a relatively decreased ristocetin cofactor activity (VWF:RCo), and IIB, with an increased ristocetin-induced platelet agglutination (RIPA) at low concentrations of ristocetin [7,8]. These variants were later shown to be clinically different, at least with respect to the incidence of spontaneous and DDAVP (1-deamino-8-D-arginine vasopressin)(desmopressin)-induced thrombocytopenia (Figure 6.2) [9].

Von Willebrand Disease, 1st edition. Edited by Augusto B. Federici, Christine A. Lee, Erik E. Berntorp, David Lillicrap, Robert R. Montgomery. © 2011 Blackwell Publishing Ltd.

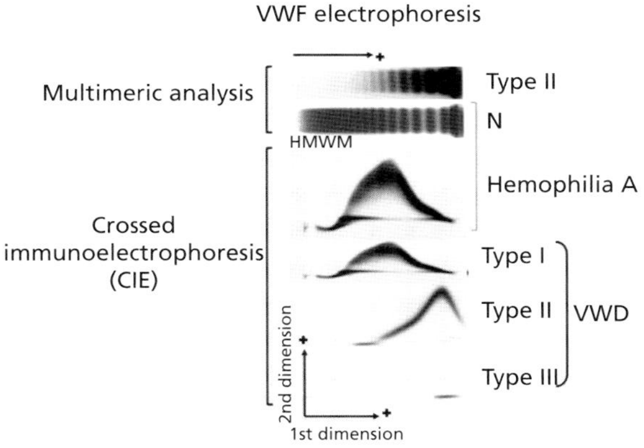

Figure 6.1 Electrophoresis of von Willebrand factor (VWF) using crossed immunoelectrophoresis (CIE) and by multimeric analysis. HMWM indicates high-molecular-weight multimers of VWF. The arrows indicate the direction of the electrophoretic separation; in the case of CIE, the protein is subjected to a first run (first dimension) followed by a second run (second dimension) with migration toward the anode (+). Several plasma samples are compared: a normal individual (N), a patient with hemophilia A, and patients with type I, II, and III von Willebrand disease (VWD) (from the initial classification). Type I shows a decreased VWF with normal mobility, type II shows a shift of the VWF toward the anode because of the absence of the HMWM, and type III shows a virtual absence of VWF.

A few years later, a new, abnormal VWF was reported in a family with recessive VWD with a variant and aberrant multimeric pattern, named type IIC VWD (Figure 6.2) [10,11]. Since then, an explosion of observations of different abnormalities in multimeric patterns has led to the classification of many additional subtypes of type II VWD (IID, IIE, IIG, IIF) [12–14]. Different abnormalities were also described within type I VWD (IB, IC, ID). The role of platelet VWF complicated the diagnosis of VWD with new forms, such as platelet-low, platelet-discordant, and platelet-normal, making their appearance [15]. Many additional subtypes have been distinguished based on the mode of inheritance, details of the VWF multimer patterns, the relationship of platelet and plasma VWF properties, and specific biochemical abnormalities. The recognition of such variations in VWD is considered to be important because it may lead to a better

understanding of its pathophysiology and to individualized treatment and genetic counseling [14].

Classification of VWD based on structural and functional abnormalities of VWF (1987)

Until 1987 there was no systematic classification of VWD. Several independent investigators had published reports describing patients with supposedly distinctive characteristics as defined by a variety of laboratory techniques. This led to the nomenclature of VWD becoming very complex and, more importantly, not very practical for the clinician. Several distinctive patterns were identified within both type I and type II, but the two groups included patients in whom the bleeding manifestations were caused by different pathogenetic mechanisms. Patients with similar features were also reported by independent investigators under different designations, adding to the confusion of the many existing subtypes.

To afford a more systematic classification, in 1987 Ruggeri and Zimmerman [14] proposed the first attempt to classify VWD into categories identified by well-defined parameters and presumably common pathogenetic mechanism (Table 6.1). They clustered the different subtypes previously reported into types I and II. To avoid further confusing terminology, they retained the nomenclature proposed by the authors who had originally described each new form of VWD. Type III was considered a separate group (no longer a severe manifestation of type I) because of the recessive modality of genetic transmission and because in some cases the trace amounts of VWF present in plasma and platelets showed evidence of structural abnormalities. At that time, some mutations were characterized in several types I, II, and III VWD [15].

Table 6.1 Classification of von Willebrand disease (VWD) based on structural and functional abnormalities of the von Willebrand factor (VWF) (1987).

Quantitative abnormalities and no evidence of intrinsic functional abnormality of VWF
VWF with low ristocetin cofactor activity
Patients with enhanced responsiveness to ristocetin
Patients with type III (severe) VWD

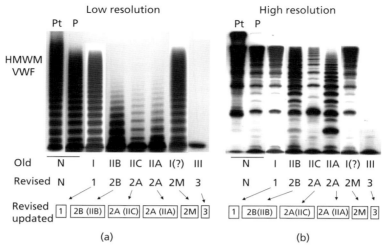

Figure 6.2 von Willebrand factor (VWF):Ag in sodium dodecyl sulfate (SDS)-agarose gels. Multimeric analysis of VWF in a normal patient and patients with von Willebrand disease (VWD). The presence of all the multimers is observed in normal plasma (N). In platelet lysate, super-large multimers (arrow) are seen when compared with the corresponding plasma. Plasma from patients with types 2A (IIA), 2A (IIC), 2B (IIB), 2M, and 3 VWD (current type and in brackets the old designation) are also included. In the low-resolution gels the absence of the high-molecular-weight multimers (HMWMs) of VWF is seen in types 2A (IIA), 2A (IIC), and 2B (IIB). In contrast, HMWM of VWF is normal in 2M. A virtual absence of VWF is seen in type 3. In the high-resolution gel, different complex satellite banding patterns are observed: 2A (IIA) and 2B (IIB) show an increase in the relative proportion of the outer satellite bands in each multimer, while type 2A (IIC) shows an aberrant multimeric banding pattern is seen.

The revised classification of VWD (1994)

To achieve more consensus in this complex field, a new classification of VWD was proposed based on criteria developed by the VWF Subcommittee of the International Society on Thrombosis and Haemostasis (ISTH SCC VWF) [16].

It is true that the previous nomenclature had several advantages. The primary categories (types I, II, and III) had a clear relationship to pathopysiology, type of genetic abnormality, and clinical behavior. Assignment to these major categories was relatively easy based on the patient's history and the results of the laboratory tests. Certain subcategories were easy to recognize and were clinically useful. There were, however, difficulties involving the use of many subcategories.

The original distinction between qualitative and quantitative VWF deficiency was blurred by the sporadic use of the multimer pattern alone as the primary criterion for the separation of type I from type II VWD. As a consequence of identifying some qualitative disorders as "type I" variants, this major category did not correlate well with clinical behavior or type of genetic abnormality. For example, type I VWD New York and also type I VWD Malmö had a normal multimeric pattern, but the clinical and laboratory features were otherwise very similar to type IIB [17,18] and were caused by the same missense mutation very near to all known mutations that cause type IIB VWD [16]. Similarly, variants with abnormal factor VIII binding, also referred to as VWD Normandy [19,20], had a normal multimer pattern but did not behave in any other way like a VWF deficiency. These examples demonstrated the limited precision and clinical utility of the previous nomenclature.

It was agreed that a reclassification of VWD should be compatible with the problems caused by compound heterozygosity for a multimeric protein and should exhibit a clear correlation with pathophysiology, type of genetic abnormality, clinical response to therapy, and genetic counseling. It should be simple, easily recognized, not confused with previous classifications, and the number of formal subcategories should be as few as feasible. It should be flexible, allowing more precise classification of individual patients as more information becomes available, without requiring significant renaming. It was designed to be conceptually independent of specific laboratory testing procedures, although most of the VWD types could be assigned by using tests that were widely available. Accordingly, a hierarchical scheme was determined to be most suitable. It reserved the designation of VWD for disorders caused by mutations within the *VWF* gene.

In accordance with these principles, Sadler [16], on behalf of the ISTH VWF SCC, published the revised classification of VWD in 1994. There is no doubt this was a work of the utmost importance and a positive step forward for clarifying such a complex situation. The different types or subtypes previously described were now grouped into new and simpler classifications and definitions as indicated in Table 6.2 and Figure 6.2. The molecular defects causing VWD became part of the tertiary level of classification categories with the two first levels being the major categories essential in the classification. The subsidiary categories are appropriate only in certain specific contexts.

Most of the VWD variants were amalgamated into type 2A in this classification. However, a separate new classification was created for type 2B (formerly IIB). In addition, a new type (2M, with "M" representing "multimer") was created to include those variants with decreased platelet-dependent function (VWF:RCo) but no significant decrease of HMWM of VWF (which may or may not have another aberrant structure). Type 2N VWD, with "N" representing "Normandy" where the first individuals were identified, was defined to include cases with a secondary decreased FVIII owing to VWF defects of FVIII binding.

Current classification. The updated revised classification (2006)

Subsequent added knowledge of VWF required that the ISTH SCC VWF updated the classification of VWD to better incorporate these advances into the conceptual framework for understanding the patho-

Table 6.2 Revised classification of von Willebrand disease (VWD), 1994.

All VWD is caused by mutations at the von Willebrand factor (VWF) locus

Type 1 refers to partial quantitative deficiency of VWF

Type 3 VWD refers to virtually complete deficiency of VWF

Type 2 VWD refers to qualitative deficiency of VWF

Type 2A VWD refers to qualitative variants with decreased platelet-dependent function that is associated with the absence of high-molecular-weight (HMW) VWF multimers

Type 2B VWD refers to all qualitative variants with increased affinity for platelet glycoprotein Ib (GPIb)

Type 2M VWD ("M" for "multimer") refers to qualitative variants with decreased platelet-dependent function that is not caused by the absence of HMW VWF multimers

Type 2N VWD ("N" for Normandy") refers to all qualitative variants with markedly decreased affinity for factor VIII

When recognized, a mixed phenotype caused by compound heterozygosity is indicated by separate classification of each allele separated by a slash (/)

For the description of mutations, amino acid residues are numbered 1–2813 from the initiator methionine to the carboxyl-terminus of pre-pro-VWF

According to Sadler, 1994 [17].

physiology of VWD [21]. The purposes of the classification remained primarily clinical to facilitate the diagnosis, treatment, and counseling of patients with VWD (Table 6.3).

Nomenclature and abbreviations

The abbreviations for VWF and its activities and the conventions for describing mutations in this newer system adhere to recommendations in previous VWF Subcommittee reports. Nucleotides of the human VWF cDNA sequence are numbered sequentially, beginning with "+1" assigned to the "A" of the initiation codon. The encoded amino acid residues are numbered from 1 to 2813, beginning with the initiator methionine. The database of mutations and polymorphisms in the *VWF* gene is maintained at the University of Sheffield and is accessible at http://www.shef.ac.uk/vwf/index.html.

Table 6.3 Updated revised classification of von Willebrand disease (VWD), 2006.

Type	Description
1	Partial quantitative deficiency of von Willebrand factor (VWF)
2	Qualitative VWF defects
2A	Decreased VWF-dependent platelet adhesion and a selective deficiency of high-molecular-weight (HMW) VWF multimers
2B	Increased affinity for platelet glycoprotein Ib (GPIb)
2M	Decreased VWF-dependent platelet adhesion without a selective deficiency of HMW VWF multimers
2N	Markedly decreased binding affinity for factor VIII
3	Virtually complete deficiency of VWF

According to Sadler, 2006 [22].

Table 6.4 Changes in the revised and updated classifications of von Willebrand disease (VWD).

1994 Revision	2006 Updated revision
VWD is caused by mutations at the von Willebrand factor (VWF) locus	VWD is not restricted to VWF gene mutations
Type 1 VWD includes partial quantitative deficiency of VWF. The multimers distribution and structure of plasma VWF is indistinguishable from normal	Type 1 VWD includes partial quantitative deficiency of VWF. Plasma VWF may contain mutant subunits, but has normal functional activity relative to antigen level. The proportion of large multimers is not decreased significantly

Phenotypic classification of VWD

Classification is not restricted to mutations within the *VWF* gene (Table 6.4) [21] because no generally available method can identify or exclude VWF mutations in a significant percentage of patients; thus, any requirement for identification of a mutation can rarely be satisfied in practice. Locus heterogeneity

cannot be excluded for VWD, and mutations in other genes could conceivably produce a similar disease indistinguishable from the VWD that is caused by intragenic VWF mutations.

Processing of VWF

The processing of VWF involves various different mechanisms: synthesis, assembly, secretion, proteolysis, and clearance. VWD mutations cause abnormalities of one of these mechanisms, although in some mutations more than one abnormality is simultaneously involved (Figure 6.3).

Type 1 VWD

Type 1 VWD is by far the most frequent form [21,22]. The principal change in classification of type 1 was intended to include patients whose proportion of HMWM in plasma VWF is decreased slightly, but not enough to prevent the achievement of a hemostatically effective level of large multimers after desmopressin (Table 6.4). In addition, the plasma VWF multimers may or may not contain mutant VWF subunits. When sensitive assay methods are used, many patients with type 1 VWD have mild or minimal abormalities of multimer structure or distribution, as shown by the European Molecular and Clinical Markers for the Diagnosis and Management of Type 1 VWD study (MCMDM-1VWD) and the Canadian Type 1 VWD study [23–26].

A synthesis defect of VWF is the most common mechanism that causes type 1 VWD. However, some mutations can also decrease secretion by impairing the intracellular transport of VWF subunits, causing a severe dominant inherited form of type 1 VWD, although the phenotype is often mixed and may have features of both type 1 and type 2A VWD [21, 22,27,28]. Reduced secretion may be caused by VWF mutations affecting gene expression, although this mechanism has been difficult to demonstrate consistently. Accelerated clearance can also cause dominant type 1 VWD as in VWD Vicenza. An increased susceptibility of VWF to proteolytic cleavage may also modulate the severity of type 1 VWD (Figure 6.3) [21,22,29,30].

It is clear that several distinct mechanisms can cause type 1 VWD and that some of these can be identified by appropriate tests. For example, variants associated with rapid clearance are identified by their

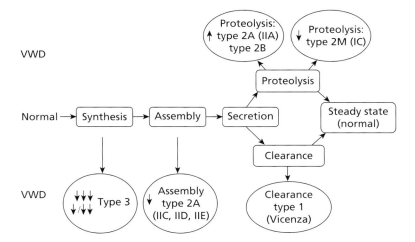

Figure 6.3 Synthesis and catabolism of von Willebrand factor (VWF) multimers. The normal processing of VWF involves different mechanisms: synthesis, assembly, secretion, proteolysis, and clearance. von Willebrand disease (VWD) mutations cause abnormalities of one of these mechanisms, although in some more than one are simultaneously involved.

characteristic response to a test dose of desmopressin. The clinical significance of this heterogeneity is under investigation and could lead to further changes in the classification of VWD.

Type 2 VWD

Bleeding symptoms in type 2 VWD are often thought to be more severe than in type 1, although this impression needs to be evaluated by suitable clinical studies [21,22,29,30].

Type 2A VWD. Type 2A VWD refers to qualitative variants in which VWF-dependent platelet adhesion is decreased because the proportion of large VWF multimers is decreased. Levels of VWF:Ag and FVIII may be normal or modestly decreased in this subtype, but VWF activity is abnormal, as shown by markedly decreased VWF:RCo. The deficiency in large multimers predisposes persons to bleed [21,22,29–31].

Type 2A VWD may be inherited as a dominant trait, although some variants are recessive. Homozygous mutations of the propeptide impair multimer assembly in the Golgi apparatus and lack the satellite bands usually associated with proteolysis. This condition was initially described as the recessive trait "type IIC" VWD [10,11]. Heterozygous mutations in the cystine knot domain can impair dimerization of pro-VWF in the endoplasmic reticulum causing a multimer pattern originally referred to as "type IID" [12]. Heterozygous mutations in cystine residues of the D3 domain also can impair multimer assembly (Figures 6.3 and 6.4),

but these mutations often also produce an indistinct or "smeary" multimer pattern referred to as "type IIE" [13].

In contrast, mutations within or near the A2 domain of VWF cause a type 2A VWD that is associated with markedly increased proteolysis of the VWF subunits [21,22]. Two subgroups of this pattern have been distinguished: group I mutations enhance proteolysis by VWF-cleaving protease (ADAMTS13) and also impair multimer assembly and group II mutations enhance proteolysis without decreasing the assembly of large VWF multimers. Thus, the location of type 2A VWD mutations can sometimes be inferred from the banding on high-resolution VWF multimer gels.

Although type 2A VWD is heterogeneous in mechanism, these distinctions are not currently employed to further subdivide type 2A VWD because their clinical utility has not been clearly demonstrated.

Type 2B VWD. Type 2B VWD is caused by mutations within or adjacent to VWF domain A1 which pathologically increase platelet membrane glycoprotein (GPIb)–VWF binding; this leads to the proteolytic degradation of VWF by ADAMTS13 and the depletion of large, functional VWF multimers (Figures 6.3 and 6.4) [21,22,29,30]. The diagnosis of type 2B VWD depends on finding abnormally increased RIPA at low concentrations of ristocetin. Although laboratory results for type 2B VWD may be similar to those in type 2A or type 2M, patients who have type 2B VWD typically have a

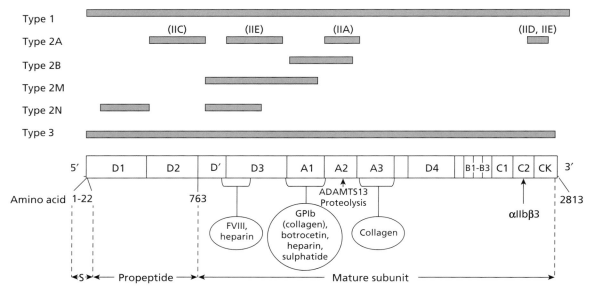

Figure 6.4 Structure of the von Willebrand factor (VWF) precursor and location of mutations in von Willebrand disease (VWD). The VWF precursor consists of a signal peptide (S), propeptide, and mature subunit. Structural domains (A, B, C, CK, and binding sites for factor VIII, platelet glycoprotein Ib, collagen, and platelet integrin αIIbβ3) are labeled. Bars show the mutation positions that cause VWD. Some type 2 VWD phenotypes are indicated in brackets.

thrombocytopenia that is exacerbated by surgery, pregnancy, or other stress.

Type 2B VWD Malmö or New York is caused by the mutation Pro1266Leu and is associated with increased RIPA at low concentrations of ristocetin, although RIPA has been found to be normal in some patients with this mutation [21,22]. The plasma multimer distribution is normal, VWF subunit proteolysis is not increased, and desmopressin does not cause thrombocytopenia. Some patients have mild bleeding, others have none. It is thought that decreased large plasma VWF multimers and increased subunit proteolysis may correlate with the occurrence of significant bleeding in patients with RIPA values consistent with type 2B VWD [22,30].

A differential diagnosis should include a phenotype similar to type 2B VWD that is caused by heterozygous gain-of-function mutations in platelet GPIbα [17,18], a disorder referred to as platelet-type pseudo-VWD [22,30].

Type 2M VWD. Type 2M VWD refers to variants with decreased VWF-dependent platelet adhesion not caused by the absence of HMWM of VWF multimers. Instead, type 2M VWD mutations reduce the interaction of VWF with platelet GPIb or with connective tissue and do not substantially impair multimer assembly. Screening laboratory results in type 2M VWD and type 2A VWD are similar, the distinction between them being determined by multimer gel electrophoresis (Figure 6.2) [21,22,30,31].

Mutations in type 2M VWD have been identified in domains D′, D3, and A1, where they interfere with binding to platelet GPIb (Figure 6.4). A study of one family found that a mutation in the VWF A3 domain reduces VWF binding to collagen, thereby reducing platelet adhesion and possibly causing type 2M VWD [32]. The detection of type 2M VWD may depend on which of the assays are used. For example, VWF:CB is insensitive to mutations that impair platelet binding and decrease VWF:RCo. Conversely, VWF:RCo cannot detect defects in collagen binding that might impair platelet adhesion *in vivo*. Most cases of type 2M VWD have been identified based upon a value for VWF:RCo that is disproportionately low compared with VWF:Ag. These patients usually have mutations within the VWF A1 domain that impair binding to platelet GPIb.

Type 2N VWD. Type 2N VWD is inherited as a recessive trait, and heterozygous relatives usually have mild or no bleeding symptoms. It is caused by VWF mutations that impair binding to FVIII, lowering FVIII levels such that type 2N VWD masquerades as an autosomal recessive form of hemophilia A [19–22,33,34]. The differential diagnosis is based on measuring the affinity of patient VWF for FVIII (VWF:FVIIIB), usually in a solid-phase immunoassay.

Most mutations that cause type 2N VWD occur within the FVIII binding site of VWF that lies between residues Ser764 and Arg1035 and spans domain D' and part of domain D3 (Figure 6.4) [21,22,30,33]. Sometimes both VWF alleles have FVIII binding mutations, but often one allele has the FVIII binding mutation while the other allele expresses little or no VWF (a so-called "null allele").

Type 3 VWD

Type 3 VWD is inherited as a recessive trait, and heterozygous relatives usually have mild or no bleeding symptoms [21,22,30,35]. It is characterized by undetectable VWF protein and activity, FVIII levels are usually very low (1–9 IU/dL), and patients seldom have a measurable response to desmopressin. Nonsense and frameshift mutations commonly cause type 3 VWD, although large deletions, splice site mutations, and missense mutations have also been found to produce this condition. Mutations are distributed throughout the *VWF* gene and most are unique to the family in which they were first identified (Figure 6.4). A small fraction of patients who have type 3 VWD develop alloantibodies to VWF in response to the transfusion of plasma products. Large deletions in the *VWF* gene may predispose patients to this complication. Virtually complete deficiency of VWF is categorized as type 3 VWD, regardless of the phenotype of heterozygous relatives.

The term "severe" VWD has sometimes been used to describe type 3 VWD and symptomatic type 1 VWD, which is characterized by very low VWF levels; however, these conditions are almost always clinically distinct [35,36]. Type 1 VWD caused by dominant heterozygous mutations is rarely associated with VWF levels as low as 10 IU/dL, and patients with dominant type 1 VWD can have therapeutically useful responses to desmopressin.

Compound heterozygosity and compound phenotypes

The phenotype of heterozygous patients depends on interactions between subunits encoded by both VWF alleles. If compound heterozygosity can be inferred from laboratory studies of the patient or relatives, then the compound phenotype can be represented by a separate designation for each allele, separated by a slash (/) [21]. For example, co-inheritance of type 2N VWD and a nonexpressing or "null" VWF allele would be described as "type 2N/3 VWD." Recognition of compound heterozygosity has implications for treatment as well as genetic counseling.

Multiple pathophysiologic mechanisms

Single mutations may cause VWD by more than one mechanism in various combinations [21,22,30]. These effects can produce type 1, type 2A, and type 2N VWD and various blended phenotypes.

A hierarchical approach to classification

There are two major levels of classification: primary (1, 2, 3) and secondary (A, B, M, N). Additional "tertiary" information that is not reflected in the defined types of VWD can be appended in parentheses (Figure 6.2) [21]. Examples of such information may include a place name that indicates a remarkable phenotype (e.g., Vicenza), the patient's mutation using standard nomenclature, or a VWF multimer pattern that suggests a specific disease mechanism (e.g., IIA, IIC, IID, IIE). In some cases, a complex phenotype with features of both type 2 and type 1 VWD should be classified as "type 2" in order to preserve the correlation with the response to desmopressin. A phenotype with prominent defects in more than one "type 2" character simultaneously, such as multimer structure and ligand binding, can be designated as "type 2 (mixed phenotype)" without further differentiation.

VWD classification—general issues

The principal difficulty in using the current VWD classification arises from how to define the boundaries among the various types through laboratory testing. Adding to the problem, some mutations have pleiotropic effects on VWF structure and function, and some individuals are compound heterozygous for mutations producing VWD by different mechanisms. Such heterogeneity can produce complex phenotypes that are difficult to categorize [21,22].

The distinction between quantitative (type 1) and qualitative (type 2) defects depends on the ability to recognize discrepancies among VWF assay results. Similarly, distinguishing between type 2A and type 2M VWD requires multimer gel analysis. Standards need to be established for using laboratory tests to make these important distinctions. The example of VWD Vicenza illustrates some of these problems. Whether VWD Vicenza is classified as type 1 VWD or type 2M VWD depends on the interpretation of laboratory test results. The abnormally large multimers and very low RIPA values have led some investigators to prefer the designation as type 2M VWD. However, the VWF:RCo/VWF:Ag ratio typically is normal, and large VWF multimers are not decreased relative to smaller multimers, leading other investigators to classify VWD Vicenza as type 1 VWD. Regardless of the classification of this variant, the markedly shortened half-life of plasma VWF in VWD Vicenza is the key clinical factor that dictates whether the individual should receive treatment with DDAVP or FVIII/VWF concentrates.

Similarly, C1149R VWD was categorized as a dominant type 1 [27]. However, some recent data would indicate that it should be considered to be type 2A (IIE) VWD [28].

Type 1 VWD versus low VWF as a risk factor for bleeding

Type 1 VWD can be hard to diagnose with confidence because the major laboratory criterion is merely a low value for the plasma VWF concentration; however, VWF levels vary widely and are continuously distributed in the human population. Bleeding risk also varies continuously with the VWF level, so there is no VWF threshold separating patients into groups with distinctly different clinical features [21,22,30,37]. Consequently, many patients diagnosed with type 1 VWD do not have a specific hemorrhagic disease at all, which limits the utility of the diagnosis. This problem may be avoided by substituting an empirical epidemiologic approach like that applied to other modest risk factors for disease, such as elevated cho-

lesterol and high blood pressure. Such a risk management strategy could be generalized to include other hemorrhagic and thrombotic risk factors.

Issues in Laboratory Testing. Subtle defects can be difficult to characterize and consequently some patients are difficult to classify. The standardized interpretation of multimer scans would be facilitated by increased availability of reference plasmas, widespread adoption of validated analytical methods and diagnostic criteria, and additional data on VWF multimer patterns associated with specific VWD mutations. Further information is needed to establish the value of particular test combinations and ratios for the classification of type 2 VWD variants [21,22,30].

Emerging issues in VWD classification

Bleeding score

Standardized assessment tools are being developed to evaluate the bleeding symptoms caused by the various defects in VWF [38,39]. There is a strong inverse correlation between the bleeding score and the VWF level. However, the relationship between the VWF level and bleeding score has a limited prognostic value for individuals, requiring future data to know how the risk of medically significant bleeding depends on the level of plasma VWF [21].

Correlation with response to therapy

The type of VWD generally correlates well with the probability of a useful therapeutic response to desmopressin, but the correlation is weaker for the intermediate VWD phenotypes that are hard to classify as either type 1 or type 2 [40–43]. Several observations suggest that the less a patient's VWD phenotype deviates from normal or type 1 VWD, the more likely it is that they will respond well to desmopressin. Therefore, the desmopressin test dose is more useful to assess potential response [21,22,30]. Those rare patients with type 2 VWD who also respond to desmopressin can also be identified with a test dose [33,42,43]. Assays of plasma VWF during a desmopressin trial can be useful to resolve ambiguities among baseline test results and to facilitate classification of some of the VWD types.

Newer tests for diagnosing VWD

Highly sensitive and reproducible assays for VWF platelet binding have been developed that use purified platelet GPIb instead of platelets. These tests could represent a substantial improvement for the diagnosis and classification of VWD [44,45]. The recently developed VWF propeptide (VWFpp) assay and the ratio of VWFpp to VWF:Ag may help in identifying mutants of VWF with a decreased half-life [29].

The role of VWF mutations

Usually, the location of VWF mutations correlates with the VWD type [21,22,29,30,46]. Detailed relationships between gene mutations and phenotype have been documented in detail for types 2A, 2B, 2M, and 2N VWD, as well as for some forms of type 1 VWD. In type 2A VWD the location of some mutations is predictable from features of the plasma VWF multimer pattern. As genetic testing strategies evolve, results from other laboratory tests for VWF combined with gene sequencing should increase our ability to predict responses to desmopressin or factor replacement therapy, which may lead to further improvements in the classification of VWD. Expression of all candidate mutations and determination of intracellular and secreted VWF will help to resolve the remaining classification issues in the near future [29].

An additional consideration for future updating of the VWD classification—is type 2M redundant?

The distinction between types 2A and 2M VWD depends on ascertaining the absence of HMW VWF multimers. Differentiation between a "normal" multimer distribution and one lacking some HMW VWF multimers can be difficult [21].

This problem is well illustrated by VWD caused by R1374C mutation [47,48]. This mutation has been classified into several categories, including 2A, 2M, 1 severe, 1B, 1B variant of 2A, and unclassified. In the MCMDM-1VWD European Study, it was categorized as type 2A VWD [23]. The mutations R1315C and R1374H also were included in the type 2A group. This study concluded that "multimer patterns observed are often so subtle that they may have been interpreted in the past as normal, and may be beyond the resolution of multimer analysis in many laboratories today, and discrimination between 2A and 2M

patterns is sometimes equivocal." In contrast, in the Canadian 1 VWD study these three mutations were considered to be type 2M [26], and the panel stressed that "type 2M VWD definition may need to be more stringent, and should be the subject of an international initiative."

Moreover, type 2B of the revised classification [16,21] includes all groups of the old type IIB with the loss of HMWM and the type I New York and I Malmö that have a normal multimeric pattern. In a similar vein, type 2A includes very distinct molecular abnormalities, such as the old type IIC with decreased proteolytic susceptibility and the classic IIA with increased proteolytic susceptibility.

It is true that there is a specific 2M molecular abnormality with a selective VWF:CB defect and a normal multimeric pattern, which is due to the mutation S1731T as described in two patients from one family [32]. The same mutation has been detected in some other patients, sometimes found by chance, and associated with no related bleeding problem. It is important to remember that deficiency in VWF:CB function is also present in type 2A.

Considering all these data suggests that differentiation of types 2A and 2M at the second hierarchical or clinical level serves to create confusion. The proposal that needs to be discussed is to combine both type 2A and 2M into a new wider type 2A group. The multimeric information, proteolytic susceptibility data, and other appropriate properties could then be used to differentiate the subtypes at the third hierarchical level for better understanding of pathophysiologic mechanisms involved and facilitation of more effective search for the underlying mutation. This would simplify classification without missing important clinical implications, thus avoiding confusion.

In summary, the 2006 revised VWD classification system has proved superior to its predecessors, although ambiguities in classification criteria remain to be resolved through future research efforts.

Acknowledgements

This work was supported by the Fondo de Investigación Sanitaria, F.I.S. Carlos III, Ministerio de Sanidad, Spain (FIS PI# 07/0229). Consellería de Innovación e Industria, Xunta de Galicia (INCITE08ENA916109ES).

References

1 Zimmerman TS, Ratnoff OD, Powell AE. Immunologic differentiation of classic hemophilia (factor 8 deficiency) and von Willebrand's disease, with observations on combined deficiencies of antihemophilic factor and proaccelerin (factor V) and on an acquired circulating anticoagulant against antihemophilic factor. *J Clin Invest* 1971; **50**: 244–54.

2 Holmberg L, Nilsson IM. Genetic variants of von Willebrand's disease. *Br Med J* 1972; **3**: 317–20.

3 Kernoff PB, Gruson R, Rizza CR. A variant of factor 8 related antigen. *Br J Haematol* 1974; **26**: 435–40.

4 Peake IR, Bloom AL, Giddings JC. Inherited variants of factor-VIII-related protein in von Willebrand's disease. *N Engl J Med* 1974; **291**: 113–17.

5 Meyer D, Obert B, Pietu G, *et al.* Multimeric structure of factor VIII/von Willebrand factor in von Willebrand's disease. *J Lab Clin Med* 1980; **95**: 590–602.

6 Zimmerman TS, Ruggeri ZM. Von Willebrand's disease. *Prog Hemost Thromb* 1982; **6**: 203–36.

7 Ruggeri ZM, Pareti FI, Mannucci PM, *et al.* Heightened interaction between platelets and factor VIII/von Willebrand factor in a new subtype of von Willebrand's disease. *N Engl J Med* 1980; **302**: 1047–51.

8 Ruggeri ZM, Zimmerman TS. Variant von Willebrand's disease: characterization of two subtypes by analysis of multimeric composition of factor VIII/von Willebrand factor in plasma and platelets. *J Clin Invest* 1980; **65**: 1318–25.

9 Holmberg L, Nilsson IM, Borge L, *et al.* Platelet aggregation induced by 1-desamino-8-D-arginine vasopressin (DDAVP) in type IIB von Willebrand's disease. *N Engl J Med* 1983; **309**: 816–21.

10 Ruggeri ZM, Nilsson IM, Lombardi R, *et al.* Aberrant multimeric structure of von Willebrand factor in a new variant of von Willebrand's disease (type IIC). *J Clin Invest* 1982; **70**: 1124–7.

11 Batlle J, Lopez Fernandez MF, Lasierra J, *et al.* von Willebrand disease type IIC with different abnormalities of von Willebrand factor in the same sibship. *Am J Hematol* 1986; **21**: 177–88.

12 Kinoshita S, Harrison J, Lazerson J, *at al.* A new variant of dominant type II von Willebrand's disease with aberrant multimeric pattern of factor VIII-related antigen (type IID). *Blood* 1984; **63**: 1369–71.

13 Zimmerman TS, Dent JA, Ruggeri ZM, *et al.* Subunit composition of plasma von Willebrand factor. Cleavage is present in normal individuals, increased in IIA and IIB von Willebrand disease, but minimal in variants with aberrant structure of individual oligomers (types IIC, IID, and IIE). *J Clin Invest* 1986; **77**: 947–51.

14 Ruggeri ZM, Zimmerman TS. von Willebrand factor and von Willebrand disease. *Blood* 1987; **70**: 895–904.

15 Ginsburg D, Sadler JE. von Willebrand disease: a database of point mutations, insertions, and deletions. For the Consortium on von Willebrand Factor Mutations and Polymorphisms, and the Subcommittee on von Willebrand Factor of the Scientific and Standardization Committee of the International Society on Thrombosis and Haemostasis. *Thromb Haemost* 1993; **69**: 177–84.

16 Sadler JE. A revised classification of von Willebrand disease. 1994; *Thromb Haemost* **71**: 520–5.

17 Weiss HJ, Meyer D, Rabinowitz R, *et al.* Pseudo-von Willebrand's disease. An intrinsic platelet defect with aggregation by unmodified human factor VIII/von Willebrand factor and enhanced adsorption of its high-molecular-weight multimers. *N Engl J Med* 1982; **306**: 326–33.

18 Miller JL, Castella A. Willebrand's disease: characterization of a new bleeding disorder. *Blood* 1982; **60**: 790–4.

19 Nishino M, Girma JP, Rothschild C, *et al.* New variant of von Willebrand disease with defective binding to factor VIII. *Blood* 1989; **74**: 1591–9.

20 Mazurier C, Dieval J, Jorieux S, *et al.* A new von Willebrand factor (vWF) defect in a patient with factor VIII (FVIII) deficiency but with normal levels and multimeric patterns of both plasma and platelet vWF. Characterization of abnormal vWF/FVIII interaction. *Blood* 1990; **75**: 20–6.

21 Sadler JE, Budde U, Eikenboom JC, *et al.* Update on the pathophysiology and classification of von Willebrand disease: a report of the Subcommittee on von Willebrand Factor. *J Thromb Haemost* 2006; **4**: 2103–14.

22 Nichols WL, Hultin MB, James AH, *et al.* von Willebrand disease (VWD): evidence-based diagnosis and management guidelines, the National Heart, Lung, and Blood Institute (NHLBI) Expert Panel report (USA). *Haemophilia* 2008; **14**: 171–232.

23 Budde U, Schneppenheim R, Eikenboom J, *et al.* Detailed von Willebrand factor multimer analysis in patients with von Willebrand disease in the European study, molecular and clinical markers for the diagnosis and management of type 1 von Willebrand disease (MCMDM-1VWD). *J Thromb Haemost* 2008; **6**: 762–71.

24 Goodeve A, Eikenboom J, Castaman G, *et al.* Phenotype and genotype of a cohort of families historically diagnosed with type 1 von Willebrand disease in the European study, Molecular and Clinical Markers for the Diagnosis and Management of Type 1 von Willebrand Disease (MCMDM-1VWD). *Blood* 2007; **109**: 112–21.

25 James PD, Notley C, Hegadorn C, *et al.* The mutational spectrum of type 1 von Willebrand disease: results from a Canadian cohort study. *Blood* 2007; **109**: 145–54.

26 James PD, Notley C, Hegadorn C, *et al.* Challenges in defining type 2M von Willebrand disease: results from a Canadian cohort study. *J Thromb Haemost* 2007; **5**: 1914–22.

27 Eikenboom JCJ, Matsushita T, Reitsma PH, *et al*. Dominant type 1 von Willebrand disease caused by mutated cysteine residues in the D3 domain of von Willebrand factor. *Blood* 1996; **88**: 2433–41.

28 Pérez-Rodríguez A, García-Rivero A, Lourés E, *et al*. Autosomal dominant C1149R von Willebrand disease (VWD): phenotypic findings and their implications. *Haematologica* 2009; **94**: 679–86.

29 Schneppenheim R, Budde U. Phenotypic and genotypic diagnosis of von Willebrand disease: a 2004 update. *Semin Hematol* 2005; **42**: 15–28.

30 Sadler J, Blinder M. Von Willebrand disease: Diagnosis, classification and treatment. In: Colman R, Marder V, Claves A, George J, Goldhaber S (eds.). *Hemostasis and Thrombosis. Basic Principles and Clinical Practice.* 5th edn, pp 905–922. Lippincott Williams & Wilkins: Philadelphia, 2006.

31 Meyer D, Fressinaud E, Hilbert L, *et al*. Type 2 von Willebrand disease causing defective von Willebrand factor-dependent platelet function. *Best Pract Res Clin Haematol* 2001; **14**: 349–64.

32 Ribba AS, Loisel I, Lavergne JM, *et al*. Ser968Thr mutation within the A3 domain of von Willebrand factor (VWF) in two related patients leads to a defective binding of VWF to collagen. *Thromb Haemost* 2001; **86**: 848–54.

33 Mazurier C, Goudemand J, Hilbert L, *et al*. Type 2N von Willebrand disease: clinical manifestations, pathophysiology, laboratory diagnosis and molecular biology. *Best Pract Res Clin Haematol* 2001; **14**: 337–47.

34 Lopez-Fernandez MF, Blanco-Lopez MJ, Castiñeira MP, *et al*. Further evidence for recessive inheritance of von Willebrand disease with abnormal binding of von Willebrand factor to factor VIII. *Am J Hematol* 1992; **40**: 20–7

35 Eikenboom JC. Willebrand disease type 3: clinical manifestations, pathophysiology and molecular biology. *Best Pract Res Clin Haematol* 2001; **14**: 365–79.

36 Eikenboom JC, Reitsma PH, Peerlinck KM, *et al*. Recessive inheritance of von Willebrand's disease type I. *Lancet* 1993; **341**: 982–6.

37 Sadler JE. Von Willebrand disease type 1: a diagnosis in search of a disease. *Blood* 2003; **101**: 2089–93.

38 Rodeghiero F, Castaman G, Tosetto A, *et al*. The discriminant power of bleeding history for the diagnosis of type 1 von Willebrand disease: an international, multicenter study. *J Thromb Haemost* 2005; **3**: 2619–26.

39 Tosetto A, Rodeghiero F, Castaman G, *et al*. A quantitative analysis of bleeding symptoms in type 1 von Willebrand disease: results from a multicenter European study (MCMDM-1 VWD). *J Thromb Haemost* 2006; **4**: 766–73.

40 Federici AB, Mazurier C, Berntorp E, *et al*. Biologic response to desmopressin in patients with severe type 1 and type 2 von Willebrand disease: results of a multicenter European study. *Blood* 2004; **103**: 2032–8.

41 Mannucci PM. Treatment of von Willebrand's Disease. *N Engl J Med* 2004; **351**: 683–94.

42 Michiels JJ, van de Velde A, van Vliet HH, *et al*. Response of von Willebrand factor parameters to desmopressin in patients with type 1 and type 2 congenital von Willebrand disease: diagnostic and therapeutic implications. *Semin Thromb Hemost* 2002; **28**: 111–32.

43 Castaman G, Lethagen S, Federici AB, *et al*. Response to desmopressin is influenced by the genotype and phenotype in type 1 von Willebrand disease (VWD): results from the European Study MCMDM-1VWD. *Blood* 2008; **111**: 3531–9.

44 Caron C, Hilbert L, Vanhoorelbeke K, *et al*. Measurement of von Willebrand factor binding to a recombinant fragment of glycoprotein Ibalpha in an enzyme-linked immunosorbent assay based method: performances in patients with type 2B von Willebrand disease. *Br J Haematol* 2006; **133**: 655.

45 Federici AB, Canciani MT, Forza I, *et al*. A sensitive ristocetin cofactor activity assay with recombinant glycoprotein Ibα for the diagnosis of patients with low von Willebrand factor levels. *Haematologica* 2004; **89**: 77–85.

46 James P, Lillicrap D. The role of molecular genetics in diagnosing von Willebrand disease. *Semin Thromb Hemost* 2008; **34**: 502–8.

47 Batlle J, Pérez-Rodríguez A, Franqueira MD, *et al*. Type 2M von Willebrand disease: a variant of type 2A? *J Thromb Haemost* 2008; **6**: 388–90.

48 Penas N, Pérez-Rodríguez A, Torea JH, *et al*. von Willebrand disease R1374C: type 2A or 2M? A challenge to the revised classification. High frequency in the northwest of Spain (Galicia). *Am J Hematol* 2005; **80**: 188–96.

7 The epidemiology of von Willebrand disease

Giancarlo Castaman and Francesco Rodeghiero
Department of Hematology and Hemophilia and Thrombosis Center, San Bortolo Hospital, Vicenza, Italy

Introduction

von Willebrand disease (VWD) is the most frequent inherited bleeding disorder, with a prevalence up to 1% estimated in *ad hoc* epidemiologic investigations [1,2] by using conservative criteria. However, most of these cases present with only mild bleeding symptoms and diagnosis would have otherwise remained elusive since they rarely require referral-based investigations by specialized centers. Furthermore, a significant proportion of these cases fails to show a clear linkage with von Willebrand factor (VWF) locus [3]. Thus, it has been suggested that the prevalence of clinically relevant cases is at least tenfold lower than previously realized [4].

Usually, VWD is classified into three types [5,6]. Type 1 and 3 represent the spectrum of quantitative VWF deficiencies, while type 2 VWD includes qualitative variants owing to the presence of an abnormally functioning VWF. Most, if not all, of the identified cases through epidemiologic studies show a type 1 VWD phenotype, while the majority of cases referred to specialized centers for the frequency or severity of bleeding manifestations are represented by types 2 and 3 VWD. As a consequence, increased effort should be put toward the identification of diagnostic tools that better identify those patients for whom a definite diagnosis of a genetic disorder confers advantages rather than unnecessarily cause them alarm and anxiety.

Von Willebrand Disease, 1st edition. Edited by Augusto B. Federici, Christine A. Lee, Erik E. Berntorp, David Lillicrap, Robert R. Montgomery. © 2011 Blackwell Publishing Ltd.

Historical studies on the prevalence of VWD

Two population-based studies have approached with firmly established diagnostic criteria the epidemiology of VWD (Table 7.1). The first study evaluated 1218 schoolchildren aged 11–14 years in the Vicenza province in northern Italy [1,7]. Two types of diagnosis of VWD were considered: (i) "probable," in children with low VWF levels (VWF:RCo below an ABO-adjusted reference range) belonging to a family with two or more members, including or not the individual under investigation, referring a bleeding history with two or more symptoms; (ii) "definite" if in addition to these criteria at least one other family member on the hemorrhagic side had a low VWF level. Ten children (four with probable and six with definite VWD) were classified as affected (0.82%). This figure could range from seven (0.57%) to 14 (1.15%) taking into account the 90% confidence interval for the lower limit of the normal range. All these children had at least one bleeding symptom. This translates into a prevalence of 5700 to 11,500 cases per million. The large majority of these individuals had mildly reduced VWF levels and had never been referred before for specific investigations. Even though their VWF levels could simply represent a "risk factor" for bleeding [11], the consistency of VWF reduction within the family in association with bleeding suggests a true inheritance of the abnormality.

The second study investigated the prevalence of VWD in a population of 600 American schoolchildren aged 12–18 years examined at the pediatric ambulatory clinics of the hospitals located in Virginia, Ohio, and Mississippi [2]. The diagnostic criteria

Table 7.1 Epidemiologic investigations of prevalence of von Willebrand disease.

Study	Methodology	Population	Prevalence (%)	Number with VWF <30 IU/dL
Rodeghiero et al. [1]	Anamnesis + VWF:RCo[a] Family study	White children	0.82	1/14
Rodeghiero et al. [7]	As above + VWF:Ag instead of VWF:RCo	As above	0.7	1/14
Miller et al. [9]	VWF:RCo	Adult blood donors	1.6 (0.2% bleeder)	n.s.
Meriane et al. [10]	Anamnesis + VWF:RCo Family study	Arabic–Turkish Adult students	1.23	n.s.
Werner et al. [2]	Anamnesis + VWF:RCo Family study	White people, black people Children	1.3 (1.15 white people; 1.81 black people)	1/8 3/9
Bowman et al. [8]	Anamnesis + VWF:Ag, VWF:RCo, and FVIII:C	Canadian primary care patients	0.09	

n.s., not stated.
[a] von Willebrand Factor ristocetin cofactor activity.

included all three of the following: at least one bleeding symptom, a family member with at least one bleeding symptom, and low VWF. The overall prevalence was estimated at 1.3%, with no racial difference (1.15% among white people and 1.8% among black people).

These data have been confirmed in two additional studies, not reported as full papers [9,10], using the same functional test (VWF:RCo) and separate normal ranges according to blood groups. The prevalence of VWD appears to be similar in different ethnic groups. Even though these figures appear high, the prevalence could be probably even higher since the sensitivity of the functional test is about 50% [12]. Even though in some cases several different symptoms were reported, information about the severity of each symptom has been poorly investigated in these studies and no standardized assessment was provided.

All the reported cases had type 1 VWD diagnosis, also demonstrated by the normal multimeric pattern observed [1]. Interestingly, in about half of the diagnosed families from this investigation linkage was not subsequently demonstrated [3]. In keeping with the data purported by Sadler [4] of a prevalence of 1:1,000 clinically significant VWD, only one out of the 14 cases identified by Rodeghiero et al. [1] had a clear-cut evidence of a strong FVIII, VWF reduction, and relevant bleeding symptoms within the family that often required specific treatment. These patients

turned out to carry the R1205H mutation, associated with VWD Vicenza [5], which is quite common in the north-east of Italy (Castaman and Rodeghiero, unpublished observation). As a further confirmation, a recent evaluation of a large population of adults attending primary care physicians in Canada has demonstrated that the prevalence of clinically significant VWD is approximately 1:1000 [8].

Prevalence of bleeding patients in the general population

When assessing the prevalence of a mild bleeding disorder in a given population, it should be taken into consideration that even normal individuals refer hemorrhagic symptoms fairly frequently (Table 7.2) [13–15]. By using a self-reported questionnaire, Friberg et al. [16] found that about 25% of Swedish girls reported three or more hemorrhagic symptoms, whereas using a questionnaire guided by a physician, Rodeghiero et al. [17] observed three or more hemorrhagic symptoms in less than 1% of normal controls. Stringent criteria and clinical expertise are therefore always advisable in collecting a bleeding history, and the use of appropriate tools may ensure interobserver reproducibility of the process [18].

By using the results of a physician interview, 49 families (at least two members within a family with

Table 7.2 Frequency of self-reported hemorrhagic symptoms in the general population [12,13].

Investigated symptom	Frequency (%)
Profuse menstruation	44
Nosebleeds	5–36
Bleeding at delivery	19.5–23
Bleeding after tonsillectomy	2–11
Bleeding after surgery	6
Bleeding from small wounds	2
Various symptoms (one or more)	40–50 in men; 50–60 in women

Table 7.3 Frequency of hemorrhagic symptoms in the 107 family members with two or more bleeding symptoms (total 268) identified in the study by Rodeghiero et al. [1].

Investigated symptom	Frequency (%)
Nosebleeds	38
Bleeding after tooth extraction	20
Menorrhagia	18
Postpartum hemorrhage	8
Bleeding after tonsillectomy or adenoidectomy	4.5
Bleeding from small wounds	4
Bleeding after surgery	3.5
Easy bruising	2
Other manifestations	1

This research was originally published in *Blood*. Rodeghiero F, Castaman G, Dini E. Epidemiological investigation of the prevalence of von Willebrand disease. *Blood* 1987; **69**: 454–9. © the American Society of Hematology.

at least two hemorrhagic symptoms) in the epidemiologic investigation by Rodeghiero et al. [1] were classified as bleeders, with a prevalence of about 4.5%, while 2% of the investigated children had two or more bleeding symptoms. Table 7.3 summarizes the type of bleeding reported. The main limitations about this figure are represented by the lack of a grading of the severity of bleeding symptoms reported by the investigated individuals. Nevertheless, although rough, this figure represents the sole estimation of the prevalence of family bleeding tendency in the general population.

Bleeding score: a new diagnostic tool to assess clinically relevant VWD

Until recently, no quantitative description of bleeding symptoms in VWD has been available to fully appreciate the diagnostic relevance of bleeding symptoms for VWD or to discriminate between a significant bleeding history and trivial symptoms in VWD. Obtaining a clear picture of the clinical presentation of VWD and comparing the bleeding symptoms reported by patients and normal individuals is the first step toward a more precise definition of the prevalence of VWD and selection for treatment. A bleeding score was designed to evaluate whether an index accounting for both the number and the severity of each bleeding symptom could actually improve the sensitivity and specificity for the identification of obligatory carriers of VWD [17]. The bleeding score is generated by summing the severity of all bleeding symptoms reported by an individual and graded according to an arbitrary scale. In a subsequent refinement, the number of possible grades for each bleeding symptom was increased, ranging from −1 to 4 [19] to further appreciate subtle changes in patients with VWD with wide heterogeneity of their bleeding tendency.

The problem of diagnosing mild VWD

In a recent multicenter survey, we demonstrated that the pretest probability (likelihood ratio) of VWD is significantly increased only when a clinically relevant history of hemorrhage is present (at least two hemorrhagic symptoms in the proband or a bleeding score >3 in males and >5 in females) [17]. Moreover, at least two (but preferably three) family members should be present in a family to reasonably suspect VWD in cases with mild VWF reduction or dubious bleeding symptoms [20]. Therefore, every laboratory assessment should be undertaken only in individuals presenting with significant bleeding symptoms as graded above, or in those who have two first-degree relatives with hemorrhagic symptoms or a VWF level <40 IU/dL. In a pediatric setting, these criteria could be more relaxed and family investigation becomes more important.

It has been shown that the more severe the VWF reduction, the more severe the bleeding history, particularly with VWF levels below 30 IU/dL [19].

According to this threshold applied to our epidemiologic investigation, it would turn out that the prevalence of VWD would be around 1:1300.

Recently, a Bayesian model to better appreciate the level of uncertainty in situations with mild deficiency and mild VWF reduction has been developed by our group [20]. Using this approach, the bleeding history in the patient (summarized in the bleeding score) and VWF measurements in the patient and as many first-degree relatives as possible is translated into likelihood ratios, thereby producing a "final probability" of having VWD. Since we do not have a "gold standard" for diagnosing clinically significant VWD, it has been provisionally assumed that cases with proven autosomal dominant hemorrhagic disease should be taken as the VWD paradigm [20]. Identifying additional family members with reduced VWF greatly increases the final VWD probabilities, and family investigations should always be performed for borderline patients, especially when the patient is too young to have experienced significant hemostatic challenge. At present, the probability cut-off that best discriminates those patients who may benefit from receiving a diagnosis from those who may not is unknown. Thus, prospective studies on patients with VWD who are diagnosed with graded criteria are needed to confirm a prognostic significance in the context of the diagnosis. Our group has proposed the following minimal criteria for VWD diagnosis: a bleeding score >3 in males and >5 in females and a VWF:RCo <40IU/dL. It is reasonable to assume that the individuals and families identified by the suggested criteria are also those who are more likely to benefit from an appropriate therapy (e.g., desmopressin treatment or prophylaxis).

Prevalence of intermediate VWD

This is a group of patients in whom VWD presents with high penetrance and expressivity of the clinical and laboratory phenotype. Usually, their VWF levels range from 10–30IU/dL and their bleeding tendency is evident. This group includes most patients with type 2A and 2B, some patients with type 2M and 2N, and patients with type 1 VWD with clearcut dominant negative mutations or peculiar phenotypes (VWD Vicenza). There is no formal estimation of their prevalence in the general population, even though indirect estimation could set the prevalence around 1/1000–10,000 inhabitants. Generally, phenotypic diagnosis is relatively easy. These patients usually need treatment and are diagnosed at specialized centers as they have a lifelong bleeding tendency.

Prevalence of severe VWD

Unlike mild VWF deficiency, type 3 VWD is characterized by a recessive inheritance, moderate to severe bleeding tendency, and severely reduced FVIII and VWF measurements. As a consequence, all these individuals are usually diagnosed during infancy and no cases go unrecognized. Hence, the prevalence of type 3 VWD is usually extrapolated taking into account the series of patients followed up at specialized centers. These patients are very rare, with an estimated prevalence ranging from 0.1 to 5.3 per million [21]. On the basis of the reports from 195 referral centers worldwide, a prevalence of 1.53 and 1.38 per million of severe VWD has been documented in Europe and North America, respectively [22]. By using a highly sensitive method (immunoradiometric assay) to measure VWF:Ag, a subsequent re-evaluation of these subjects showed a prevalence of severe VWD (defined by an antigen level below 1IU/dL) of 0.45 per million [20]. Significant differences in the prevalence of severe VWD were present in different countries, notably with a higher prevalence in Scandinavian countries (2.4–3.12 per million) [23]. The highest prevalence of type 3 VWD was, however, observed by Berliner *et al.* [24] in Arabs, in whom consanguinity is rather frequent, with an estimated prevalence of 5.3 per million. For the same reasons, a high number of patients with type 3 VWD is also present in the Iranian population, even though no formal estimation of VWD prevalence is available [25].

Conclusions

The prevalence of VWD in the general population may vary depending on the diagnostic criteria used and the availability of standardized clinical and laboratory methodologies. However, the diagnostic criteria should always be used considering the clinical utility of the diagnosis in a given patient [26]. The genetic determinants of the patients with "low VWF" and a mild bleeding tendency not caused by specific *VWF* gene mutations remains to be elucidated by future studies.

References

1 Rodeghiero F, Castaman G, Dini E. Epidemiological investigation of the prevalence of von Willebrand's disease. *Blood* 1987; **69**: 454–9.

2 Werner EJ, Broxson EH, Tucker EL, *et al.* Prevalence of von Willebrand disease in children: A multiethnic study. *J Pediatr* 1993; **123**: 893–8.

3 Castaman G, Eikenboom JCJ, Bertina R, Rodeghiero F. Inconsistency of association between type 1 von Willebrand disease phenotype and genotype in families identified in an epidemiologic investigation. *Thromb Haemostas* 1999; **82**: 1065–70.

4 Sadler JE, Mannucci PM, Berntorp E, *et al.* Impact, diagnosis and treatment of von Willebrand disease. *Thromb Haemost* 2000; **84**: 160–74.

5 Castaman G, Federici AB, Rodeghiero F, Mannucci PM. Von Willebrand's disease in the year 2003: towards the complete identification of gene defects for correct diagnosis and treatment. *Haematologica* 2003; **88**: 94–108.

6 Sadler JE, Budde U, Eikenboom JC, *et al*; Working Party on von Willebrand Disease Classification. Update on the pathophysiology and classification of von Willebrand disease: a report of the Subcommittee on von Willebrand Factor. *J Thromb Haemost* 2006; **4**: 2103–14.

7 Rodeghiero F, Castaman G, Tosetto A. von Willebrand factor antigen is less sensitive than ristocetin cofactor for the diagnosis of type I von Willebrand disease—results based on a epidemiological investigation. *Thromb Haemostas* 1990; **64**: 349–52.

8 Bowman M, Hopman WM, Rapson D, Lillicrap D, James P. The prevalence of von Willebrand disease in primary care practice. *J Thromb Haemost* 2010; **8**: 213–16.

9 Miller CH, Lenzi R, Breen C. Prevalence of von Willebrand's disease among U.S. adults. *Blood* 1987; **70** (Suppl. 1): 377 (Abstract).

10 Meriane F, Sultan Y, Arabi H, *et al.* Incidence of a low von Willebrand factor activity in a population of Algerian students. *Blood* 1991; **78** (Suppl. 1): 484 (Abstract).

11 Sadler JE. Von Willebrand disease type 1: a diagnosis in search of a disease. *Blood* 2003; **101**: 2089–93.

12 Miller CH, Graham JB, Goldin LR, Elston RC. Genetics of classic von Willebrand's disease. I. Phenotypic variation within families. *Blood* 1979; **54**: 117–36.

13 Sramek A, Eikenboom JC, Briet E, Vandenbroucke JP, Rosendaal FR. Usefulness of patient interview in bleeding disorders. *Arch Intern Med* 1995; **155**: 1409–15.

14 Wahlberg T, Blomback M, Hall P, Axelsson G. Application of indicators, predictors and diagnostic indices in coagulation disorders. I. Evaluation of a self-administered questionnaire with binary questions. *Methods Inf Med* 1980; **19**: 194–200.

15 Mauser Bunschoten EP, van Houwelingen JC, Sjamsoedin Visser EJ, van Dijken PJ, Kok AJ, Sixma JJ. Bleeding symptoms in carriers of hemophilia A and B. *Thromb Haemost* 1988; **59**: 349–52.

16 Friberg B, Orno AK, Lindgren A, Lethagen S. Bleeding disorders among young women: a population-based prevalence study. *Acta Obstet Gynecol Scand* 2006; **85**: 200–6.

17 Rodeghiero F, Castaman G, Tosetto A, *et al.* The discriminant power of bleeding history for the diagnosis of von Willebrand disease type 1: an international, multicenter study. *J Thromb Haemost* 2005; **3**: 2619–26.

18 Tosetto A, Castaman G, Rodeghiero F. Bleeding scores in inherited bleeding disorders: clinical or research tools? *Haemophilia* 2008; **14**: 415–22.

19 Tosetto A, Rodeghiero F, Castaman G, *et al.* Impact of plasma von Willebrand factor levels in the diagnosis of type 1 von Willebrand disease: results from a multicenter European study (MCMDM-1VWD). *J Thromb Haemost* 2006; **4**: 766–73.

20 Tosetto A, Castaman G, Rodeghiero F. Evidence-based diagnosis of type 1 von Willebrand disease: a Bayes theorem approach. *Blood* 2008; **111**: 3998–4003.

21 Mannucci PM, Bloom AL, Larrieu MJ, Nilsson IM, West RR. Atherosclerosis and von Willebrand factor. I. Prevalence of severe von Willebrand's disease in Western Europe and Israel. *Br J Haematol* 1984; **57**: 163–9.

22 Weiss HJ, Ball AP, Mannucci PM. Incidence of severe von Willebrand's disease. *N Engl J Med* 1982; **307**: 127.

23 Nilsson IM. Von Willebrand disease from 1926 to 1983. *Scand J Haematol* 1984; **33** (Suppl. 40): 21–43.

24 Berliner SA, Seligsohn U, Zivelin A, Zwang E, Sofferman G. A relatively high frequency of severe (type III) von Willebrand's disease in Israel. *Br J Haematol* 1986; **62**: 535–43.

25 Lak M, Peyvandi F, Mannucci PM. Clinical manifestations and complications of childbirth and replacement therapy in 385 Iranian patients with type 3 von Willebrand disease. *Br J Haematol* 2000; **111**: 1236–9.

26 Rodeghiero F. von Willebrand disease: still an intriguing disorder in the era of molecular medicine. *Haemophilia* 2002; **8**: 292–300.

Clinical aspects of von Willebrand disease: bleeding history

Paula D. James[1] *and Alberto Tosetto*[2]

[1]Etherington Hall, Queen's University, Kingston, ON, Canada
[2]Department of Hematology, San Bortolo Hospital, Vicenza, Italy

Introduction

A diagnosis of von Willebrand disease (VWD) requires fulfillment of three criteria: (i) a personal history of excessive bleeding, mainly mucocutaneous; (ii) laboratory tests that confirm quantitative or qualitative defects in von Willebrand factor (VWF); and (iii) a positive family history (in most cases). Satisfying the first criterion can present significant challenges, and a careful appraisal of bleeding symptoms is critical in making an accurate diagnosis. The number and quality of symptoms reported by a patient may be influenced by his or her education, family background, and personality, as well as by the type of data ascertainment because bleeding histories are subject to physicians' interpretation. All these factors contribute to the great deal of overlap between the mild mucocutaneous bleeding symptoms reported by patients with VWD and those reported by the general population.

The first description of the bleeding symptoms seen in VWD can be found in the seminal paper "Hereditary Pseudohemophilia," published in 1931 [1]. In this manuscript, Dr Erik von Willebrand described the bleeding symptoms he observed in a large family from the Åland Islands of Finland, including nose bleeds, bleeding from trivial wounds, bleeding after dental extractions, mouth bleeding, and female gynecologic bleeding. He recognized and highlighted the fact that hemarthrosis was rare and commented on the range of severity of bleed-

ing symptoms between affected individuals. This original description maintains its relevance today and helps to underscore the importance of a careful assessment of the clinical impact of the disease.

Bleeding history in VWD

In a general sense, a bleeding history should include a discriminant approach to the assessment of the reported symptoms. Details such as the timing and frequency of bleeding episodes should be noted, as well as whether the onset was associated with a hemostatic challenge. Measures used to treat or alleviate the symptoms are important, as are potential contributing factors such as the use of medications including aspirin, nonsteroidal anti-inflammatory drugs (NSAIDS), or anticoagulants.

The characteristic bleeding symptoms in VWD involve the skin and mucous membranes and include easy bruising, epistaxis, menorrhagia, excessive bleeding from minor wounds, dental extractions, surgery, or childbirth, and bleeding from the oral cavity or gastrointestinal tract. Musculoskeletal bleeding such as hemarthrosis and intramuscular hematomas are rare and usually only occur only in severe forms of VWD. Severe, life-threatening bleeding can occur in type 3 VWD and in some individuals with type 2; however, this is rare in individuals with type 1 VWD. Intracerebral hemorrhage is also rare and is usually only described in those with type 3 VWD [2]. Given the overall predominance of type 1 VWD, symptoms are typically of mild to moderate severity, although there is evidence that even this degree of

Von Willebrand Disease, 1st edition. Edited by Augusto B. Federici, Christine A. Lee, Erik E. Berntorp, David Lillicrap, Robert R. Montgomery. © 2011 Blackwell Publishing Ltd.

symptomatology can significantly interfere with quality of life [3].

The clinical evaluation of these bleeding symptoms presents a number of challenges including the degree of overlap of mild symptoms with those reported by normal individuals, the fact that symptoms may only become apparent following hemostatic challenge (such as menses, surgery, or trauma) making it particularly difficult to assess young children and men, and that coexisting illnesses or medications can modify symptoms. Perhaps the most difficult of these challenges is the overlap with normal individuals; in many instances healthy controls report bleeding symptoms as frequently as individuals with VWD, particularly those with type 1. A review of the information presented in Table 8.1 highlights this issue. As a result, significant effort has been focused on the development of tools to distinguish between normal and abnormal bleeding; these assessment tools will be discussed later in this chapter.

Bleeding symptoms in VWD

Cutaneous symptoms

Patients with VWD typically report bruising that occurs with minimal or no recalled trauma; in some cases the frequency of bruising among patients with VWD is as high as 100% [4]. Ecchymoses are often described as larger than normal and are more often associated with cutaneous hematoma. A distinctive characteristic may be appearance of ecchymoses in areas unexposed to trauma, such as the abdomen and trunk. Petechiae are also sometimes described by patients with VWD, but less commonly than bruising and are more frequently associated with thrombocytopenia-related bleeding [9]. Prolonged bleeding following minor wounds was one of the classic symptoms of VWD described in the 1931 paper, and patients often describe prolonged bleeding following puncture wounds such as venipuncture for phlebotomy or after injections and injuries [4].

Epistaxis

Epistaxis is a commonly reported symptom that may occur spontaneously or following challenge [10]. von Willebrand himself described patients who experienced nosebleeds if they worked in a bent posture for long periods of time [1] and other descriptions of nosebleeds occurring following vigorous physical exertion have been reported [4]. Patients with VWD often describe the need to seek medical attention for

Table 8.1 Incidence (%) of bleeding symptoms both in patients with von Willebrand disease (VWD) and in healthy individuals (normal).

Symptoms	Normal n = 500 [4] n = 341 [5][a] n = 215 [6]	All types of VWD n = 264 [4]	Type 1 VWD n = 671 [7] n = 84 [6]	Type 2 VWD n = 497 [7]	Type 3 VWD n = 348 [8] n = 66 [7]
Epistaxis	5–11	63	54–61	63	66–77
Menorrhagia	17–44	60	32–67	32	56–69
Post dental extraction bleeding	5–11	52	31–72	39	53–77
Hematoma	12	49	13	14	33
Bleeding from minor wounds	0.2–5	36	36–46	40	50
Gum bleeding	7–37	35	31	35	56
Postsurgical bleeding	1–6	28	20–38	23	41
Postpartum bleeding	3–23	23	17–61	18	15–26
Gastrointestinal bleeding	1	14	5	8	19.2
Joint bleeding	6	8	3	4	37–45
Hematuria	1–8	7	2	5	1–12
Cerebral bleeding	n.r.	n.r.	1	2	9

[a] 341 controls were sent a questionnaire. Exact number of respondents is not reported (n.r.).

nosebleeds and sometimes require treatment with nasal packing or cautery. In some cases, particularly in more severe forms of VWD, epistaxis can be profuse, requiring treatment with clotting factor concentrates or even blood transfusion. In rare instances, life-threatening nosebleeds can occur.

Gynecologic bleeding

Menorrhagia is one of the most common symptoms reported by women with VWD and can be accompanied by anemia and/or iron deficiency. Women describe menstrual periods that are longer than normal and are associated with profuse flow. These symptoms can range from being quite mild to being severe enough to require urgent surgical intervention with hysterectomy [11]. Hemorrhagic ovarian cysts are also reported in women with VWD and can be a cause of significant mid-menstrual cycle pain [4]. Postpartum hemorrhage also occurs, but perhaps at a lower frequency than might be expected. This is presumably because of the increase in VWF that occurs during pregnancy. Delayed postpartum hemorrhage is a particular concern as it can occur when the VWF levels fall to baseline after delivery [8]. Prolonged vaginal bleeding following childbirth is frequently described by women with VWD.

Oral cavity bleeding

Gingival bleeding, particularly following brushing or flossing, is commonly described by patients with VWD, particularly if coexisting gingivitis or periodontal disease is present. Bleeding associated with trauma to the lips and oral cavity is reported, particularly during childhood, as is bleeding during the eruption and shedding of baby teeth. Rare reports of tonsillar bleeding can be found; these are typically associated with tonsillitis and can be severe [4].

Postoperative bleeding

Significant bleeding can occur at the time of surgery or during the postoperative period [4]. In some cases, particularly in males, surgery may represent the first hemostatic challenge experienced and can lead to the diagnosis in previously unrecognized cases. Bleeding may be particularly severe for interventions on mucous tissues where surgical hemostasis may be more difficult, such as nose, pharynx, or prostate. Bleeding after tooth extraction is a particular issue, with several patients suffering from VWD experiencing delayed bleeding that occurs several hours after extraction.

Gastrointestinal bleeding

Gastrointestinal bleeding is reported by patients with VWD, predominantly adults, and can be severe [4]. The source of bleeding can sometimes be difficult to identify. Small bowel or colon angiodysplasia has been associated with VWD, particularly in those forms that lack of high molecular weight multimers [12].

Other bleeding symptoms

Other bleeding symptoms reported by patients with VWD include conjunctival or eye bleeding, postcoital bleeding, bleeding from dental or other abscess, and retroperitoneal bleeding.

Specific situations

Pediatrics—value of a positive family history

Evaluating a child for VWD can be particularly difficult. Although bruising and epistaxis are common among children with VWD, these symptoms are also frequently reported by healthy children. Some of the classic symptoms of VWD in adults, such as menorrhagia and postsurgical bleeding, are clearly not prevalent or evaluable in the pediatric population. A child with a bleeding disorder may not have had surgery or, in the case of girls, reached the age of menarche but may still have symptoms that cause difficulty and merit treatment. The pattern of hemorrhagic symptoms in children with VWD is different from that of children affected by more severe bleeding disorders, particularly in the newborn period, as symptoms such as cephalohematoma, bleeding from the umbilical stump, or following circumcision are usually rare. The true incidence of these pediatric-specific symptoms in children affected with VWD is not known.

The challenges faced when evaluating a pediatric patient are significant and it is in this situation that the value of a positive family history becomes apparent. Assuming an autosomal dominant model, the most frequent genetic model for VWD, the likelihood of VWD increases exponentially the more first-degree relatives have a low level of VWF [13]. Unfortunately, positive family histories are not always present, particularly in cases of mild VWD where penetrance and expression may be issues. Therefore, in some cases a careful clinical assessment is all that is available to direct management. Bleeding assessment tools specific to pediatrics have been developed [9,10,14,15] and work to develop quantitative scoring systems that are consistent between pediatric and adult populations has been recently completed [16,17].

Women—value of gynecologic assessment

Several studies have reported VWD prevalence rates of ~15% in women with menorrhagia [18–21]. As can be seen in Table 8.1, women with VWD frequently report menorrhagia; however, so do normal women. Menorrhagia can therefore be considered a sensitive, but not specific, sign of VWD. Menorrhagia (defined as >80 mL of blood loss per menstrual period) is one of the most important clinical issues faced by women with VWD and therefore a careful gynecologic assessment is a critical component in the evaluation of a female patient for VWD. Clinical features on a gynecologic history that have been identified as being predictive of VWD include menorrhagia since menarche and higher pictorial bleeding assessment chart (PBAC) scores [18]. PBAC scores of >100 have been shown to correlate with menstrual blood loss of >80 mL [22]; features such as clots of >1 inch, low serum ferritin, and changing sanitary protection more than hourly have also been shown to correlate with menstrual blood loss >80 mL [23].

Additionally, a number of studies have reported an increased incidence in gynecologic abnormalities such as endometriosis, polyps, and fibroids in VWD [11]. This may not reflect a true increase in incidence, rather these conditions may come to medical attention more readily if there is an underlying bleeding disorder. Therefore, examination of the pelvis is an important part of the gynecologic assessment; however, structural abnormalities do not rule out the possibility of VWD.

Standard treatment modalities used in the general population for menorrhagia, such as oral contraceptives or fibrinolytic inhibitors, are also effective in treating menorrhagia in women with underlying VWD; however, it is important to recognize the effect that these treatments might have not only on the laboratory testing for VWD, but also on the other mucocutaneous bleeding symptoms reported by patients. A careful history must therefore include an assessment of severity of symptoms before the introduction of such medications.

Bleeding assessment tools

Over the years, multiple investigators have made attempts to standardize bleeding histories by identifying questions that best distinguish between affected and unaffected individuals. In 1995, Sramek and colleagues [5] published their experience with a bleeding questionnaire that was administered to both patients known to have a bleeding disorder and a group of normal controls. The most informative questions in terms of discrimination were about bleeding after traumatic events such as tonsillectomy or dental extraction (but not childbirth) and the presence of a bleeding disorder in a family member. Interestingly, these questions were only discriminatory in a screening setting, not in a referral setting, perhaps because a referral population comprises a preselected group of individuals with highly prevalent symptoms. A number of other tools to assess hemorrhagic symptoms exist; details can be found in Table 8.2.

Recently, the value of quantifying bleeding symptoms for the diagnosis of VWD has been recognized. This approach has many potential advantages over other classification systems, including facilitating the exploration of variability in bleeding severity, informing treatment decisions, and providing an efficient means of communication between colleagues. The quantitative bleeding questionnaire that is detailed on the International Society of Thrombosis and Haemostasis (ISTH) website (http://www.isth.org/default/index.cfm/) was developed and validated by a group of investigators in Vicenza, Italy [6]. After administration of this questionnaire, the bleeding score is generated by summing the severity of all bleeding symptoms reported by a participant. Bleeding symptoms are scored from 0 (absence or trivial symptoms) to 3 (symptom requiring medical intervention). In order to improve the sensitivity and specificity of the bleeding score, this scoring system was later

Table 8.2 Published bleeding assessment tools.

Reference	Tool	Study population	Result	Scoring system	Ages studied mean/median (range)
Rodeghiero [6]	ISTH bleeding questionnaire	Type 1 VWD obligatory carriers	Score, but data analyzed based on the number of reported bleeding symptoms	Semi-quantitative	Type 1 obligatory carriers—49 years Type 1—38 years Controls 49 years
Buchanan [9]	Grading system for hemorrhage	ITP	Overall and site-specific severity grade	Semi-quantitative	5 years (8 months–17 years)
Katsanis [10]	Epistaxis severity score	Recurrent epistaxis	Mild vs. severe	Semi-quantitative	8.8 years (3–16)
Dean [14]	The Hospital for Sick Children bleeding questionnaire	VWD	Bleeder vs. nonbleeder	Semi-quantitative	9.4 years (1.5–18)
Higham [22]	Pictorial bleeding assessment chart	Menorrhagia	Score	Quantitative	n/a
Philipp [24]	Screening tool	Menorrhagia	Each symptom analyzed individually	Qualitative	39 years (13–53 years)
Castaman [25]	ISTH bleeding questionnaire	Type 3 VWD obligatory carriers	Score	Quantitative	Type 3—15 years Type 3 obligatory carriers—47 years Type 1 obligatory carriers—47 years

ISTH, International Society for Thrombosis and Haemostasis; VWD, von Willebrand disease; ITP, immune (idiopathic) thrombocytopenic purpura.

Table 8.3 Molecular and Clinical Markers for the Diagnosis and Management of Type 1 von Willebrand Disease (MCMDM-1 VWD) bleeding score.

Symptom	Score					
	−1	0	1	2	3	4
Epistaxis	—	No or trivial (<5)	>5 or >10′	Consultation only	Packing, cauterization, or antifibrinolytic	Blood transfusion, replacement therapy, or desmopressin
Cutaneous	—	No or trivial (<1 cm)	>1 cm and no trauma	Consultation only		
Bleeding from minor wounds	—	No or trivial (<5)	>5 or >5′	Consultation only	Surgical hemostasis	Blood transfusion, replacement therapy, or desmopressin
Oral cavity	—	No	Referred at least one	Consultation only	Surgical hemostasis or antifibrinolytic	Blood transfusion, replacement therapy, or desmopressin
Gastrointestinal bleeding	—	No	Associated with ulcer, portal hypertension, hemorrhoids, angiodysplasia	Spontaneous	Surgical hemostasis, blood transfusion, replacement therapy, desmopressin, antifibrinolytic	
Tooth extraction	No bleeding in at least two extractions	None done or no bleeding in one extraction	Referred in <25% of all procedures	Referred in >25% of all procedures; no intervention	Resuturing or packing	Blood transfusion, replacement therapy, or desmopressin

Surgery	No bleeding in at least two surgeries	None done or no bleeding in one surgery	Referred in <25% of all surgeries	Referred in >25% of all procedures; no intervention	Surgical hemostasis or antifibrinolytic	Blood transfusion, replacement therapy, or desmopressin
Menorrhagia	—	No	Consultation only	Antifibrinolytics, pill use	Dilation and currettage, iron therapy	Blood transfusion, replacement therapy, desmopressin, or hysterectomy
Postpartum hemorrhage	No bleeding in at least two deliveries	No deliveries or no bleeding in one delivery	Consultation only	Dilation and currettage, iron therapy, antifibrinolytics	Blood transfusion, replacement therapy, or desmopressin	Hysterectomy
Muscle hematomas	—	Never	Post trauma; no therapy	Spontaneous, no therapy	Spontaneous or traumatic, requiring desmopressin or replacement therapy	Spontaneous or traumatic, requiring surgical intervention or blood transfusion
Hemarthrosis	—	Never	Post trauma; no therapy	Spontaneous, no therapy	Spontaneous or traumatic, requiring desmopressin or replacement therapy	Spontaneous or traumatic, requiring surgical intervention or blood transfusion
Central nervous system bleeding	—	Never	—	—	Subdural; any intervention	Intracerebral; any intervention

Reproduced from Tosetto *et al.* [26], with permission from Wiely-Blackwell.

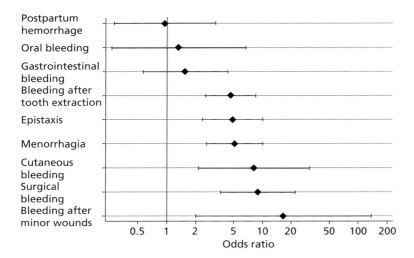

Figure 8.1 Odds ratio for type 1 von Willebrand disease associated with presence of a score of 1 or higher is presented. Reproduced from Tosetto *et al.* [26], with permission from Wiley-Blackwell.

revised to increase the range of possible grades from −1 (absence of bleeding after significant hemostatic challenge such as two dental extractions or surgeries) to 4 (symptoms requiring the most significant medical intervention such as infusion of clotting factor concentrates or surgery to control bleeding) [26].

This −1 to 4 version (Table 8.3) was used for the European Molecular and Clinical Markers for the Diagnosis and Management of Type 1 VWD (MCMDM-1VWD) study, and the resultant bleeding score was strongly related to VWF level. Higher bleeding scores were associated with an increased likelihood of VWD, and scores specifically related to spontaneous mucocutaneous bleeding predicted an increased risk of bleeding after surgery or dental extraction. Odds ratios for type 1 VWD based on this study are presented in Figure 8.1. A condensed version of this questionnaire was prospectively analyzed in the primary care setting for the diagnosis of VWD and showed a sensitivity of 100%, specificity of 87%, positive predictive value (PPV) of 0.20, and negative predictive value of 1 [27]. The poor PPV highlights the overlap in the mucocutaneous bleeding symptoms seen in VWD with those seen in other conditions such as platelet function disorders.

An additional area of interest for research involving bleeding quantitation lies in differentiating bleeding severity between subtypes of VWD. The data in Table 8.1 show that, in general, mucocutaneous bleeding symptoms are reported more frequently by patients with type 3 VWD than those with type 2 and type 1 VWD, although there is a great deal of overlap. Bleeding scores have been shown to follow the same pattern, with type 3 > type 2 > type 1 [27]. Interesting work has evaluated subtype differences even further by comparing bleeding symptoms between type 3 VWD obligate carriers and controls without VWD. Type 3 obligate carriers reported more epistaxis, cutaneous bleeding, and postsurgical bleeding than the controls [25], further highlighting the heterogeneity of symptoms in VWD.

International collaborative efforts in the area of bleeding assessments are ongoing, with efforts directed at harmonizing existing tools. A Working Party of the ISTH has been established with the objective of developing and validating a comprehensive scoring system and questionnaire not only for VWD, but for all inherited bleeding disorders.

Conclusion

Bleeding history is a critical component in the evaluation of a patient for VWD, and thus must be done carefully. Standardized bleeding assessment tools and quantitative scoring systems are useful additions to improve the accurate assessment of bleeding symptoms.

References

1 von Willebrand EA. Hereditary pseudo haemophilia. *Haemophilia* 1999; **5**: 223–31.

2 Mishra P, Naithani R, Dolai T, *et al*. Intracranial haemorrhage in patients with congenital haemostatic defects. *Haemophilia* 2008; **14**: 952–5.

3 Barr RD, Sek J, Horsman J, *et al*. Health status and health-related quality of life associated with von Willebrand disease. *Am J Hematol* 2003; **73**: 108–14.

4 Silwer J. von Willebrand's disease in Sweden. *Acta Paediatr Scand Suppl* 1973; **238**: 1–159.

5 Sramek A, Eikenboom JC, Briet E, Vandenbroucke JP, Rosendaal FR. Usefulness of patient interview in bleeding disorders. *Arch Intern Med* 1995; **155**: 1409–15.

6 Rodeghiero F, Castaman G, Tosetto A, *et al*. The discriminant power of bleeding history for the diagnosis of type 1 von Willebrand disease: an international, multicenter study. *J Thromb Haemost* 2005; **3**: 2619–26.

7 Federici AB. Clinical diagnosis of von Willebrand disease. *Haemophilia* 2004; **10** (Suppl. 4): 169–76.

8 Lak M, Peyvandi F, Mannucci PM. Clinical manifestations and complications of childbirth and replacement therapy in 385 Iranian patients with type 3 von Willebrand disease. *Br J Haematol* 2000; **111**: 1236–9.

9 Buchanan GR, Adix L. Grading of hemorrhage in children with idiopathic thrombocytopenic purpura. *J Pediatr* 2002; **141**: 683–8.

10 Katsanis E, Luke KH, Hsu E, Li M, Lillicrap D. Prevalence and significance of mild bleeding disorders in children with recurrent epistaxis. *J Pediatr* 1988; **113**: 73–6.

11 Kirtava A, Drews C, Lally C, Dilley A, Evatt B. Medical, reproductive and psychosocial experiences of women diagnosed with von Willebrand's disease receiving care in haemophilia treatment centres: a case–control study. *Haemophilia* 2003; **9**: 292–7.

12 Makris M. Gastrointestinal bleeding in von Willebrand disease. *Thromb Res* 2006; **118** (Suppl. 1): S13–S17.

13 Tosetto A, Castaman G, Rodeghiero F. Evidence-based diagnosis of type 1 von Willebrand disease: a Bayes theorem approach. *Blood* 2008; **111**: 3998–4003.

14 Dean JA, Blanchette VS, Carcao MD, *et al*. von Willebrand disease in a pediatric-based population—comparison of type 1 diagnostic criteria and use of the PFA-100 and a von Willebrand factor/collagen-binding assay. *Thromb Haemost* 2000; **84**: 401–9.

15 Hedlund-Treutiger I, Revel-Vilk S, Blanchette VS, Curtin JA, Lillicrap D, Rand ML. Reliability and reproducibility of classification of children as "bleeders" versus "non-bleeders" using a questionnaire for significant mucocutaneous bleeding. *J Pediatr Hematol Oncol* 2004; **26**: 488–91.

16 Bowman M, Riddel J, Rand ML, Tosetto A, Silva M, James PD. Evaluation of the diagnostic utility for von Willebrand disease of a pediatric bleeding questionnaire. *J Thromb Haemost* 2009; **7**: 1418–21.

17 Biss TT, Blanchette VS, Clark DS, *et al*. Quantitation of bleeding symptoms in children with von Willebrand disease: use of a standardized pediatric bleeding questionnaire. *J Thromb Haemost* 2010; **8**: 950–6.

18 Kadir RA, Economides DL, Sabin CA, Owens D, Lee CA. Frequency of inherited bleeding disorders in women with menorrhagia. *Lancet* 1998; **351**: 485–9.

19 Dilley A, Drews C, Miller C, *et al*. von Willebrand disease and other inherited bleeding disorders in women with diagnosed menorrhagia. *Obstet Gynecol* 2001; **97**: 630–6.

20 Edlund M, Blomback M, von SB, Andersson O. On the value of menorrhagia as a predictor for coagulation disorders. *Am J Hematol* 1996; **53**: 234–8.

21 Goodman-Gruen D, Hollenbach K. The prevalence of von Willebrand disease in women with abnormal uterine bleeding. *J Womens Health Gend Based Med* 2001; **10**: 677–80.

22 Higham JM, O'Brien PM, Shaw RW. Assessment of menstrual blood loss using a pictorial chart. *Br J Obstet Gynaecol* 1990; **97**: 734–9.

23 Warner PE, Critchley HO, Lumsden MA, Campbell-Brown M, Douglas A, Murray GD. Menorrhagia I: measured blood loss, clinical features, and outcome in women with heavy periods: a survey with follow-up data. *Am J Obstet Gynecol* 2004; **190**: 1216–23.

24 Philipp CS, Faiz A, Dowling NF, *et al*. Development of a screening tool for identifying women with menorrhagia for hemostatic evaluation. *Am J Obstet Gynecol* 2008; **198**: 163–8.

25 Castaman G, Rodeghiero F, Tosetto A, *et al*. Hemorrhagic symptoms and bleeding risk in obligatory carriers of type 3 von Willebrand disease: an international, multicenter study. *J Thromb Haemost* 2006; **4**: 2164–9.

26 Tosetto A, Rodeghiero F, Castaman G, *et al*. A quantitative analysis of bleeding symptoms in type 1 von Willebrand disease: results from a multicenter European study (MCMDM-1 VWD). *J Thromb Haemost* 2006; **4**: 766–73.

27 Bowman M, Mundell G, Grabell J, *et al*. Generation and validation of the Condensed MCMDM-1VWD Bleeding Questionnaire for von Willebrand disease. *J Thromb Haemost* 2008; **6**: 2062–6.

Laboratory diagnosis of von Willebrand disease: the phenotype

Ulrich Budde[1] and Emmanuel J. Favaloro[2]

[1]Hemostaseology, Medilys Laborgesellschaft mbH, c/o Asklepois Klinik Altona, Hamburg, Germany

[2]Department of Haematology, Institute of Clinical Pathology and Medical Research, Westmead Hospital, Westmead, Australia

von Willebrand disease (VWD) is one of the most common congenital bleeding disorders. Laboratory values below the reference range will be detected in about 1% of the population [1]; however, the prevalence of true VWD is much lower (between 1:3000 and 1:10,000). A prevalence of 125 cases per million of the population has been estimated for Sweden, a country with a homogeneous population and that retains excellent records for patients with a bleeding diathesis. Therefore, clinical observation is necessary for differentiation between a purely laboratory phenomenon versus a clinically relevant disease. Additionally, the concentration of circulating von Willebrand factor (VWF) depends on the ABO blood group [2]. In individuals with blood group O, VWF has a shorter half-life than in other individuals. This leads to, on average, 25% lower VWF plasma levels. Thus, for blood group O, a VWF concentration of 35% may be "normal," whereas it would be identified as reduced for other blood groups. VWF levels do not have an association with gender, but do, however, increase from the age of 40 years onwards by about 6% for each decade of life. The behavior of VWF as an acute-phase protein complicates matters further, because levels will increase in short-term "stress situations" or for longer periods during pregnancy or in the presence of malignant disease. Thus, the lack of a personal and family history of a bleeding diathesis would usually exclude a diagnosis of inherited VWD (not acquired von Willebrand syndrome [aVWS]) in an individual otherwise presenting with laboratory-defined "low VWF."

For any given individual, the differentiation between being diagnosed with mild VWD versus being identified as a healthy individual with a low plasma VWF concentration is important. On the one hand, healthy individuals may be stigmatized as "bleeders" throughout their lives (emergency card, insurance issues), while on the other, patients with true VWD who for a short period are identified with normal test parameters might wrongly be classified as healthy and denied appropriate therapy. Consequently, it is usual to undertake several investigations in order to confirm or discard a suspected diagnosis (Tables 9.1 and 9.2).

Screening diagnostic tests

Bleeding time

The bleeding time is a global test of primary hemostasis. It may be prolonged in qualitative and quantitative platelet defects, VWD, disorders of the vessel wall, and even in anemia [3]. A prolonged bleeding time is characteristic of patients with VWD and was repeatedly described in its first reports. It is, however, variable and quite often normal in mild forms of VWD. The bleeding time is becoming increasingly less important because of the application of more sensitive *in vitro* methods, which are operator independent and essentially atraumatic. Thus, the bleeding time is no longer an essential test for the diagnosis of VWD.

Von Willebrand Disease, 1st edition. Edited by Augusto B. Federici, Christine A. Lee, Erik E. Berntorp, David Lillicrap, Robert R. Montgomery. © 2011 Blackwell Publishing Ltd.

PFA-100 and other global shear stress test systems

A number of instruments are now available that measure some aspect of "global primary hemostasis." The best known of these is called the PFA-100 [4], although there are several others including the cone and plate(let) analyzer. As VWF is integral to the process of primary hemostasis, these instruments are sensitive to the presence or absence of VWF, or to VWF dysfunction, and they can therefore be used to identify VWD. The PFA-100, for example, is 100% sensitive to all severe forms of VWD including types 2A, 2M, 2B, and 3. It is variably sensitive to type 1 VWD, according to the presenting level of plasma VWF, but on average will detect around 80% of cases. However, like the bleeding time, these instruments are also sensitive to other components of primary hemostasis, such as platelet count and activity, and sometimes other blood components. They are also variably sensitive to antiplatelet medication, in particular aspirin. Accordingly, these instruments are not specific for VWD and an abnormal test result may or may not reflect presence of the disease. They are, however, potentially useful as negative predictors of VWD as a normal test result can exclude severe VWD. They are also potentially useful for monitoring desmopressin therapy, and in that context may help to functionally characterize VWD (see later section).

Activated partial thromboplastin time

The activated partial thromboplastin time (aPTT) is not a diagnostic test for VWD. It may be prolonged in patients with a clear reduction in factor (F) VIII and will detect most patients with type 2N, as well as severe cases of VWD. However, most patients with VWD will have sufficiently high FVIII activity to yield a normal aPTT. In any case, for a prolonged aPTT, deficiency of FVIII or FIX associated with hemophilia A and B, deficiency of FXI, FXII, high-molecular-weight (HMW) kininogen and prekallikrein, as well as interfering inhibitors (lupus inhibitors) must all be excluded. Furthermore, mild reduction in FXII is relatively frequent. Thus, many "irrelevant" patients will be identified during the diagnostic assessment of a prolonged aPTT. Combined FXII and VWF deficiency was previously classified as a special type (VWD San Diego). However, it was recently shown that this association is purely coincidental. It has also been shown that the aPTT is not a sensitive test for mild hemophilia because of the substantial biologic, pathologic, and analytic variation, and, similarly, the aPTT is also not suitable for identification of mild VWD.

Platelet adhesion

Because VWF is the most important protein for platelet adhesion, quantitative and/or qualitative disorders of VWF are accompanied by a defect of platelet adhesion. Assessment of platelet adherence is, like the bleeding time, a functional VWF activity test [5,6]. However, the flow chamber tests required are not suitable for routine investigations, with the exception of the high shear stress methods that measure platelet adhesion in automatic or semi-automatic devices such as the PFA-100 (see above), which may replace the bleeding time in general practice.

Platelet count

Measurement of the platelet count is a frontline test used for the exclusion of other diseases of primary hemostasis and the possible identification of patients with type 2B and platelet-type (pseudo) VWD (PT-VWD). Such patients may suffer from consistent or intermittent thrombocytopenia depending on the reactivity of the VWF, indicating increased interaction between the platelet receptor (glycoprotein Ib [GPIb]) and the A1 domain of VWF.

Extended diagnostic tests

Assay of the FVIII/VWF complex

For comparable results, laboratories are required to use assay reference standards that have been calibrated to the World Health Organization (WHO) standard [7]; each laboratory should determine its own reference ranges. Whether separate normal ranges for patients with blood group O and non-O are necessary is still a matter of controversy.

Factor VIII (FVIII)
FVIII may be low in patients with VWD, either because of a VWF binding defect (type 2N VWD) or because VWF normally acts to stabilize and protect FVIII. The most frequently used test system for the determination of FVIII coagulant (FVIII:C) is the

Table 9.1 Typical laboratory patterns in von Willebrand disease (VWD).[a]

Laboratory assay	VWD subtype					
	1	2A	2B[b]	2N	2M	3
(i) Screening tests						
Prothrombin time	Normal	Normal	Normal	Normal	Normal	Normal
APTT	Raised (/normal)	Raised (/normal)	Normal (/raised)	Raised (/normal)	Normal (/raised)	Raised
Platelet count	Normal	Normal	Low (/normal)	Normal	Normal	Normal
PFA-100® (closure time; CT)	Prolonged (/normal)	Prolonged/no closure	Prolonged/no closure	Normal	Prolonged/no closure	Prolonged/no closure
(ii) Diagnostic assays[c,d,e]						
FVIII:C	Low (/normal)	Low (/normal)	Low/normal	Proportionally low	Normal/low	Low (<20IU/dL)
VWF:Ag	Low (<50IU/dL)	Low (/normal)	Low/normal	Normal (/low)	Normal/low	Very low (<5IU/dL)
VWF:RCo	Low (/occasionally normal)	Low (<30IU/dL)	Low (occasionally normal)	Normal (/low)	Low (/normal)	Very low (<5IU/dL)
VWF:CB	Low (/occasionally normal)	Very low (<15IU/dL)	Low (<40IU/dL)	Normal (/low)	Low (/normal)	Very low (<5IU/dL)
VWF:RCo to VWF:Ag ratio[f,g,h]	Normal (>0.7)	Low (<0.7)	Low (<0.7)	Normal (>0.7)	Low/normal	Variable—don't use
VWF:CB to VWF:Ag ratio[f,g,h]	Normal (>0.7)	Low (<0.7)	Low (<0.7)	Normal (>0.7)	Low/normal	Variable—don't use

(iii) Confirmative/VWD subtyping assays

VWF:FVIII binding assay

Bound FVIII:bound VWF ratio	Normal (>0.6)	Normal (>0.6)	Normal (>0.6)	Low (<0.6)	Normal (>0.6)	Variable—don't use
RIPA—ristocetin						
Low dose (e.g., 0.5 mg/mL)	Absent	Absent	Present	Absent	Absent	Absent
1.0 mg/mL	Reduced (/normal)	Reduced	Normal	Normal	Reduced (/normal)	Absent
1.5 mg/mL	Reduced (/normal)	Reduced/(normal)	Normal	Normal	Reduced (/normal)	Absent
VWF multimer pattern	Normal pattern, VWF reduced	Large to intermediate multimers missing	Large multimers missing	Normal	Normal VWF multimer distribution (but with possible abnormal bands)	Multimers "absent"

APTT, activated partial thromboplastin time; RIPA, ristocetin-induced platelet agglutination, VWF, von Willebrand factor.

[a] Values within the table are approximate guide values only; different laboratories many derive different reference ranges.

[b] Pseudo- or "platelet-type" VWD patterns are similar to those for type 2B VWD.

[c] For VWF and FVIII: values >50IU/dL are usually considered normal; however, single or individual "normal" assay results cannot discount VWD.

[d] For VWF and FVIII: values <50IU/dL are usually considered abnormal; however, single or individual "abnormal" assay results do not diagnose VWD.

[e] Normal reference ranges vary between laboratories, tests, and methods; lower VWF values are expected in individuals with blood type O.

[f] Some workers use reciprocal ratios (i.e., VWF:Ag/functional VWF [e.g., Ag:RCo, Ag:CB]).

[g] For type 2A VWD, the CB:Ag ratio is generally lower than RCo:Ag because VWF:CB is generally more sensitive to the loss of high molecular weight VWF than VWF:RCo.

[h] For type 2M VWD, discordance in RCo:Ag or CB:Ag depends on the specific defect defined by type 2M VWD (i.e., platelet adhesion or matrix adhesion). However, most individuals with type 2M VWD so far defined show inherent VWF platelet adhesion defect (not inherent VWF–collagen adhesion defect) and so, in these cases of type 2M, the RCo:Ag ratio is lower than the CB:Ag ratio.

Table 9.2 Diagnostic tests for the phenotyping of VWD.

Screening diagnostic tests
Bleeding time
Systems with high shear stress
Partial thromboplastin time

Extended diagnostic tests
VWF antigen (VWF:Ag)
Ristocetin cofactor activity (VWF:RCo)
FVIII activity (FVIII:C)
Ratio VWF:RCo/VWF:Ag
Ratio FVIII:C/VWF:Ag

Special diagnostic tests
VWF collagen-binding capacity (VWF:CB)
VWF "activity" tests (VWF:Act)
Ristocetin-induced platelet agglutination
VWF propeptide (VWF:Ag II)
Multimer analysis
FVIII binding capacity of VWF

---

aPTT system using specific deficient plasmas. Assays using chromogenic substrates are less subject to disturbance by interfering antibodies and assay variables, but are less commonly used. The FVIII antigen can be assayed using enzyme-linked immunosorbent assay (ELISA) methods, but is of little utility for diagnostic purposes.

VWF antigen (VWF:Ag)
The determination of VWF (protein or "antigen"—VWF:Ag) concentration is indispensable for the investigation of defective primary hemostasis and proving or excluding an inherited VWD or aVWS. This test is also critical in order to distinguish between a reduction in and/or dysfunction of VWF.

The historic landmark electroimmunoassay method for VWF:Ag of Zimmerman *et al.* [8] is now very rarely used. ELISA methods, using poly- and/or monoclonal antisera, are much more sensitive and have better reproducibility at low concentrations of VWF [9]. Rapid latex-based methods have recently become available that allow a relatively cheap, quick (about 15 min), and precise assay [10] for VWF:Ag, but suffer from limitations that affect all latex tests (e.g., potential interference from rheumatoid factor and lipemia). Commercial kits from several companies are available for all the above mentioned nonradioactive VWF:Ag methods.

VWF:Ag is reduced in more than 80% of patients with VWD, but may be normal in the remainder. In mild forms of VWD the lower range of normal may sometimes be reached, especially in situations of stress [11]. Normal levels of VWF:Ag are often also observed in type 2B VWD. The blood group relationship of the FVIII–VWF complex in the so-called "gray area" between 0.4 and 0.6 IU/dL also results in diagnostic difficulties. Accordingly, investigation of suspected VWD will be incomplete if testing of VWF:Ag is not combined with a method that assesses the functional capability of VWF.

Ristocetin cofactor activity (VWF:RCo)
In vitro, platelets react with each other in the presence of ristocetin and VWF. Using washed platelets, the property of VWF to bind its receptor GPIb is facilitated by the presence of ristocetin. The principle of the VWF:RCo activity method is as follows: normal platelets, a constant quantity of ristocetin (usually at 1.0 mg/mL) and standard or patient plasma dilutions are allowed to react under suitable conditions and the resultant agglutination is assessed quantitatively [12] against that of standard plasma. Fresh and fixed, lyophilized or frozen platelets are all suitable; however, fresh platelets deteriorate after a short time. Preserved platelets are thus usually used [13] and commercial washed and fixed-test platelets are available. The reaction may take place in an aggregometer, on test plates, or in a platelet counter [14,15]. Ristocetin may be replaced by botrocetin. VWF:RCo can be automatically assayed in some coagulation analyzers.

The great variability of the available methods has been problematic since their inception and, despite much effort, cannot be eliminated. Another serious problem in general diagnostic laboratories is the poor reported sensitivity of the assay for low levels of VWF [16]. An ELISA method potentially enabling better standardization and lower level VWF sensitivity comparable to VWF:Ag was recently published [17] where binding of VWF takes place on immobilized recombinant GPIb. However, this test is not yet commercially available.

VWF:RCo behaves only somewhat like VWF:Ag (see above). For patients with a mild form of VWD, it is generally more sensitive in the lower normal range. Patients with type 2 VWD are often detected by the constellation VWF:Ag > VWF:RCo, even if both test results are in the normal range. Since VWF:RCo detects the interaction between VWF and GPIb, it is an indispensable test for the diagnosis of type 2M VWD.

Special and/or newer diagnostic tests and processes

Collagen-binding capacity (VWF:CB)

The collagen-binding capacity (VWF:CB) is typically performed by ELISA, although a flow cytometry-based method has been described [18]. VWF:CB ELISA assays are technically similar to VWF:Ag ELISA assays but rely on the ability of VWF to adhere to collagen. Although the potential significance of this as an *in vivo* correlate has yet to be fully evaluated, VWF binding to tissue matrix proteins including collagen is a primary hemostatic mechanism after injury. It also needs to be recognized that this adhesive activity is distinct to the functional activity identified by VWF:RCo.

An optimized VWF:CB selectively detects primarily HMW VWF (i.e., most functional, adhesive, and hemostatically potent forms of VWF) and may be more sensitive to these than VWF:RCo, although efficacy depends on various factors and not all VWF:CB assays behave identically. This standardization issue has delayed the more general incorporation of this assay into laboratory practice. In brief, the following can be emphasized: (i) type I/III collagen mixture preparations (from equine or bovine tendon) are generally better able to preferentially detect HMW VWF than either purified human-derived type III collagen or purified animal-derived type I collagen; (ii) the purified human-derived type III collagen systems appear to bind VWF too well, and thus may not show selective discrimination of HMW VWF, whereas the purified type I collagen systems appear to bind VWF too poorly, leading to poor reproducibility issues, particularly at low levels of VWF; (iii) HMW VWF discrimination findings from factor concentrate studies seem to mimic those in plasma systems. A number of different commercial ELISA-based kits are available, but most are generally based on type III collagen and have yet to be proved effective in discriminating HMW VWF.

In interlaboratory studies, optimized VWF:CB assays are better at identifying type 2A and 2B VWD

than VWF:RCo, and the additional use of a VWF:CB will reduce many errors in VWD misidentification [19]. However, the VWF:RCo is still a necessary diagnostic test in VWD and must be utilized to identify the major forms of type 2M VWD. Accordingly, the VWF:CB should not be seen as an alternative to VWF:RCo, but rather as a supplementary assay.

New and emerging "activity" assays for VWF

A number of assays are now available (distinct to both VWF:RCo and VWF:CB) that identify themselves as VWF "activity" (VWF:Act) assays. These may be performed by ELISA or by a latex immunoassay and are typically based on monoclonal antibodies directed against a functional domain on VWF [18]. However, the premise that this therefore engenders some functional property to these assays is flawed. These assays do have some ability to preferentially detect HMW VWF, and thus possess some sensitivity to dysfunctional forms of VWD such as types 2A and 2B, but this is likely due to affinity or avidity properties of the antibody rather than a functional property per se. In any case, in comparative studies, an optimized VWF:CB assay tends to be more sensitive to HMW VWF loss and thus to qualitative VWD variants.

Comparative utility of functional VWF–antigen ratios

As mentioned previously, qualitative defects in VWF are represented by type 2 VWD variants, with the specific defect characterizing the "subtype" (i.e., 2A = loss of HMW VWF; 2B = hypersensitive to VWF; 2M = dysfunction not caused by loss of HMW VWF; 2N = VWF FVIII binding defect). In contrast, types 1 and 3 are quantitative defects characterized by loss of (type 1) or absence of (type 3) VWF. Although VWF is low in type 1 VWD, the residual VWF is functionally normal; therefore, plasma VWF results as measured by any assay tend to be similar to one another. Thus, VWF:Ag, VWF:CB, and VWF:RCo test results will tend to be "concordant." In contrast, type 2 VWD variants, reflecting functional defects, will show discordance in test results between VWF:Ag and functional test parameters, with the type of discordance reflecting the subtype.

105

As a result, VWF:RCo and VWF:CB assay results tend to be lower than those of VWF:Ag in types 2A and 2B VWD because of the absence of HMW VWF. The use of functional VWF–antigen ratios (i.e., VWF:RCo/VWF:Ag [RCo:Ag] and VWF:CB/VWF:Ag [CB:Ag]) permits some objective quantification in these assessments [18]. In summary, both CB:Ag and RCo:Ag ratios are reduced in types 2A and 2B VWD (because of the loss of HMW VWF), whereas in type 2M VWD, most cases to date are reflected by a selective loss of VWF binding to GPIb, and may thus show only a reduced RCo:Ag. The use of functional VWF–antigen ratios, together with an assessment of the level of plasma VWF, can thus be used to help discriminate types 1, 2A, 2M, 2B, and 3 VWD from one another. Similarly, the use of FVIII/VWF:Ag ratios can help identify type 2N VWD and hemophilia, which can then be differentiated using the VWF:FVIII binding assay. While this process is now being better utilized in routine laboratory diagnosis, there remains uncertainty regarding ideal cut-off values, although most laboratories use either 0.6 or 0.7. The use of these functional VWF–antigen ratios can be supplemented with the use of a desmopressin challenge to better functionally characterize patients with VWD (see below).

Ristocetin-induced agglutination in platelet-rich plasma (RIPA)

The main goal of the ristocetin-induced agglutination in platelet-rich plasma (RIPA) test is to identify an increased interaction between VWF and GPIb (i.e., type 2B VWD and PT-VWD [20]). Patients with type 2A and 2M may show a decreased reactivity, but this is somewhat inconsistent and the RIPA test is not an obligatory test for the distinction between types 2A and 2M from type 1. Patients with Bernard–Soulier syndrome (BSS) and absent/dysfunctional GPIb and those with type 3 VWD (absent plasma VWF) show no agglutination even with high ristocetin concentrations. Because the reaction takes place in the patient's platelet-rich plasma (PRP), RIPA has to be performed in a local laboratory and not in a remote center.

It is important to use graded ristocetin concentrations (final concentrations between 0.1 and 1.5 mg/mL) [21]. While all patients with type 2B have increased ristocetin sensitivity (by definition of this subtype), the behavior in type 2 VWD subtypes is variable and often cannot be differentiated from that in healthy individuals or patients with type 1 VWD.

RIPA mixing studies with washed platelets can be used to differentiate patients with type 2B from those with PT-VWD [22], and plasma VWF testing plus other characteristic features of BSS can be used to differentiate BSS from type 3 VWD.

Botrocetin-induced aggregation in platelet-rich plasma (BIPA)

The snake venom botrocetin induces binding of VWF to GPIb, which is, unlike ristocetin, independent of the degree of multimerization of the molecule. Thus, botrocetin-induced aggregation in platelet-rich plasma (BIPA) theoretically allows differentiation between types 2A and 2M VWD [23] as type 2M is characterized by normal BIPA and abnormal RIPA, whereas abnormal results are found with both reagents in type 2A VWD. However, whether this holds true for all cases of 2A and 2M has not been thoroughly tested, and BIPA is not widely performed and is only available in specialized laboratories.

Binding studies with washed platelets

Patients with very low platelet counts cannot undergo RIPA, and some laboratories find it difficult to utilize RIPA to differentiate type 2B and PT-VWD. In such cases, the high-affinity binding of type 2B VWF and the low-affinity binding of VWF from patients with type 2A VWD and PT-VWD to platelets can be assessed [24]. While VWF from patients with type 2B VWD binds at very low ristocetin concentrations, often spontaneously, the VWF from patients with type 2A and PT-VWD does not bind or binds only at high ristocetin concentrations. Conversely, platelets from patients with PT-VWD bind normal VWF with much higher affinity than normal platelets or platelets from other VWD subtypes (including types 2A and 2B VWD).

To a mixture of washed and fixed normal (patient) platelets and patient (normal) plasma, increasing concentrations of ristocetin (0–1.2 mg) are added. After an incubation time of at least 30 min at room temperature, the platelets are separated from the plasma by centrifugation and the VWF:Ag not bound to platelets is assayed from the supernatant. Because of the complexity of this test, it is rarely used routinely and is performed only by a few specialized laboratories.

VWF propeptide (VWF:Ag II)

During synthesis of the VWF, the propeptide is cleaved after multimerization is complete and is secreted together with the mature VWF. The elimination of the propeptide is independent from that of VWF and is not influenced by the patient's blood group, nor does it undergo changes in patients with aVWS. In any case with an enhanced elimination of VWF (either inherited or acquired), the ratio between von Willebrand factor propeptide (VWFpp) and VWF:Ag will rise [25]. Thus, the determination of VWFpp may be helpful for detecting patients with a short half-time of VWF in plasma [26,27]. However, of 11 patients with an aVWS as result of a lymphoproliferative disorder only six showed a higher ratio, although all had clear evidence of a short VWF residence time in plasma [28]. Accordingly, the test may not be 100% sensitive. This has also been suggested by Millar *et al.* [29].

VWF:Ag II is assayed using a sandwich ELISA system with specific polyclonal or monoclonal antibodies as capture and detection antibodies. A commercial fluorescence test has recently become available.

Qualitative changes in VWF

VWF multimers

The purpose of multimer analysis is to (sub)type patients with inherited VWD or aVWS. In special cases, VWD can be diagnosed only by performing multimer analysis. There are other diseases, such as thrombotic thrombocytopenic purpura (TTP), hemolytic uremic syndrome (HUS), or sepsis, where the VWF structure may provide clinically helpful information.

The principle of the method follows closely that used by Lämmli [30] and first published by Ruggeri and Zimmerman [31]. The individual oligomers of VWF are separated by electrophoresis in a large-pore agarose gel in the presence of sodium dodecylsulfate (SDS) as an ionic detergent. Affinity-purified ^{125}I-labeled antibodies to VWF are then allowed to

diffuse in and the individual bands are mapped autoradiographically. Agarose gels of different concentration allow low, medium, and high resolutions of the banding pattern. The original radioactive method has been modified several times, because radioactive methods have become unpopular and the thickness of gels of more than 1 mm causes technical difficulties (extremely long diffusion times during washing and antibody incubation procedures). The turnover or turnaround time of these gels is at least 5 days. This time can be considerably shortened by transfer from the gel on to suitable membranes (e.g., nitrocellulose or nylon). Because of the extraordinary HMW of some VWF multimers of more than 10,000 kd, special precautions are required in order to transfer the whole set of multimers quantitatively. Modifications of all known techniques have been described: diffusion, vacuum blot, semi-dry blot, and tankblot. The disadvantage of nonradioactive methods is the lower sensitivity of the usual enzymatic methods (e.g., alkaline phosphatase- or peroxidase-labeled antibodies together with their classic substrates). This cannot be overcome by using more protein because a sufficiently high dilution of plasma is a prerequisite for optimal results. Plasma dilutions of less than 1:10 lead to abnormal distribution patterns of the bands and subbands, which may resemble congenital defects of the molecule. Besides attempts to increase sensitivity, for example with streptavidine/biotin, the use of luminescence achieves a sensitivity that is as good as, or better than, the sensitivity of radioactive methods [32]. The short-lived nature of the light reaction has also been improved so that modern substrates are active for more than 24 hours. The next logical step was to move from X-ray film as a medium to video detection with highly sensitive charge-coupled device (CCD) cameras that have optimally improved both sensitivity and ease of gel evaluation. The superior performance of these camera systems allows detection of many more variants than those obtained using X-ray films although, given this new information, retrospective analysis of old films can also identify these previously "hidden" abnormalities. The validity of this method can best be demonstrated through the detection of specific mutations. In the Molecular and Clinical Markers for the Diagnosis and Management of Type 1 VWD (MCMDM-1VWD) study [33], abnormal multimer mutations could be detected that segregated within all affected family members in all families (i.e., >98% specificity; the mutation(s) in three families were detected after publication). The same usefulness could be shown for patients with aVWS [28]. Comparable performance cannot be achieved with any other method or even a combination of methods.

For optimal results, there is a need to show the absence or presence of multimers within the complete set of multimers, as well as to evaluate the structure of the subbands generated post-translationally by the action of shear forces and ADAMTS13. Gels of low resolution allow the VWF to migrate better than gels with higher agarose concentrations. This facilitates very good differentiation between samples with loss of the large multimers, supranormal multimers, or with a normal picture (Figure 9.1). However, the variants with structural abnormalities remain undetected. Thus, to use a gel of medium resolution as the standard gel has the advantage that, in addition to sufficiently good visualization of the large multimers, structural defects are recognized to such an extent that gels of higher resolution are rarely needed (Figures 9.2 and 9.3).

Although the eye can visually recognize a loss of large multimers or an abnormal quantitative distribution within a lane, an objective quantitative assessment of the bands is desirable. Although densitometers can be used for the results of any method, they are most suited to video camera results stored on a microchip. The following division into oligomers is now widely accepted (Figure 9.4): 1–5 = small multimers, 6–10 = medium multimers, and >10 = large multimers.

VWF fragments

The size of the VWF molecule in plasma is regulated by ADAMTS13. ADAMTS13-induced proteolysis results in a loss of the ultralarge multimer fraction and the generation of specific fragments—the sub-

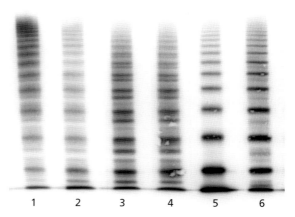

Figure 9.2 Normal plasma and von Willebrand disease (VWD) variants in a discontinuous gel of medium (1.6% LGT-agarose) resolution. The dye front is at the bottom of the gel and the large multimers are found in the upper part of the gel. Lane 1 = normal plasma (pool of 30); lane 2 = type 2A with all multimers but a relative loss of the largest multimers; lane 3 = type 2A with a loss of the large multimers and increased proteolytic subbands; lane 4 = type 2B with a loss of the large multimers and increased proteolytic subbands (note that types 2A and 2B may show the same multimer pattern depending on the responsible mutations); lane 5 = type 2A (IIC) with a severe loss of the large multimers, increased protomer, and no proteolysis; lane 6 = type 2A (IID) with a loss of the large multimers, intervening bands representing odd numbered oligomers and not proteolysis.

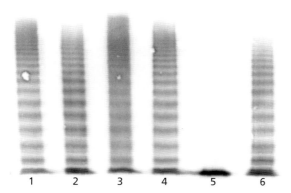

Figure 9.1 Normal plasma and variants of von Willebrand disease (VWD) in a discontinuous gel of low (1.2% LGT-agarose) resolution. The dye front is at the bottom of the gel and the large multimers are found in the upper part of the gel. Lane 1 = normal plasma (pool of 30); lanes 2, 4, and 6 = type 2A VWD with clearly visible but small losses of the large multimers. Lane 3 = type 1 VWD with a smeary pattern; lane 5, plasma from a patient with severe acquired von Willebrand syndrome caused by a monoclonal gammopathy of unknown significance of the IgG kappa type. Only the protomer is present.

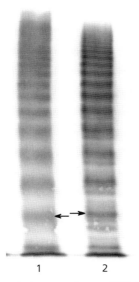

Figure 9.3 Normal plasma and a von Willebrand disease variant in a discontinuous gel of medium (1.6% LGT-agarose) resolution. The dye front is at the bottom of the gel and the large multimers are found in the upper part of the gel. Lane 1 = normal plasma (pool of 30), lane 2 = type 1 showing all plus supranormal multimers. The normally "von Willebrand factor-free" space between the oligomers is filled with amorphous material and there are no proteolytic subbands (smeary pattern), and the oligomers run faster through the gel (arrows). The responsible cysteine mutation in the carboxyterminus creates a new intramolecular loop that hinders unfolding of the molecule (faster velocity) and makes it less accessible for ADAMTS13 (severely reduced proteolytic bands).

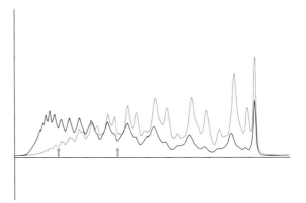

Figure 9.4 Densitometric visualization of von Willebrand factor multimers in a medium-resolution gel. The running direction is from left to right (i.e., the large multimers are in the left part). Red = normal plasma; black = plasma from a patient with type 2A. The left arrow marks the limit between the large (>10) and medium (6–10) multimers; the right arrow marks the limit between the medium and small (1–5) multimers. The proteolytic changes in the triplet structure are also well visualized.

bands of the quintuplet. Because every qualitative abnormal VWF (with the exception of type 2N) shows alterations of the subband pattern, the evaluation of the VWF subunits can theoretically be helpful in the diagnosis of variants of VWD. Different inherited abnormalities of the VWF lead to variants with increased ("classic" type IIA and 2B) or decreased (types IIC, IID, IIE) proteolysis. Augmented proteolysis may also be clinically relevant in pathologic states with increased shear stress. Disorders with elevated platelet counts also show increased fragmentation compared with normal plasma. Alternatively, enhanced clearance owing to antibodies against VWF

in acquired VWS may lead to decreased proteolytic fragmentation. The methods for subunit isolation, sizing, and detection are cumbersome [34] and have to date not been utilized in routine diagnosis of patients with suspected VWD.

FVIII binding capacity of VWF (VWF : FVIIIB)

This assay assesses the ability of VWF to bind FVIII and is used to differentially diagnose type 2N VWD, generally from hemophilia rather than other types of VWD [35–37]. In type 2N VWD, VWF binding to FVIII is dysfunctional, and hence the circulating half-life of factor VIII is severely reduced, lowering the plasma concentration. This assay is typically performed as an ELISA procedure and may also involve a chromogenic assay step. Although various test modifications have been described, they all follow the principle shown in Table 9.3. A disproportionate amount of bound VWF and bound FVIII identified in this assay (i.e., FVIII : VWF ratio <0.6) is suggestive of a type 2N VWD defect. This assay should always be performed for newly identified individuals who give a clinical presentation of hemophilia, particularly

109

Table 9.3 Test principles for the determination of von Willebrand factor (VWF):FVIIIB.

The FVIII–VWF complex is immobilized on a microtiter plate with monoclonal or polyclonal anti-VWF antibodies

The endogenous FVIII is removed from the complex by incubation and subsequent washings with high $CaCl_2$ concentrations

The binding capacity for FVIII is tested by incubation with defined amounts of rFVIII

The amount of bound FVIII is measured with tests for FVIII:C (chromogenic) or by incubation with enzyme-labeled anti-FVIII antibodies

The amount of immobilized VWF is measured with labeled anti-VWF antibodies

The amount of bound FVIII by a defined unit of VWF is calculated

---

where the genetic inheritance does not fit the classic pattern (sex-linked, whereas type 2N VWD is not).

VWF antibodies/inhibitors

In contrast to the situation in hemophila A and B, the formation of alloantibodies against VWF is a rare event in patients with type 3 VWD. In patients with aVWS, those with lymphoproliferative disorders show a response that is typical for antibody action: low recovery and short residence time in plasma. However, an antibody will be detected in only a minority of these patients (about 10%). Thus, current methods appear to show poor sensitivity to such antibodies. Because the testing of such antibodies is now compulsory for the license process of new VWF concentrates, better tests will need to be developed in the future.

Indirect methods

Altered recovery and residence time in plasma after therapy with VWF-containing concentrates, desmopressin, or potentially high-dose immunoglobulins may provide some evidence for the presence of an inhibitor against VWF, although such patterns will occur also in some forms of congenital VWD. Similarly, a high ratio of the VWF propeptide to VWF:Ag also suggests an enhanced turnover indicative of an inhibitor should an inherited VWD be excluded.

Direct methods

For antibodies that reduce the functional properties of VWF, tests analogous to the Bethesda assay for FVIII and FIX are used: VWF:CB, VWF:RCo, VWF:Act, VWF:FVIIIB, and VWF:Ag [38]. In a first step, suitable dilutions of the patient plasma are mixed with normal plasma and incubated for a defined time at a defined temperature. Because the antibodies are much less time and temperature dependent than FVIII/FIX antibodies, incubation time and temperature are not critical. Usually, the temperature is set to 37°C and the incubation times between 15 min and 1 h. The reference sample and positive and negative controls are incubated together with the patient samples. At the end of the incubation step, the residual activity of the samples is determined according to the chosen test(s). The inhibitor titer is determined as per the Bethesda assay (i.e., using a normogram between 0.5 and 2 BU and corrected for the dilution factor).

An ELISA test with immobilized, purified VWF has been described repeatedly [28,39,40]. ELISA tests, however, are hampered by a very high background (especially using antihuman IgM as the detecting antibody, but also with antihuman IgG). The reason for this is that VWF bears ABO blood group antigens, and every human plasma has at least some antibodies against ABO blood group determinants. This may be overcome by using recombinant VWF from nonhuman species that are not able to form ABO blood groups. In any case, because of this high background the test should be controlled rigorously by appropriate positive and negative controls. Because VWF is a large protein with multiple functions, it may be necessary to perform each and every possible test to identify the potential antibody [41,42].

Diagnosis in neonates and young children

This provides for some additional challenges. First, there is limited clinical information available regarding personal history because of lack of hemostatic challenge. In mild forms of type 1, diagnosis in neonates is often difficult because, physiologically, neonates have high VWF levels. False-normal levels may be obtained in very excited, screaming small children as a result of stress-induced release. Therefore, reliable levels can be obtained only from the sixth month of life onward. However, neonates and young children with a type 2 VWD will only rarely show a normal phenotype. Similarly, severe type 3 VWD should be easy to diagnose even in neonates because of the absolute deficiency of VWF. For this purpose, blood sampling from cord blood or the placenta can be used. It is important to recognize the possibility of a false diagnosis of hemophilia A in patients with type 3 VWD, particularly in young children, if testing is performed for FVIII:C without also testing for VWF.

In newborns with thrombocytopenia, after differential exclusion of the more common reasons, consideration should always also be given to a potential diagnosis of type 2B VWD or TTP in order to avoid errors in treatment.

Diagnosis in pregnancy

During pregnancy, VWF increases more than twofold, especially in the late stages. In type 1 VWD this results in diagnostic problems (normalization), but potentially not a complete therapeutic solution, because VWF rapidly falls to its original level after birth and late bleeding may then possibly occur. A currently unexplained phenomenon is the fact that about 30% of pregnant women are noted to have loss of the large multimers [43]. However, this loss does not apparently lead to clinical problems.

Desmopressin trials as an aid to the diagnosis and functional characterization of VWD

Desmopressin is a nontransfusional form of therapy for VWD and causes release of endogenous endothelial-stored VWF. Desmopressin is effective for treating only certain types of VWD, usually type 1, but also some cases of type 2. In addition to therapy, or to assess potential therapeutic responses, a desmopressin challenge can also be used to functionally characterize VWD. Desmopressin causes the release of VWF into plasma, with peak concentrations within 30 min that will subsequently decrease with time as a result of clearance and proteolysis mechanisms including ADAMTS13. In VWD, the patterns of release and clearance, as differentially detected using different assays, can help to characterize particular types of VWD. For example, the pattern in mild type 1 is fairly characteristic, with VWF reaching levels around 2–4 times baseline, reducing over time and reaching approximate baseline values within 24 h. The VWF initially detected by the VWF:CB tends to increase more so than that detected by VWF:Ag and VWF:RCo, as the VWF:CB best reflects the ultra-HMW VWF initially released by desmopressin [44]. Put another way, post desmopressin, the VWF:CB/VWF:Ag ratio tends to rise to a higher level (generally >1.0) than that of VWF:RCo/VWF:Ag. The pattern for type 2A is different, with desmopressin tending to increase VWF:Ag to much higher levels than either VWF:RCo or VWF:CB. Thus, neither the VWF:CB/VWF:Ag or VWF:RCo/VWF:Ag ratio tend to rise, remaining <0.7 for most cases. The pattern for type 2M VWD (GPIb binding defect) is different again, with VWF:CB/VWF:Ag ratios remaining normal post desmopressin and VWF:RCo/VWF:Ag ratios remaining low (generally <0.7).

Future perspectives

The VWF:RCo assay will hopefully be substituted by tests that use specific GPIb fragments that may be made more reactive by introducing specific mutations. While ELISA tests have a limit of detection well below 1 IU/dL, latex tests have their lower limit at 2–3 IU/dL. In contrast to most ELISA tests, they can be fully automated and performed in urgent cases within 15 min. Having these tests in the repertoire means that ratios between VWF:RCo over VWF:Ag will become much more reliable. Recently [45], a llama-derived antibody fragment (AU/VWFa-11) was described that specifically recognizes the GPIb binding conformation. It does not bind VWF in solution, but interacts efficiently with activated VWF. Thus, it could become a valuable tool for the characterization of patients with VWF in an activated state such as type 2B and TTP.

References

1 Rodeghiero F, Castaman GC, Dini E. Epidemiological investigation of the prevalence of von Willebrand's disease. *Blood* 1987; **69**: 454–9.

2 Gill JC, Endres-Brooks J, Bauer PJ, *et al.* The effect of ABO blood group on the diagnosis of von Willebrand disease. *Blood* 1987; **69**: 1691–5.

3 Ivy AC, Shapiro PF, Melnick P. The bleeding tendency in jaundice. *Surg Gynecol Obstet* 1935; **60**: 781–4.

4 Favaloro EJ. Clinical utility of the PFA-100. *Semin Thromb Hemost* 2008; **34**: 709–33.

5 Sakariassen KS, Nieuwenhuis K, Sixma JJ. Differentiation of patients with subtype IIB-like von Willebrand's disease by means of perfusion experiments with reconstituted blood. *Br J Haematol* 1985; **59**: 459–70.

6 Ruggeri ZM, Orje JN, Habermann R, *et al.* Activation-independent platelet adhesion and aggregation under elevated shear stress. *Blood* 2006; **108**: 1903–10.

7 Hubbard AR, Rigsby P, Barrowcliffe TW. Standardisation of factor VIII and von Willebrand factor in plasma: Calibration of the 4th International Standard (97/586). *Thromb Haemost* 2001; **85**: 634–8.

8 Zimmerman TS, Hoyer LW, Dickinson, Edgington TS. Determination of the von Willebrand's disease antigen (factor VIII-related antigen) in plasma by immunoelectrophoresis. *J Lab Clin Med* 1975; **86**: 152–9.

9 Cejka J. Enzyme immunoassay for factor VIII-related antigen. *Clin Chem* 1982; **28**: 1356–8.

10 Veyradier A, Fressinaud E, Sigaud M, *et al.* A new automated method for von Willebrand factor antigen measurement using latex particles. *Thromb Haemost* 1999; **81**: 320–1.

11 Tosetto A, Rodeghiero F, Castaman G, *et al.* Impact of plasma von Willebrand factor levels in the diagnosis of type 1 von Willebrand disease: results from a multicenter European study (MCMDM-1VWD). *J Thromb Haemost* 2007; **5**: 715–21.

12 Weiss HJ, Hoyer LW, Rickles F, *et al.* Quantitative assay of a plasma factor in von Willebrand's disease that is necessary for platelet aggregation. *J Clin Invest* 1973; **52**: 2701–16.

13 Macfarlane DE, Stibbe J, Kirby EP, *et al.* A method for assaying von Willebrand factor (ristocetin cofactor). *Thromb Diath Haemorrh* 1975; **34**: 306–8.

14 Brinkhous KM, Graham JE, Cooper HA, *et al.* Assay of von Willebrand factor in von Willebrand's disease and hemophilia: Use of a macroscopic platelet aggregation test. *Thromb Res* 1975; **6**: 267–72.

15 Brinkhous KM, Read MS. Preservation of platelet receptors for platelet aggregation factor/von Willebrand factor by air drying, freezing or lyophilization: New stable platelet preparations for von Willebrand factor assays. *Thromb Res* 1987; **13**: 591–5.

16 Favaloro EJ, Bonar R, Marsden K (on behalf of the RCPA QAP Haemostasis Committee). Lower limit of assay sensitivity: an under-recognised and significant problem in von Willebrand disease identification and classification. *Clin Lab Sci* 2008; **21**: 178–85.

17 Vanhoorelbeke K, Cauwenbergs N, Vauterin S, *et al.* A reliable and reproducible ELISA method to measure ristocetin cofactor activity of von Willebrand factor. *Thromb Haemost* 2000; **83**: 107–13.

18 Favaloro EJ. An update on the von Willebrand factor collagen binding assay: 21 years of age and beyond adolescence, but not yet a mature adult. *Semin Thromb Hemost* 2007; **33**: 727–44.

19 Favaloro EJ, Bonar R, Kershaw G, *et al.* Reducing errors in identification of von Willebrand disease: The experience of the Royal College of Pathologists of Australasia Quality Assurance Program. *Semin Thromb Hemost* 2006; **32**: 505–13.

20 Ruggeri ZM, Pareti FI, Mannucci PM, *et al.* Hightened interaction between platelets and factor VIII/von Willebrand factor in a new subtype of von Willebrand's disease. *N Engl J Med* 1980; **302**: 1047–51.

21 Federici AB, Mannucci PM, Castaman G, *et al.* Clinical and molecular predictors of thrombocytopenia and risk of bleeding in patients with von Willebrand disease type 2B: a cohort study of 67 patients. *Blood* 2009; **113**: 526–34.

22 Favaloro EJ. Phenotypic identification of Platelet Type-von Willebrand disease and its discrimination from Type 2B von Willebrand disease: A question of 2B or not 2B? A story of non-identical twins? Or two-sides of a multi-denominational or multi-faceted primary haemostasis coin? *Semin Thromb Hemost* 2008; **34**: 113–27.

23 Fujimura Y, Miyata S, Nishida S, *et al.* The interaction of botrocetin with normal or variant von Willebrand factor (type-IIA and type-IIB) and its inhibition by monoclonal antibodies that block receptor binding. *Thromb Haemost* 1992; **68**: 464–9.

24 De Marco L, Mazzuccato M, Del Ben MG, *et al.* Type IIB von Willebrand factor with normal sialic acid content induces platelet aggregation in the absence of ristocetin. *J Clin Invest* 1987; **80**: 475–82.

25 Vischer UM, Ingerslev J, Wollheim CB, *et al.* Acute von Willebrand factor secretion from the endothelium *in vivo*: Assessment through plasma propeptide (vWf: AgII) levels. *Thromb Haemost* 1997; **77**: 387–93.

26 de Romeuf C, Mazurier C. Comparison between von Willebrand factor (vWF) and vWF antigen II in normal individuals and patients with von Willebrand disease. *Thromb Haemost* 1998; **80**: 37–41.

27 Haberichter SL, Castaman G, Budde U, *et al.* Identification of type 1 disease patients with reduced von Willebrand factor (VWF) survival by assay of the VWF propeptide in the European study, Molecular and Clinical Markers for the Diagnosis and Management of Type 1 von Willebrand Disease (MCMDM-1VWD). *Blood* 2008; **111**: 4979–85.

28 Thiede A, Priesack J, Werwitzke S, *et al.* Diagnostic workup of patients with acquired von Willebrand

syndrome: a retrospective single-centre cohort study. *J Thromb Haemost* 2008; **6**: 569–76.

29 Millar CM, Riddell AF, Brown SA, *et al*. Survival of von Willebrand factor released following DDAVP in a type 1 von Willebrand disease cohort: influence of glycosylation, proteolysis and gene mutations. *Thromb Haemost* 2008; **99**: 916–24.

30 Lämmli UK. Cleavage of structural proteins during the assembly of the head of bacteriophage T4. *Nature* 1979; **227**: 680–5.

31 Ruggeri ZM, Zimmerman TS. Variant von Willebrand's disease. Characterization of two subtypes by analysis of multimeric composition of factor VIII/von Willebrand factor in plasma and platelets. *J Clin Invest* 1980; **65**: 1318–25.

32 Budde U, Schneppenheim R, Plendl H, *et al*. Luminographic detection of von Willebrand factor multimers in agarose gels and on nitrocellulose membranes. *Thromb Haemost* 1990; **63**: 312–15.

33 Budde U, Schneppenheim R, Eikenboom J, *et al*. Detailed von Willebrand factor multimer analysis in patients with von Willebrand disease in the European study, Molecular and Clinical Markers for the Diagnosis and Management of Type 1 von Willebrand Disease (MCMDM-1VWD). *J Thromb Haemost* 2008; **6**: 762–71.

34 Zimmerman TS, Dent JA, Ruggeri ZM, Nannini LH. Subunit composition of plasma von Willebrand factor. Cleavage is present in normal individuals, increased in IIA and IIB von Willebrand disease, but minimal in variants with aberrant structure of individual oligomers (types IIC, IID and IIE). *J Clin Invest* 1986; **77**: 947–51.

35 Nishino M, Girma JP, Rothschild C, *et al*. New variant of von Willebrand disease with defective binding to factor VIII. *Blood* 1989; **74**: 1591–9.

36 Mazurier C. Von Willebrand disease masquerading as haemophilia A. *Thromb Haemost* 1992; **67**: 391–6.

37 Casonato A, Pontara E, Sartorello F, *et al*. Identifying carriers of type 2N von Willebrand disease: procedures and significance. *Clin Appl Thromb Hemost* 2007; **13**: 194–200.

38 van Genderen PJJ, Vink T, Michiels JJ. Acquired von Willebrand disease caused by an autoantibody selectively inhibiting the binding of von Willebrand factor to collagen. *Blood* 1994; **84**: 3378–84.

39 Stewart MW, Etches WS, Shaw ARE, Gordon PA. VWF inhibitor detection by competitive ELISA. *J Immunol Meth* 1997; **200**: 113–19.

40 Siaka C, Rugeri L, Caron C, Goudemand J. A new ELISA assay for diagnosis of acquired von Willebrand syndrome. *Haemophilia* 2003; **9**: 303–8.

41 Guerin V, Ryman A, Velez F. Acquired von Willebrand disease: potential contribution of the von Willebrand factor collagen binding to the identification of functionally inhibiting auto-antibodies to von Willebrand factor: a rebuttal. *J Thromb Haemost* 2008; **6**: 1051–2.

42 Coleman R, Favaloro EJ, Soltani S, Keng TB. Acquired von Willebrand disease: potential contribution of the VWF:CB to the identification of functionally inhibiting auto-antibodies to von Willebrand factor. *J Thromb Haemost* 2006; **4**: 2085–8.

43 Bergmann F, Rotmensch S, Rosenzweig B, *et al*. The role of von Willebrand factor in pre-eclampsia. *Thromb Haemost* 1991; **66**: 525–8.

44 Favaloro EJ. Towards a new paradigm for the identification and functional characterization of von Willebrand disease. *Semin Thromb Hemost* 2009; **35**: 60–75.

45 Hulstein JJJ, de Groot PG, Silence K, *et al*. A novel nanobody that detects the gain-of-function phenotype of von Willebrand factor in ADAMTS13 deficiency and von Willebrand disease type 2B. *Blood* 2005; **106**: 3035–42.

113

Molecular diagnosis of von Willebrand disease: the genotype

Anne C. Goodeve[1,2] *and Reinhard Schneppenheim*[3]

[1]Sheffield Diagnostic Genetics Service, Sheffield Children's NHS Foundation Trust, Sheffield, UK

[2]Haemostasis Research Group, Faculty of Medicine, Dentistry and Health, University of Sheffield, Sheffield, UK

[3]Department of Paediatric Haematology and Oncology, University Medical Center Hamburg-Eppendorf, Hamburg, Germany

Introduction

von Willebrand factor (VWF) has two main functions. Under shear forces, binding to collagen in damaged, and exposed subendothelium allows the surface-bound VWF molecule to extend and expose binding sites for platelet glycoprotein Ib (GPIb), which contributes to platelet plug formation at sites of vascular damage [1]. Additionally, the molecule binds factor VIII (FVIII), thereby protecting it from proteolysis and delivering it to sites where it is required in the coagulation cascade [2].

The large VWF gene (*VWF*) encodes VWF, which is situated on the short arm of chromosome 12 and which spans 178 kb of DNA. *VWF* is flanked by *CD9* 76 kb to the 5′ (centromeric) end and *ANO2* 2.6 kb to the 3′ (telomeric) end. The region controlling VWF production may stretch several kb from the transcription start site and remains relatively poorly characterized. *VWF* comprises 52 exons, with protein coding initiating in exon 2. Most exons are small, ranging from 41 to 342 bp. However, exon 28 is somewhat larger at 1379 bp [3]. The VWF protein has a repeated domain structure, with domains in the order S-D1-D2-D′-D3-A1-A2-A3-D4-B1-B2-B3-C1-C2-CK (Figure 10.1).

Deficiency of plasma VWF leading to von Willebrand disease (VWD) can be divided into partial (type 1) and virtually complete (type 3) quantitative

defects and qualitative defects (type 2), which are then further subdivided into four subtypes dependent on function perturbed. Laboratory analysis of VWD requires an initial array of determinations of quantity (VWF:Ag)—ability to bind platelets (VWF:RCo), and FVIII coagulant activity (FVIII:C), followed by specialist tests to subtype the disorder; ability to bind to FVIII (VWF:FVIIIB) and collagen (VWF:CB), ristocetin-induced platelet aggregation (RIPA), and analysis of the VWF multimeric structure using gel electrophoresis (multimer profile)—that includes determining the presence of any excessively large (supranormal) multimers or loss of high-molecular-weight (HMW) multimers.

This chapter will describe the range of mutation types that contribute to VWD and their location. Methods available for genetic analysis are described, along with advantages and disadvantages of their use. Utility of mutation analysis in the different disease types is discussed and the methods for the interpretation of possible pathogenicity of sequence variants identified are also examined.

Molecular analysis

Phenotype analysis is often sufficient for diagnosis of VWD in patients who have reduced VWF and FVIII levels and a multimeric profile that readily fits into the standard VWD classification [4]. Molecular genetic analysis is useful where this is not the case, and clarification of the cause of bleeding or of reduced clotting factor levels is required. Genetic analysis can be used to clarify VWD type so that appropriate treatment can be

Von Willebrand Disease, 1st edition. Edited by Augusto B. Federici, Christine A. Lee, Erik E. Berntorp, David Lillicrap, Robert R. Montgomery. © 2011 Blackwell Publishing Ltd.

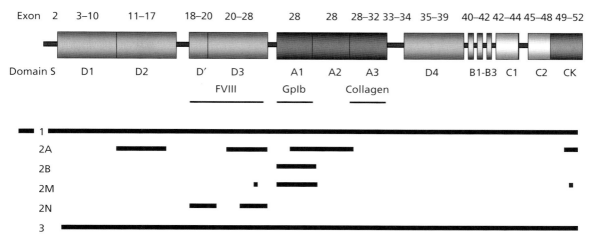

Figure 10.1 Organization of the von Willebrand factor (VWF) protein, its' binding activities and mutation location. The top panel indicates *VWF* exons that encode protein domains, along with ligand binding sites. The lower panel illustrates reported mutation location in different von Willebrand disease (VWD) types.

offered and the risk of the same disease type in family members can be understood. It can be challenging to differentiate between male sufferers of and (symptomatic) female carriers of mild hemophilia A and those with type 2N VWD. Similarly, platelet-type VWD can be difficult to discriminate from type 2B VWD. Without access to the full range of phenotypic analysis, it can be challenging to discriminate types 2A, 2B, and 2M from one another. The disorders can be differentiated using genetic analysis. Families with severe type 3 VWD may request carrier diagnosis that is not reliably assessed by phenotypic studies or prenatal diagnosis (PND) and may wish to investigate the possibility of pre-implantation genetic diagnosis (PGD), although the latter has yet to be described for VWD. Knowledge of the mutation(s) responsible for the disease in the family can help to facilitate these processes.

Range of genetic defects that contribute to VWD

Missense mutations

The replacement of an amino acid by a different residue can lead to a specific VWF function being perturbed; such mutations are responsible for the majority of type 2 VWD. They can result in, for example, an increase (type 2B) or decrease (types 2A and 2M) in binding affinity for platelet glycoprotein GPIb or decrease in affinity for FVIII (type 2N) and additionally can interfere with intra- and intermolecular interactions required for dimer and multimer formation, particularly through loss/gain of cysteine residues. Missense mutations can also lead to VWF that is retained within the cell [5–10]; this can contribute to the qualitative type 1 and 3 variants of VWF or VWF that is more rapidly cleared from the circulation in type 1 VWD [11–13].

Null mutations

A number of mutation types can result in a lack of VWF protein secretion. These include nonsense, some splice, insertion, and deletion mutations that disrupt the protein reading frame. Heterozygous null alleles alone often cause no symptoms of VWD; Nichols *et al.* compiled data from eight studies on 190 heterozygous carriers of type 3 VWD and reported that 15% had some bleeding symptoms while 62% had a VWF level of <50 IU/dL [14]. Null mutations comprise up to 90% of the molecular defects in type 3 VWD (Table 10.1) [19].

Nonsense mutations

Nonsense mutations can lead to premature termination of the VWF protein and a mismatch in length

115

Table 10.1 Mutation detection and null allele proportion in type 3 VWD.

Study	No. IC	Ethnicity (no.)	Screening method	No. alleles	No. mutation detected	% mutation detected	No. null	% null
Sutherland [15]	20	British (11), Asian (9)	Seq 2–52 & RNA	40	38	95	37	97
Gupta [16]	27	Indian (21), Greek (6)	Seq 2–52	54	45	83	40	89
Baronciani [17]	40	Italian (12), Iranian (14), Indian (14)	SSCP 1–52	80	80	100	66	83
Zhang [18]	24	Swedish	Seq Pro-52	48	42	88	38	90
TOTAL	111	—	—	222	205	92	181	88

IC, index cases.

between the protein and its mRNA template. In some circumstances, this can lead to nonsense-mediated decay [20–22] whereby residual mRNA is degraded. Recent analysis of patient platelet mRNA suggests that this mechanism does not always occur for VWF [23]. Nonsense mutations lead to lack of VWF expression from the affected allele. They are commonly seen in recessive VWD types (types 3, 2N, 2A) and more rarely in dominant type 1 VWD [24,25].

Splice

Disruption of the invariant GT and AG dinucleotides at the 5′ and 3′ ends of each intron generally results in complete lack of recognition of these signals. Mutation away from the GT and AG dinucleotides can also result in aberrant splicing [26]. In *VWF* to date, candidate pathogenic alterations are reported from −4 bp to +7 bp from intron/exon boundaries [17,27]. Mutation can lead to exonic sequence being omitted from the mRNA (exon skipping, a common result of splice site mutation), activation of cryptic splice sites, creation of a pseudo-exon from intronic sequence, or intron retention [28].

Insertion/deletion

Most insertion/deletion mutations are of a single nucleotide, but some affect a small number of nucleotides and these alterations are often at repeated

sequence motifs [17]. A single C deletion (c.2435delC; p.P812fs) has been reported as the most frequent central/northern European mutation in type 3 VWD and was found on 50%, 75%, and 20% of type 3 VWD alleles in the Swedish, Polish, and German populations, respectively [29,30]. More rarely reported mutations result in deletion of one or more exons. Where present in the homozygous form, the latter can readily be detected owing to lack of PCR amplification of affected exons. In heterozygotes, a technique to detect altered exon dosage/copy number is required. Recombination between Alu repeat sequences is often implicated in the pathogenesis of these mutations [31–33]. Large deletions have been reported in patients with type 3 VWD [27] and also recently in type 1, where the same inframe deletion of exon 4–5 can result in homozygous/compound heterozygous type 3 and in heterozygous type 1 VWD [33,34]. Deletions may be quite frequent in particular populations as a result of founder effect; a deletion of exons 1–3 is the most frequent mutation (25% alleles) in type 3 VWD in Hungary [30] and a large deletion of 253 kb including the complete *VWF* sequence and part of the neighboring *ANO2* locus has been repeatedly identified in German and Italian patients with type 3 VWD [35]. There is a single report of a multi-exon inframe deletion in type 2 VWD (subtype not defined) [36]. Similar deletion/insertion mutations that maintain the reading frame may result in a smaller or larger VWF protein being produced, with the effect of the mutation being dependent on the missing/additional amino acids. Splice mutations resulting in exon skipping may also result in inframe deletions and have been reported in type 1 and 2 VWD [25,37].

Promoter mutations

There were few reports on sequence variation in the *VWF* proximal promoter region (~3 kb 5′ to the translation start site) until three recent type 1 VWD studies were published [24,25,38]. The region back as far as c.–2813 was analyzed and several variants were identified. Few had previously been described as single nucleotide polymorphisms (SNPs), but analysis of ethnically matched healthy controls demonstrated presence of several variants in the control population [27,39], making their pathogenicity less likely. A small number of single nucleotide variants were absent from healthy controls and warrant further investigation. A 13 bp deletion (c.1522_1510del13) disrupting transcription factor binding sites is likely responsible for type 1 VWD in a Canadian patient with type 1 VWD [40].

Gene conversion

Mutation of *VWF* may result from a stretch of the pseudogene (*VWFP*) sequence invading *VWF* and replacing it [41]. Stretches of up to 335 bp of converted sequence have been reported. Gene conversion can be recognized where a number of sequential residues equivalent to the pseudogene rather than the gene sequence are present within sequence flanked by wild-type *VWF*. The resulting phenotype depends upon the pseudogene sequence(s) incorporated. c.3835G>A resulting in p.P1266L has been reported a number of times in type 2B VWD [42,43] and c.3931C>T resulting in p.Q1311X in type 3 VWD [16,44,45], in each case along with varied flanking sequence alterations [46].

VWF mutation analysis

Type 1

Type 1 VWD is a partial quantitative VWF deficiency where plasma VWF can contain mutant subunits but has normal function relative to VWF:Ag level. The proportion of HMW multimers is not decreased significantly [4]. Mutations have been identified in approximately 65% of patients with type 1 VWD in recent studies by analysis of the proximal promoter plus exons 2–52 [24,24,38]. Mutations were predominantly missense (80%), with splice, promoter, small insertion, deletion, and nonsense mutations constituting the remainder. Mutations were reported in codons 19–2804. Additionally, an inframe exon 4–5 deletion has recently been reported in patients from the UK [33], and this and similar copy number mutations may also contribute to type 1 VWD. Just over half of the point mutations were located in the central region of VWF encoded by exons 18–28; others were found throughout the remainder of the coding region. Most patients with type 1 VWD in whom candidate mutations were identified had a single heterozygous mutation. However, ~5% of patients with the lowest VWF levels (VWF:Ag < 15 IU/dL; FVIII:C < 40 IU/dL) were compound heterozygous for two different mutations [6,25]. Full ascertainment of mutations in patients with type 1 VWD may require analysis of the full coding region and flanking intronic and promoter sequences, along with dosage analysis to seek copy number changes (Figure 10.1; Table 10.2).

Genetic analysis can be useful where the etiology of the disorder is unclear. It has particular utility in cases with VWF levels below ~30 IU/dL where mutations usually can be detected [24,25]. Mutation identification can highlight the cause of the disease and recurrence risks in family members. Some mutations, such as p.R1205H, demonstrate rapid clearance from the circulation [12,48–51]. Their identification indicates that desmopressin treatment may have limited utility and that clotting factor concentrate may be the treatment of choice in some clinical circumstances. Patients with higher VWF levels (~45 IU/dL) often have incompletely penetrant disease, and mutations have been detected in only ~50% of these cases [24,25]. Incompletely penetrant mutations do not fully explain why the patient has symptoms of VWD, although blood group O contributes to reduced VWF level in this group. Mutation analysis is less useful in these cases, where it may be difficult both to attribute symptoms to a particular sequence variant and to predict the risk of VWD to family members inheriting the same variant [52].

Table 10.2 Summary of possible mutation analysis strategies in patients investigated for von Willebrand disease (VWD).

VWD type	Initial analysis of exons	Extended analysis of exons	Additional gene
1	18–28	2–17, 29–52, promoter, dosage analysis	—
2A	28	11–15, 52, remainder of gene	—
2B	28	None	*GPIBA* exons 1–2
2M	28	29–32, remainder of gene	—
2N	18–20	17, 24–25, 27 (remainder of gene only to seek null mutation)	*F8* exons 1–26, inversions & dosage analysis [47]
3	18–28	2–17, 29–52, dosage analysis	—

Types 2A, 2B, and 2M

Molecular analysis can be useful in clarifying the disease phenotype. Although analysis of VWF multimers is ideal, many laboratories distant from specialist centers do not perform this test and may use only VWF:Ag and a VWF "activity assay," for example a monoclonal antibody that binds a functional epitope of the A1 loop, rather than VWF:RCo or VWF:CB. Ristocetin-induced platelet aggregation (RIPA) may not always be available to help distinguish type 2B VWD. Analysis of exon 28, where the majority of mutations in these subtypes are located, can identify the defect and be used to confirm and subtype a dominant form of VWD. This includes differential diagnosis of 2A and 2M, where VWF:RCo is very much lower than VWF:Ag and multimers have not been analyzed, and between 2A and 2B, where HMW multimers are absent but RIPA has not been determined (Figure 10.1).

Type 2A

Patients with the type 2A VWD subtype have decreased VWF-dependent platelet adhesion plus a selective deficiency of HMW multimers. The majority of mutations lie in the A2 domain, encoded by the central portion of exon 28. Mutations are clustered around the ADAMTS13 cleavage site at p.Y1605-M1606, with the major location being amino acids 1458–1672. These all lead to dominantly inherited disease and comprised ~80% of reported 2A mutations [27] and patients diagnosed with 2A VWD in a large French study [53]. A small proportion are found in the A1 domain (p.1272–1383), encoded by the 5′ end of exon 28. Further groups of patients with type 2A have mutations in the D2 domain (exons 11–15; codons 404–625), the majority of which are recessively inherited and where patients are either homozygous for a missense change or compound heterozygous with a null second allele. Dominant mutations in the CK domain (exon 52; codons 2771–2773 plus 2801) cause dimerization defects of VWF monomers and subsequently a lack of HMW multimers [54]. An important new group of mutations in the D3 domain has recently been identified, resulting in type 2A (IIE) VWD (a subgroup defined by its distinct multimeric profile). This is reported to comprise 29% of all type 2A patients analyzed by the authors. Missense mutations affecting amino acids 956–1278 lie in exon 22 and 25–28, and a large proportion replace/introduce cysteine residues [55]. Where good quality multimer analysis is available, VWF mutation location is highlighted by differences in multimer profile [56].

Type 2M

This category comprises patients who have decreased VWF-dependent platelet adhesion without a selective deficiency of HMW multimers and includes mutations that disrupt VWF binding to platelets or to subendothelium [4]. Most of the relatively small number of reported 2M mutations lie in the GPIb binding site in the A1 domain (codons 1266–1467; Figure 10.1) and can be detected by sequencing the 5′ end of exon 28. A small number of mutations have been reported in exons 30–31 (codons 1731–1784) within the collagen-binding A3 domain [57,58]. Although fitting the 2M category, authors argued against inclusion of these changes under the 2M descriptor. Extension of mutation analysis to the A3 domain (exons 29–32), rarely analyzed in type 2 VWD, may identify further such mutations.

Type 2B/PT-VWD

Patients with type 2B VWD have an increased affinity for platelet GPIb but do not always have good phenotypic clues as to their disease etiology. Whereas in some cases VWF:Ag and VWF:RCo are reduced, along with HMW multimer loss and thrombocytopenia, in others enhanced RIPA is the only clue to their disease type. Genetic analysis can be useful to confirm/diagnose the phenotype. All reported 2B mutations are missense alterations or inframe insertions encoded by the 5′ end of exon 28 between codons 1266 and 1461 (Figure 10.1) [27,43]. This region can be amplified in a single amplicon and sequenced. Where mutations are absent, the phenocopy platelet-type (pseudo) VWD (PT-VWD) may be present [59]. This disorder leads to platelets that have a spontaneous affinity for VWF's GPIb binding site. Differential diagnosis can be achieved by identification of variants in exons 1–2 of the *GP1BA* gene, where missense mutations and an inframe deletion have been described [60,61].

Type 2N

Type 2N VWD includes variants with a markedly decreased binding affinity for FVIII. This is the main area for genetic analysis in VWD. Patient phenotype is frequently insufficient to distinguish type 2N from mild hemophilia A in males and (symptomatic) carriership for hemophilia A in females [62], where hemophilia carriership may be accompanied by skewed X-chromosome inactivation (Lyonization), unless there is sufficient history of bleeding in the family to determine inheritance pattern. The VWF:FVIIIB assay can identify patients with type 2N VWD but is not widely available and there is no current external quality assessment for the assay.

Type 2N VWD can result from three different inheritance patterns: homozygosity for a single missense 2N mutation; compound heterozygosity for two different 2N missense mutations; and compound heterozygosity for a 2N missense mutation plus a null allele, which can be anywhere in *VWF*. Although most patients with type 2N VWD have normal VWF multimers, abnormal multimers have been reported several times, particularly, but not only, in patients with loss or gain of a cysteine residue (Table 10.3). The effect on multimer profile ranges from partial or complete loss of HMW multimers to presence of supranormal multimers, and the pattern often appears smeary. Analysis of *VWF* in patients presenting with this mixed phenotype of reduced FVIII and abnormal multimers may be required to understand the phenotype. This is particularly true in cases such as p.C788R/Y, p.D879N, and p.C1225G, where mutations also result in intracellular retention, very reduced levels of VWF:Ag, and discrepantly low VWF:RCo [63–65].

There appears to be little consensus regarding exons that should be analyzed for type 2N VWD. The International Society on Thrombosis and Haemostasis Scientific and Standardization Committee on VWF (ISTH SSC VWF) mutation database (VWFdb) lists 25 different missense mutations in exons 17–20, 24, 25, and 27 in patients with type 2N VWD (Table 10.3; Figure 10.1) [27]. p.R924Q in exon 21 has also been associated with type 2N VWD, but appears not to result in an FVIII-binding defect [66]. Approximately 75% of mutations are in exons 18–20 [27,53]. p.R854Q is found in the heterozygous form in 2% of white people [67] and is by far the most frequent type 2N change. A large French study found this change in 40 of 51 (78%) patients with type 2N equally distributed between homozygous and compound heterozygous cases [53]. Where analysis of exons 17–20, 24, 25, and 27 identifies no candidate 2N mutation, it is unlikely that the patient has type 2N VWD. However, in compound heterozygous cases the second mutation may not be identified by analysis of only these exons, and 2N status may have to be inferred from a single missense mutation plus phenotype if the remaining exons are not analyzed. Where the second mutation leads to lack of VWF expression, VWF:Ag levels are typically ≤50 IU/dL [62]. *F8* gene analysis can be undertaken when no 2N missense *VWF* mutations are identified in patients originally analyzed for possible type 2N VWD [52].

Type 3

The laboratory phenotype of virtually undetectable VWF is often sufficient to diagnose this disorder.

Table 10.3 Type 2N von Willebrand disease mutations and their association with multimer profile.

Exon no.	Mutation	Cysteine change	AbM	Multimer profile
17	R760C	Yes	Yes	Supranormal, smeary
18	R763G	No	Yes	Supranormal, smeary
18	R782W	No	No	Normal
18	G785E	No	No	Normal
18	E787K	No	No	Normal
18	C788R	Yes	Yes	Absent HMW
18	C788Y	Yes	Yes	Absent HMW, smeary
18	T789P	No	No	Normal
18	A789P	No	No	Normal
18	T791M	No	No	Normal
18	Y795C	Yes	Yes	Supranormal, smeary
18	M800V	No	No	Normal
18	C804F	Yes	Yes	Slightly reduced HMW
18	P812L	No	No	Normal
19	R816W	No	No	Normal
19	R816Q	No	No	Normal
19	H817Q	No	No	Normal
20	R854W	No	No	Normal
20	R854Q	No	No	Normal
20	C858F	Yes	No	Normal
20	D879N	No	Yes	Reduced HMW
24	Q1053H	No	Yes	Supranormal
24	C1060R	Yes	Yes	Slightly reduced HMW
25	E1078K	No	No	Normal
27	C1225G	Yes	Yes	Absent HMW

AbM, abnormal multimers; HMW, high molecular weight.

Genetic analysis may be requested to identify unaffected mutation carriers among family members and to enable prenatal diagnosis (PND). Analysis requires sequencing/mutation scanning of the entire VWF coding region and intron–exon boundaries (exons 2–52; Figure 10.1) and the seeking of large heterozygous deletions. However, in particular European populations (Scandinavia, Germany, Eastern Europe) the high frequency of c.2435delC allows easy pre-screening for this mutation [30]. Mutations are currently found on approximately 90% of alleles (Table 10.1). Where two mutations are identified in the index case, one inherited from each parent, PND can be offered by seeking the mutations in a fetus. This is often undertaken by chorionic villus analysis at 11–13 weeks' gestation. Where both mutations are not identified, linkage analysis can be used to track inheritance of the affected alleles in the family instead [52].

Laboratory analysis

Many laboratories undertake analysis of mutations responsible for type 2 VWD as very limited VWF regions can be targeted. Minimal analysis of exons 18–20 for type 2N VWD and exon 28 for 2A, 2B, and 2M are offered, often with further analysis for exons harboring 2A and 2N mutations.

For types 1 and 3, the full protein-coding region (exons 2–52) requires analysis. Most mutation detection uses direct DNA sequencing, although other strategies including specific analysis for common point mutations and mutation scanning, including conformation sensitive gel electrophoresis (CSGE), denaturing high-performance liquid chromatography (dHPLC), and single-strand conformation polymorphism (SSCP) analysis have been used [17,25,68–70]. Services are listed on laboratories' own websites and on genetic testing directories such as GeneTests [71] and Orphanet [72].

Where DNA sequence analysis is used, primers designed to amplify using a single set of conditions in a 96-well format [73], possibly along with use of polymerase chain reaction (PCR) primers tailed with a common sequence such as M13 to facilitate DNA sequencing using single common forward and reverse primers, simplify laboratory work [52,69]. Where sequence quality is reliably good, initial analysis can be in a single direction only [73]. Confirmation of any candidate mutation is always achieved by fresh PCR amplification from the original sample and sequencing in both orientations [52].

Dosage analysis

Identification of partial or complete gene deletions can be achieved by use of dosage analysis. When a particular deletion has been identified, a mutation-specific "gap" PCR can be designed [32,35,74]. Alternatively, a screening technique such as multiplex ligation-dependant probe amplification (MLPA) can be used to seek unknown deletion/duplication mutations [75–77].

Platelet VWF mRNA analysis

Although genomic DNA (gDNA), generally isolated from blood leukocytes, is the main template used for *VWF* genetic analysis, *VWF* mRNA can be readily obtained from platelets as an alternative template. mRNA is considerably less robust than gDNA, but once used to generate cDNA (complementary DNA) has the advantages of requiring a much smaller number of amplicons (about 14) [15,78] than gDNA (56), lacking amplification of the pseudogene, and the potential to identify splice mutations through both aberrantly sized amplicons on gel electrophoresis and by DNA sequence analysis.

Mutation detection challenges

The *VWF* gene can be taxing to analyze for several reasons:
1 *VWF* is large, with 51 protein-coding exons. The majority of exons can be amplified and sequenced in a single amplicon, or sometimes together where inter-

vening introns are small [73]. However, exon 28 is 1.4 kb and requires overlapping amplicons (typically 2–6) for its analysis.
2 The pseudogene, *VWFP*, has a 97% sequence similarity to *VWF* across exons 23–34. PCR primer design must incorporate gene–pseudogene mismatches to prevent amplification of both *VWF* and *VWFP*, severely restricting PCR primer locations.
3 The gene is highly polymorphic, with more than 1458 variants described in *VWF* and immediately flanking the 5′ and 3′ sequence [27,79]. SNPs beneath the 3′ end of PCR primers can reduce or prevent amplification of an allele with a mismatch to the primer, leading to mono-allelic amplification. This can result in mutations being missed [80,81] or patients appearing to be homozygous for a mutation when they are actually heterozygous [82]. This again restricts PCR primer locations.
4 The high number of polymorphisms limits the utility of mutation scanning methods, which only identify that an amplicon has a sequence variant within it. Most individuals are heterozygous for SNPs throughout *VWF* and will thus generate several amplicons that require subsequent DNA sequencing. CSGE analysis of *VWF* required subsequent sequencing for an average of 16 of 56 (29%) amplicons [68]. Exon 28 has too many SNPs for any mutation scanning strategy to be useful (currently 38 reported [27]) and is usually only sequenced.
5 The entire *VWF* gene has been investigated for mutations in a relatively small number of individuals and knowledge of the extent of its "normal" variation, particularly in non-white populations, is not yet well understood. It can be challenging to determine whether novel sequence variants are likely to be pathogenic or neutral.

Mutation analysis resources

To counteract some of the challenges described above, a plethora of online resources is available.
1 A UK guideline provides a framework for the best laboratory practice in VWD genetic diagnosis [52].
2 Standard reference sequences, which should remain stable over a number of years, are available for many genes through the National Center for Biotechnology Information (NCBI) Reference Sequence (RefSeq)

collection [83]. RefSeq for genomic DNA, cDNA, and protein can be used to compare any sequence variants identified in patients.

3 A standard system has been devised by the Human Genome Variation Society (HGVS) for numbering DNA and protein sequences from the common start point of the initiator methionine codon. The website [84] describes how all sequence variants can be described using the standardized system. Use of HGVS nomenclature is recommended by the ISTH SSC VWF [85].

4 Several previously published *VWF* primer sets are available in the literature, but these may incorporate recently described SNPs. The SNPCheck tool [86] can be used to seek unwanted SNPs within proposed primer sequences. The SNP database (dbSNP) [79] and VWF database (VWFdb) [27] both list *VWF* SNPs along with their population frequency where known.

5 A variety of sequence analysis packages are available to help discriminate variant sequences from reference sequences and to identify the location and nature of any variant present, including the freeware Staden [15,87] and Mutation Surveyor (Soft Genetics, State College, Pennsylvania, USA; www.softgenetics.com/2/mutationSurveyor.html) [69].

6 A guideline from UK and Dutch molecular genetics societies recommends a systematic examination of all the available evidence to try and reach a conclusion regarding pathogenicity of novel sequence variants [88].

7 Previously described mutations in *VWF* are listed on VWFdb [27]; mutations in *GP1BA* resulting in PT-VWD are listed on the PT-VWD registry [60], while mutations in these and other genes are also listed on the human gene mutation database (HGMD) [89]. Polymorphism and mutation databases are the first resources used in determining whether a newly identified sequence variant has been previously reported. Where a variant is not listed on these online resources, a literature search using both standard tools such as PubMed as well as those that interrogate literature content such as Google and Google Scholar can be used to search for mention of the variant. Both current and previous VWF numbering are required (legacy cDNA numbering initiated at the start of the mRNA, 250 nucleotides 5′ to the HGVS ATG start site. Protein numbering was from the start of the mature VWF sequence, 764 amino acids from the first

methionine). For variants that have been reported previously on databases or in the literature, examination of the rationale by which pathogenicity or neutrality was decided can sometimes lead to alternative conclusions.

8 Where there is no evidence for the variant having been previously reported or evidence is inconclusive, splice site and protein prediction tools plus other online resources can be used to help reach a conclusion regarding likely pathogenicity [88]. Recent analysis in *BRCA* genes suggests that combined use of a number of *in silico* tools can reasonably accurately predict whether a sequence variant is likely to affect mRNA splicing [90]. It is more difficult to predict what the exact effect will be, however, particularly where a number of different transcripts may be generated as a result of mutation. Tools that predict exonic and intronic splice enhancer sequences are not yet considered sufficiently well developed to use in diagnostic work [88].

Several tools are available for amino acid substitution analysis. These use sequence and/or structure to predict the likelihood of an effect on protein function [91,92]. Packages such as Alamut mutation interpretation software [93] combine several of the above analyses into a single tool, speeding up variant interpretation.

Laboratory analysis of unclassified variants

For possible SNPs, availability of data on population frequency in healthy controls can help to verify whether the variant is part of normal variation. Where these data are unavailable, analysis of an ethnically matched population for the presence of the variant can help to indicate its status [88].

In vitro mutation analysis

Where *in silico* tools are uninformative as to pathogenicity, *in vitro* analysis may help to determine whether a sequence variant is pathogenic or not. These analyses are generally outside the scope of diagnostic service provision, but may sometimes be adopted where resources are available.

Splice site analysis

Where patient platelet mRNA is not available for analysis of the effect of a putative splice site mutation, cloning of the exon plus surrounding flanking intronic sequences containing the variant into a minigene vector can allow *in vitro* expression of a short chimeric mRNA. cDNA sequence analysis can indicate whether the candidate mutation is likely to influence splicing, for example by leading to exon skipping [25].

Protein expression

For candidate missense mutations, cloning of only the single nucleotide variant into a full-length *VWF* cDNA in an expression vector followed by transfection into a mammalian cell line can be utilized. Basic analysis consists of determining the quantity of both secreted and intracellular (cell lysate) VWF protein and analysis of multimer profile compared with that obtained for wild type and for 1:1 mutant:wild-type vector ratios (to mimic the heterozygous state). Similarity of VWF levels and multimer profiles obtained to those in patient plasma confirms likely pathogenicity. Such investigation has been used for many type 2 VWD missense mutations [27], a small number of type 3 missense changes [7,10], and type 1 VWD alterations [5,94]. This work has also illustrated that some sequence variants are unlikely to be pathogenic as missense mutations (p.G19R, p. P2063S, p.R2313H) [5].

Acknowledgements

The authors acknowledge support from the European Community Fifth Framework Programme (QLG1-CT-2000–00387) and National Institutes of Health Zimmerman Program for Molecular and Clinical Biology of VWD (HL-081588).

References

1 Ruggeri ZM. Von Willebrand factor, platelets and endothelial cell interactions. *J Thromb Haemost* 2003; **1**: 1335–42.

2 Sadler JE. Biochemistry and genetics of von Willebrand factor. *Annu Rev Biochem* 1998; **67**: 395–424.

3 Mancuso DJ, Tuley EA, Westfield LA, *et al.* Structure of the gene for human von Willebrand factor. *J Biol Chem* 1989; **264**: 19514–27.

4 Sadler JE, Budde U, Eikenboom JC, *et al.* Update on the pathophysiology and classification of von Willebrand disease: a report of the Subcommittee on von Willebrand Factor. *J Thromb Haemost* 2006; **4**: 2103–14.

5 Eikenboom J, Hilbert L, Ribba AS, *et al.* Expression of 14 von Willebrand factor mutations identified in patients with type 1 von Willebrand disease from the MCMDM-1VWD study. *J Thromb Haemost* 2009; **7**: 1304–12.

6 Eikenboom JC, Castaman G, Vos HL, *et al.* Characterization of the genetic defects in recessive type 1 and type 3 von Willebrand disease patients of Italian origin. *Thromb Haemost* 1998; **79**: 709–17.

7 Schneppenheim R, Budde U, Obser T, *et al.* Expression and characterization of von Willebrand factor dimerization defects in different types of von Willebrand disease. *Blood* 2001; **97**: 2059–66.

8 Tjernberg P, Vos HL, Castaman G, *et al.* Dimerization and multimerization defects of von Willebrand factor due to mutated cysteine residues. *J Thromb Haemost* 2004; **2**: 257–65.

9 Tjernberg P, Vos HL, Spaargaren-van Riel CC, *et al.* Differential effects of the loss of intrachain- versus interchain–disulfide bonds in the cystine-knot domain of von Willebrand factor on the clinical phenotype of von Willebrand disease. *Thromb Haemost* 2006; **96**: 717–24.

10 Baronciani L, Federici AB, Cozzi G, *et al.* Expression studies of missense mutations p.D141Y, p.C275S located in the propeptide of von Willebrand factor in patients with type 3 von Willebrand disease. *Haemophilia* 2008; **14**: 549–55.

11 Castaman G, Lethagen S, Federici AB, *et al.* Response to desmopressin is influenced by the genotype and phenotype in type 1 von Willebrand disease (VWD): results from the European Study MCMDM-1VWD. *Blood* 2008; **111**: 3531–9.

12 Casonato A, Pontara E, Sartorello F, *et al.* Reduced von Willebrand factor survival in type Vicenza von Willebrand disease. *Blood* 2002; **99**: 180–4.

13 Davies JA, Collins PW, Hathaway LS, *et al.* von Willebrand factor: evidence for variable clearance in vivo according to Y/C1584 phenotype and ABO blood group. *J Thromb Haemost* 2008; **6**: 97–103.

14 Nichols WL, Hultin MB, James AH, *et al.* von Willebrand disease (VWD): evidence-based diagnosis and management guidelines, the National Heart, Lung, and Blood Institute (NHLBI) Expert Panel report (USA). *Haemophilia* 2008; **14**: 171–232.

15 Sutherland MS, Keeney S, Bolton-Maggs PH, Hay CR, Will A, Cumming AM. The mutation spectrum associated with type 3 von Willebrand disease in a cohort of patients from the north west of England. *Haemophilia* 2009; **15**: 1048–57.

16 Gupta PK, Saxena R, Adamtziki E, *et al.* Genetic defects in von Willebrand disease type 3 in Indian and Greek patients. *Blood Cells Mol Dis* 2008; **41**: 219–22.

17 Baronciani L, Cozzi G, Canciani MT, *et al.* Molecular defects in type 3 von Willebrand disease: updated results from 40 multiethnic patients. *Blood Cells Mol Dis* 2003; **30**: 264–70.

18 Zhang ZP, Blomback M, Egberg N, *et al.* Characterization of the von Willebrand factor gene (VWF) in von Willebrand disease type III patients from 24 families of Swedish and Finnish origin. *Genomics* 1994; **21**: 188–93.

19 Eikenboom JC. Congenital von Willebrand disease type 3: clinical manifestations, pathophysiology and molecular biology. *Best Pract Res Clin Haematol* 2001; **14**: 365–79.

20 Silva AL, Romao L. The mammalian nonsense-mediated mRNA decay pathway: to decay or not to decay! Which players make the decision? *FEBS Letters* 2009; **583**: 499–505.

21 Rebbapragada I, Lykke-Andersen J. Execution of nonsense-mediated mRNA decay: what defines a substrate? *Curr Opin Cell Biol* 2009; **21**: 394–402.

22 Nicholson P, Yepiskoposyan H, Metze S, *et al.* Nonsense-mediated mRNA decay in human cells: mechanistic insights, functions beyond quality control and the double-life of NMD factors. *Cell Mol Life Sci* 2009; **67**: 677–700.

23 Plate M, Duga S, Baronciani L, *et al.* Premature termination codon mutations in the Von Willebrand factor gene are associated with allele-specific and position-dependent mRNA decay. *Haematologica* 2009; **95**: 172–4.

24 James PD, Notley C, Hegadorn C, *et al.* The mutational spectrum of type 1 von Willebrand disease: Results from a Canadian cohort study. *Blood* 2007; **109**: 145–54.

25 Goodeve A, Eikenboom J, Castaman G, *et al.* Phenotype and genotype of a cohort of families historically diagnosed with type 1 von Willebrand disease in the European study, Molecular and Clinical Markers for the Diagnosis and Management of Type 1 von Willebrand Disease (MCMDM-1VWD). *Blood* 2007; **109**: 112–21.

26 Gallinaro L, Sartorello F, Pontara E, *et al.* Combined partial exon skipping and cryptic splice site activation as a new molecular mechanism for recessive type 1 von Willebrand disease. *Thromb Haemost* 2006; **96**: 711–16.

27 ISTH-VWF-SSC. International Society on Thrombosis and Haemostasis Scientific and Standardization Committee VWF Information Homepage. www.vwf.group. shef.ac.uk [Accessed October 2009]

28 Rogan PK, Faux BM, Schneider TD. Information analysis of human splice site mutations. *Hum Mutat* 1998; **12**: 153–71.

29 Zhang ZP, Falk G, Blomback M, *et al.* A single cytosine deletion in exon 18 of the von Willebrand factor gene is the most common mutation in Swedish vWD type III patients. *Hum Mol Genet* 1992; **1**: 767–8.

30 Schneppenheim R, Budde U. Phenotypic and genotypic diagnosis of von Willebrand disease: a 2004 update. *Semin Hematol* 2005; **42**: 15–28.

31 Xie F, Wang X, Cooper DN, *et al.* A novel Alu-mediated 61-kb deletion of the von Willebrand factor (VWF) gene whose breakpoints co-locate with putative matrix attachment regions. *Blood Cells Mol Dis* 2006; **36**: 385–91.

32 Mohl A, Marschalek R, Masszi T, *et al.* An Alu-mediated novel large deletion is the most frequent cause of type 3 von Willebrand disease in Hungary. *J Thromb Haemost* 2008; **6**: 1729–35.

33 Sutherland MS, Cumming AM, Bowman M, *et al.* A novel deletion mutation is recurrent in von Willebrand disease types 1 and 3. *Blood* 2009; **114**: 1091–8.

34 Goodeve AC. When 1 plus 1 equals 3 in VWD. *Blood* 2009; **114**: 933–4.

35 Schneppenheim R, Castaman G, Federici AB, *et al.* A common 253-kb deletion involving VWF and TMEM16B in German and Italian patients with severe von Willebrand disease type 3. *J Thromb Haemost* 2007; **5**: 722–8.

36 Bernardi F, Patracchini P, Gemmati D, *et al.* In-frame deletion of von Willebrand factor A domains in a dominant type of von Willebrand disease. *Hum Mol Genet* 1993; **2**: 545–8.

37 James PD, O'Brien LA, Hegadorn CA, *et al.* A novel type 2A von Willebrand factor mutation located at the last nucleotide of exon 26 (3538G>A) causes skipping of 2 nonadjacent exons. *Blood* 2004; **104**: 2739–45.

38 Cumming A, Grundy P, Keeney S, *et al.* An investigation of the von Willebrand factor genotype in UK patients diagnosed to have type 1 von Willebrand disease. *Thromb Haemost* 2006; **96**: 630–41.

39 Hickson N. Molecular and Clinical Biology of Type 1 VWD [PhD thesis]. University of Sheffield, 2009.

40 Othman M, Chirinian Y, Brown C, *et al.* Functional characterisation of 13-bp deletion mutation (−1255_− 1510del13) in the promoter of the von Willebrand factor gene in type 1 von Willebrand disease. *Blood* 2010. doi: blood-2009-12-261131[pii]10.1182/blood-2009-12-261131.

41 Chen JM, Cooper DN, Chuzhanova N, *et al.* Gene conversion: mechanisms, evolution and human disease. *Nat Rev Genet* 2007; **8**: 762–75.

42 Baronciani L, Federici AB, Castaman G, *et al.* Prevalence of type 2B "Malmo/New York" von Willebrand disease in Italy: the role of von Willebrand factor gene conversion. *J Thromb Haemost* 2008; **6**: 887–90.

43 Federici AB, Mannucci PM, Castaman G, *et al.* Clinical and molecular predictors of thrombocytopenia and risk of bleeding in patients with von Willebrand disease type 2B: a cohort study of 67 patients. *Blood* 2009; **113**: 526–34.

44 Gupta PK, Adamtziki E, Budde U, *et al.* Gene conversions are a common cause of von Willebrand disease. *Br J Haematol* 2005; **130**: 752–8.

45 Surdhar GK, Enayat MS, Lawson S, *et al.* Homozygous gene conversion in von Willebrand factor gene as a cause of type 3 von Willebrand disease and predisposition to inhibitor development. *Blood* 2001; **98**: 248–50.

46 Goodeve A. von Willebrand disease: molecular aspects. In: Lee C, Berntorp E, Hoots K (eds.). *Textbook of Haemophilia*. 2nd edn. John Wiley and Sons Ltd, 2010, pp. 278–85.

47 Keeney S, Mitchell M, Goodeve A. The molecular analysis of haemophilia A: a guideline from the UK haemophilia centre doctors' organization haemophilia genetics laboratory network. *Haemophilia* 2005; **11**: 387–97.

48 Haberichter SL, Balistreri M, Christopherson P, *et al.* Assay of the von Willebrand factor (VWF) propeptide to identify patients with type 1 von Willebrand disease with decreased VWF survival. *Blood* 2006; **108**: 3344–51.

49 Haberichter SL, Castaman G, Budde U, *et al.* Identification of type 1 von Willebrand disease patients with reduced von Willebrand factor survival by assay of the VWF propeptide in the European study: molecular and clinical markers for the diagnosis and management of type 1 VWD (MCMDM-1VWD). *Blood* 2008; **111**: 4979–85.

50 Lenting PJ, Westein E, Terraube V, *et al.* An experimental model to study the in vivo survival of von Willebrand factor. Basic aspects and application to the R1205H mutation. *J Biol Chem* 2004; **279**: 12102–9.

51 Castaman G, Tosetto A, Rodeghiero F. Reduced von Willebrand factor survival in von Willebrand disease: pathophysiologic and clinical relevance. *J Thromb Haemost* 2009; **7** (Suppl. 1): 71–4.

52 Keeney S, Bowen D, Cumming A, *et al.* The molecular analysis of von Willebrand disease: a guideline from the UK Haemophilia Centre Doctors' Organisation Haemophilia Genetics Laboratory Network. *Haemophilia* 2008; **14**: 1099–111.

53 Meyer D, Fressinaud E, Gaucher C, *et al.* Gene defects in 150 unrelated French cases with type 2 von Willebrand disease: from the patient to the gene. INSERM Network on Molecular Abnormalities in von Willebrand Disease. *Thromb Haemost* 1997; **78**: 451–6.

54 Schneppenheim R, Brassard J, Krey S, *et al.* Defective dimerization of von Willebrand factor subunits due to a Cys->Arg mutation in type IID von Willebrand disease. *Proc Natl Acad Sci U S A* 1996; **93**: 3581–6.

55 Schneppenheim R, Michiels JJ, Obser T, *et al.* A cluster of mutations in the D3 domain of von Willebrand factor correlates with a distinct subgroup of von Willebrand disease: type 2A/IIE. *Blood* 2010. **115**: 4894–901.

56 Budde U, Pieconka A, Will K, *et al.* Laboratory testing for von Willebrand disease: contribution of multimer analysis to diagnosis and classification. *Semin Thromb Hemost* 2006; **32**: 514–21.

57 Ribba AS, Loisel I, Lavergne JM, *et al.* Ser968Thr mutation within the A3 domain of von Willebrand factor (VWF) in two related patients leads to a defective binding of VWF to collagen. *Thromb Haemost* 2001; **86**: 848–54.

58 Riddell AF, Gomez K, Millar CM, *et al.* Characterization of W1745C and S1783A: 2 novel mutations causing defective collagen binding in the A3 domain of von Willebrand factor. *Blood* 2009; **114**: 3489–96.

59 Enayat MS, Guilliatt AM, Lester W, *et al.* Distinguishing between type 2B and pseudo-von Willebrand disease and its clinical importance. *Br J Haematol* 2006; **133**: 664–6.

60 PT-VWD-Registry. Registry on platelet type von Willebrand disease. http://www.pt-vwd.org/ [Accessed October 2009]

61 Franchini M, Montagnana M, Lippi G. Clinical, laboratory and therapeutic aspects of platelet-type von Willebrand disease. *Int J Lab Hematol* 2008; **30**: 91–4.

62 Schneppenheim R, Budde U, Krey S, *et al.* Results of a screening for von Willebrand disease type 2N in patients with suspected haemophilia A or von Willebrand disease type 1. *Thromb Haemost* 1996; **76**: 598–602.

63 Allen S, Abuzenadah AM, Blagg JL, *et al.* Two novel type 2N von Willebrand disease-causing mutations that result in defective factor VIII binding, multimerization, and secretion of von Willebrand factor. *Blood* 2000; **95**: 2000–7.

64 Jorieux S, Fressinaud E, Goudemand J, *et al.* Conformational changes in the D' domain of von Willebrand factor induced by CYS 25 and CYS 95 mutations lead to factor VIII binding defect and multimeric impairment. *Blood* 2000; **95**: 3139–45.

65 Jorieux S, Gaucher C, Goudemand J, *et al.* A novel mutation in the D3 domain of von Willebrand factor markedly decreases its ability to bind factor VIII and affects its multimerization. *Blood* 1998; **92**: 4663–70.

66 Hickson N, Hampshire DJ, Winship PR, *et al.* Associations between the von Willebrand factor gene (VWF) variant c.2771G>A (p.R924Q), von Willebrand factor antigen (VWF:Ag) and FVIII activity (FVIII:C) levels and its role as a risk factor for type 1 von Willebrand disease (VWD). *J Thromb Haemost* 2010; **8**: 1986–93.

67 Eikenboom JC, Reitsma PH, Peerlinck KM, *et al.* Recessive inheritance of von Willebrand's disease type I. *Lancet* 1993; **341**: 982–6.

68 Soteh MH, Peake IR, Marsden L, *et al.* Mutational analysis of the von Willebrand factor gene in type 1 von Willebrand disease using conformation sensitive gel electrophoresis: a comparison of fluorescent and manual techniques. *Haematologica* 2007; **92**: 550–3.

69 Kakela JK, Friedman KD, Haberichter SL, *et al.* Genetic mutations in von Willebrand disease identified by DHPLC and DNA sequence analysis. *Mol Genet Metab* 2006; **87**: 262–71.

70 Baronciani L, Cozzi G, Canciani MT, *et al.* Molecular characterization of a multiethnic group of 21 patients with type 3 von Willebrand disease. *Thromb Haemost* 2000; **84**: 536–40.

71 GeneTests. GeneTests Website. www.ncbi.nlm.nih.gov/sites/GeneTests/?db=GeneTests [Accessed November 2009]

72 Orphanet. The portal for rare diseases and orphan drugs. www.orpha.net/consor/cgi-bin/index.php?lng=EN [Accessed October 2009]

73 Corrales I, Ramirez L, Altisent C, *et al.* Rapid molecular diagnosis of von Willebrand disease by direct sequencing. Detection of 12 novel putative mutations in VWF gene. *Thromb Haemost* 2009; **101**: 570–6.

74 Sutherland MS, Cumming AM, Bowman M, *et al.* A novel deletion mutation is recurrent in von Willebrand disease types 1 and 3. *Blood* 2009; **114**: 1091–8.

75 MRC-Holland. MRC-Holland MLPA homepage. http://www.mlpa.com/pages/indexpag.html [Accessed October 2009]

76 Schouten JP, McElgunn CJ, Waaijer R, *et al.* Relative quantification of 40 nucleic acid sequences by multiplex ligation-dependent probe amplification. *Nucl Acids Res* 2002; **30**: e57.

77 Acquila M, Bottini F, M DI Duca M, Vijzelaar R, Molinari AC, Bicocchi MP. Multiplex ligation-dependent probe amplification to detect a large deletion within the von Willebrand gene. *Haemophilia* 2009; **15**: 1346–8.

78 Berber E, James PD, Hough C, *et al.* An assessment of the pathogenic significance of the R924Q von Willebrand factor substitution. *J Thromb Haemost* 2009; **7**: 1672–9.

79 NCBI. db SNP. http://www.ncbi.nlm.nih.gov/projects/SNP/ [Accessed October 2009]

80 Thomas MR, Cutler JA, Savidge GF. Diagnostic and therapeutic difficulties in type 2A von Willebrand disease: resolution. *Clin Appl Thromb Hemost* 2006; **12**: 237–9.

81 Hampshire DJ, Burghel GJ, Goudemand J, *et al.* Polymorphic variation within the VWF gene contributes to the failure to detect mutations in patients historically diagnosed with type 1 VWD from the MCMDM-1VWD cohort. *Haematologica* 2010; doi: 10.3324/haematol.2010.027177.

82 Eikenboom JC, Reitsma PH, Briet E. Seeming homozygosity in type-IIB von Willebrand's disease due to a polymorphism within the sequence of a commonly used primer. *Ann Hematol* 1994; **68**: 139–41.

83 NCBI. RefSeq. http://www.ncbi.nlm.nih.gov/RefSeq/ [Accessed October 2009]

84 HGVS. Nomenclature for the description of sequence variations homepage. http://www.hgvs.org/mutnomen/ [Accessed October 2009]

85 Goodeve AC, Eikenboom JC, Ginsburg D, *et al.* A standard nomenclature for von Willebrand factor gene mutations and polymorphisms. On behalf of the ISTH SSC Subcommittee on von Willebrand factor. *Thromb Haemost* 2001; **85**: 929–31.

86 NGRL. SNPCheck. http://ngrl.manchester.ac.uk/SNPCheckV2/snpcheck.htm [Accessed October 2009]

87 Staden R. Staden Package. http://staden.sourceforge.net/ [Accessed November 2009]

88 Bell J, Bodmer D, Sistermans E, *et al.* Practice guidelines for the interpretation and reporting of unclassified variants (UVs) in clinical molecular genetics. http://cmgsweb.shared.hosting.zen.co.uk/BPGs/Best_Practice_Guidelines.htm [Accessed October 2009]

89 HGMD. The human gene mutation database at the Institute of Medical Genetics in Cardiff. http://www.hgmd.cf.ac.uk/ac/index.php [Accessed October 2009]

90 Vreeswijk MP, Kraan JN, van der Klift HM, *et al.* Intronic variants in BRCA1 and BRCA2 that affect RNA splicing can be reliably selected by splice-site prediction programs. *Hum Mutat* 2009; **30**: 107–14.

91 Ng PC, Henikoff S. Predicting the effects of amino acid substitutions on protein function. *Annu Rev Genomics Hum Genet* 2006; **7**: 61–80.

92 Thusberg J, Vihinen M. Pathogenic or not? And if so, then how? Studying the effects of missense mutations using bioinformatics methods. *Hum Mutat* 2009; **30**: 703–14.

93 Biosoftware I. Alamut—Mutation Interpretation Software. www.interactive-biosoftware.com/ [Accessed October 2009]

94 Eikenboom JC, Matsushita T, Reitsma PH, *et al.* Dominant type 1 von Willebrand disease caused by mutated cysteine residues in the D3 domain of von Willebrand factor. *Blood* 1996; **88**: 2433–41.

11 Clinical, laboratory, and molecular markers of type 1 von Willebrand disease

David Lillicrap[1], Francesco Rodeghiero[2], and Ian Peake[3]

[1]Department of Pathology and Molecular Medicine, Richardson Laboratory, Queen's University, Kingston, Canada

[2]Department of Hematology, San Bortolo Hospital, Vicenza, Italy

[3]Department of Cardiovascular Science, University of Sheffield Medical School, Sheffield, UK

Introduction

Since its original description in 1926, knowledge of the clinical and basic pathophysiologic aspects of von Willebrand disease (VWD) has advanced significantly. Overall, we now recognize that this common inherited bleeding disease represents a complex collection of quantitative and qualitative anomalies affecting the platelet-dependent and factor VIII (FVIII) binding functions of the plasma adhesive protein, von Willebrand factor (VWF).

Until the 1970s, aside from the obvious distinction of severe (type 3) forms of the condition, little was known about specific variant forms of the disease. However, through a variety of approaches, initially showing abnormal electrophoretic mobility of VWF, and later through the determination of abnormal binding to glycoprotein Ib (GPIb) and FVIII, it became apparent that, in addition to the common quantitative variants of VWD, there were a number of dysfunctional forms of the protein that also resulted in bleeding.

Currently, type 1 VWD is regarded as the most common form of the disease, with 60–80% of cases representing this quantitative trait. In the most recent version of the VWD classification scheme proposed by the International Society on Thrombosis and Haemostasis Subcommittee on von Willebrand Factor, the following features define type 1 disease (Table 11.1) [1]:

1 A partial quantitative deficiency of VWF.

2 Plasma VWF may contain mutant subunits, but has a normal function.

3 The proportion of large VWF multimers is not significantly reduced.

The epidemiology of type 1 VWD

While there is little doubt that VWD is the most common inherited bleeding disorder, there has not been a systematic evaluation of the prevalence of the various subtypes of the disease. Furthermore, the prevalence of VWD varies significantly depending on the design of the study. In two often quoted prospective epidemiologic studies performed on >1800 children, 0.8–1.3% of the participants showed evidence that was compatible with a diagnosis of VWD [2,3]. The disease definition required a personal and family history of excessive mucocutaneous bleeding and a VWF activity level, measured as the ristocetin cofactor, below the normal range. Without access to additional tests for VWF (e.g., VWF : Ag and VWF multimer analysis), the subtype determination of these cases remains uncertain. However, what is clear is that some of the ascertained cases showed sufficiently mild disease that, in the time since these original studies, very few of the participants originally diagnosed with VWD have had significant bleeding problems [4].

In a more recent study aiming to evaluate the impact of symptomatic VWD in primary care (family)

Von Willebrand Disease, 1st edition. Edited by Augusto B. Federici, Christine A. Lee, Erik E. Berntorp, David Lillicrap, Robert R. Montgomery. © 2011 Blackwell Publishing Ltd.

Table 11.1 Definition of type 1 von Willebrand disease (VWD).

Definition of type 1 VWD (ISTH SSC recommendation 2006)

Partial quantitative deficiency of VWF

Plasma VWF may contain mutant subunits but has normal function

The proportion of large VWF multimers is not significantly reduced

---

ISTH SSC, International Society on Thrombosis and Haemostasis Scientific and Standardization Committee; VWF, von Willebrand factor.

practice, a prevalence of VWD of ~0.1% was found in a review of 10,000 individuals [5]. Seven of the nine cases determined in this study showed features of type 1 VWD.

In surveys of patients with VWD seen at tertiary care inherited bleeding disorder clinics, type 1 VWD comprises 70–80% of cases enrolled [6].

Clinical features of type 1 VWD

Type 1 VWD presents with a highly variable range of mucocutaneous bleeding symptoms. While all of the influences regulating the bleeding phenotype in type 1 VWD have yet to be defined, the plasma level of VWF, gender, and age certainly contribute to this outcome. Bleeding symptoms are more likely with lower levels of VWF, and females and adults are more likely to report positive bleeding histories owing, at least in part, to the increased opportunities for manifesting symptoms in these two groups.

The range of mucocutaneous bleeding symptoms in type 1 VWD includes the following: easy bruising, menorrhagia, epistaxis, prolonged bleeding from wounds, bleeding post tooth extraction and surgery, and postpartum bleeding. Bleeding into soft tissues and joints can occur, but is very infrequent and is usually related to trauma. Owing principally to the relative lack of exposure to hemostatic challenges (particularly the avoidance of menses and childbirth), bleeding in type 1 VWD is less apparent in males and children.

Recently, the utility of formal bleeding scores has been reassessed in the context of type 1 VWD [7].

Given the fact that a personal history of excessive mucocutaneous bleeding is a key component of this diagnosis and that some of these symptoms are also reported by many unaffected individuals, a means of differentiating pathologic bleeding from normal variation would be helpful. Two studies in populations with type 1 VWD have provided support for the use of a standardized questionnaire and bleeding score to discriminate between unaffected individuals and those with VWD.

In the first study, 42 obligate carriers of type 1 VWD (individuals with affected offspring and at least one other first-degree relative with type 1 VWD) were compared with 215 healthy control individuals using a standardized bleeding questionnaire and scoring system [8]. In this study, individual bleeding symptoms were assigned scores of between 0 and 3 based on severity (no symptoms to hospitalization or transfusion therapy). The results of qualitative analysis from this study showed that, whereas 77% of the controls had never suffered from bleeding, 12% of the obligate carriers of type 1 VWD reported an absence of bleeding. The most common bleeding symptoms reported by the obligate carriers were bruising and bleeding after surgery. When three or more bleeding symptoms were present, the sensitivity and specificity for type 1 VWD diagnoses were 50% and 99.5%, respectively. In terms of the quantitative bleeding scores, in the controls a score of below or equal to 3 for males and 5 for females corresponded to the 98.8 and 99.2 percentiles, respectively. Use of an algorithm in which reports of bleeding post tooth extraction and cutaneous bleeding are assessed produced a positive predictive value of 8.9% and a negative predictive value of 99.8% for type 1 VWD in this report.

The second study to systematically evaluate bleeding symptoms in type 1 VWD accompanied the European Union-sponsored Molecular and Clinical Markers for the Diagnosis and Management of Type 1 VWD (MCMDM-1VWD) study. In this analysis, 907 participants (417 with type 1 VWD and 490 unaffected) were evaluated with the same standardized bleeding questionnaire used in the study described above [9]. The scoring system in this study was slightly modified to incorporate negative values for a lack of bleeding after events associated with a high risk of bleeding (tooth extractions, surgery, and post partum). The symptoms that showed the strongest association with type 1 VWD in this study were bleeding from minor wounds, surgical bleeding, cutaneous bleeding, and menorrhagia. In contrast, postpartum bleeding, oral bleeding, and gastrointestinal bleeding were documented as frequently in unaffected individuals as in those with type 1 VWD.

In the MCMDM-1VWD study there was a strong inverse correlation between all quintiles of the quantitative bleeding score and VWF:Ag, VWF:RCo, and FVIII:C. In addition, the bleeding score was higher in index cases of type 1 VWD than in other affected family members (scores 9 vs. 5; $P<0.0001$) despite the fact that the levels of VWF:Ag, VWF:RCo, and FVIII:C were similar in the two groups. This finding suggests that, in the context of a study setting, index cases are more likely to be diagnosed as a result of bleeding symptoms while other affected family members may be diagnosed based upon their laboratory evaluations. The other significant finding from this study was the observation that a mucocutaneous bleeding score, derived from the incidence of spontaneous bleeding events, predicted bleeding after surgery or tooth extraction at least as well as the plasma VWF and FVIII levels.

In summary, the recent literature indicates that the use of a standardized and validated bleeding questionnaire and scoring system provides significant benefit in making the diagnosis of type 1 VWD and also in predicting for future procedure-related bleeding in individuals with type 1.

The laboratory diagnosis of type 1 VWD

Type 1 VWD is defined as a partial deficiency state for plasma VWF. As such, it ought to be relatively easy to define the VWF threshold level below which this state exists. However, despite this seemingly straightforward criterion, the definition of the cut-off value for defining type 1 VWD continues to generate widespread debate and disagreement [10–12].

The use of screening tests of primary hemostasis, such as the bleeding time and PFA-100 (Siemens, Deerfield, IL, USA), may aid in the initial identification of individuals who potentially have type 1 VWD, but the key laboratory tests required to make this diagnosis are the VWF:Ag and VWF:RCo studies. In

type 1 VWD, these values should be both low and proportionately reduced such that the VWF:RCo to VWF:Ag ratio is >0.6 (although this value may vary between 0.5 and 0.7 depending upon individual laboratory reagents and testing protocols). The methodologies for the quantification of VWF:Ag levels are relatively robust and consistent, but the determination of VWF functional levels with the ristocetin cofactor assay is well recognized to be problematic in terms of standardization. There is no clear benefit from using another test for VWF function, such as collagen binding, in this context. In addition to the methodologic challenges posed by VWF, there are a number of environmental and genetic factors that also complicate the interpretation of VWF assay results [13]. These include the following:

1 transient elevations of VWF associated with acute physical stress;
2 elevations of VWF associated with prolonged periods of "stress," for example pregnancy;
3 fluctuations of VWF levels during the normal menstrual cycle;
4 elevations of VWF associated with estrogenic hormone use;
5 abnormal levels of thyroid hormones;
6 elevations of VWF associated with systemic pathologic states, for example infection or malignancy;
7 increases of VWF with increasing age; and
8 different normal ranges for VWF based on ABO blood type.

The environmental influences that regulate VWF levels cause significant fluctuations in plasma VWF levels and demand that repeat testing be performed when there is a significant clinical suggestion of VWD. Most clinicians would repeat testing 2–3 times when the clinical evidence for VWD is strong.

The cause of these variable VWF increments is, in most instances, unresolved, although the acute stress-related elevations of protein almost certainly result from the release of stored VWF from endothelial Weibel–Palade bodies. The cause of the chronic VWF elevations seen with estrogens and with increasing age likely relates to either transcriptional influences or to changes in the clearance rate of the protein.

Variations in VWF and FVIII levels during the menstrual cycle have been documented by several groups [14,15]. The lowest levels occur during menses and peak levels during the late follicular phase. These variances need to be kept in mind, but recommendations as to which levels represent the true baseline have differed.

Another factor that can influence VWF levels is ethnicity. African American individuals have VWF:Ag levels that are 15–20% higher than white individuals, but their VWF:RCo levels are similar [16].

As suggested above, there is no consensus on the VWF threshold level that defines a diagnosis of type 1 VWD. The main controversy centers on how one classifies individuals with VWF levels between 0.50 and 0.30 IU/mL. In most laboratories, these values would be below the normal range (2.5 lower percentile), but the association of these mildly reduced levels of VWF and bleeding is inconsistent, and VWF levels <0.40 IU/mL are more strongly associated with a diagnosis of type 1 VWD [17]. Spontaneous bleeding with mild deficiency of VWF would be expected to be very rare, but excessive postprocedural bleeding is still likely. Acceptance of the diagnosis of type 1 VWD with plasma VWF levels <0.30 IU/mL is less contentious, although some investigators have even suggested that this threshold is still too high [10].

While the measurement of VWF:Ag, VWF:RCo, and FVIII:C is routine in most tertiary care centers, appropriate quality assurance measures and the application of certified plasma standards must be ensured to validate the assay results.

Aside from the measurement of VWF:Ag, VWF:RCo, and FVIII:C levels, the initial evaluation of a potential case of type 1 VWD might also involve an evaluation of the VWF multimer pattern to rule out type 2 variant forms of the disease. However, if the VWF:RCo to VWF:Ag ratio is consistently >0.7, further investigation for a type 2 variant is probably not warranted. Recent studies in a large European population with type 1 VWD demonstrated multimer abnormalities in 38% of cases [18]. However, in most instances the abnormalities documented were subtle (usually subtle loss of the highest molecular-weight multimers) and only very rarely was there a more obvious loss of high-molecular-weight (HMW) VWF. It is anticipated that in most laboratories this level of discrimination will not be possible or diagnostically relevant.

The other plasma VWF assay that is beginning to be applied to VWD diagnosis is the VWF propeptide assay (VWFpp). The VWFpp is cleaved from the VWF mature monomer in the golgi apparatus and secreted into plasma as dimers. Recent studies have shown that comparison of VWFpp with VWF:Ag levels can be used as a surrogate for VWF survival time [19,20]. Thus, ratios of VWFpp to VWF:Ag >2 are suggestive of accelerated clearance of VWF from plasma, one of the pathogenetic mechanisms responsible for type 1 VWD. However, the VWFpp assay is still in the early phases of application, and widespread clinical testing will require additional validation on larger populations both with and without VWD.

The genetics of type 1 VWD

In most previous textbooks, type 1 VWD is defined as a classic autosomal dominant trait. However, recent evidence indicates that although the disease phenotype does manifest in the heterozygous state, the condition is more accurately described as a complex genetic trait in which multiple genetic and environmental modifiers influence the phenotypic outcome.

As an inherited disease, there is an expectation that a positive family history will be identified in most cases of type 1 VWD. However, the occurrence of this documentation is variable and likely relates to several phenomena: (i) penetrance of the type 1 VWD phenotype is incomplete; (ii) the phenotype shows variable expressivity; and finally (iii) the milder forms of the disease may be relatively asymptomatic, especially in males and children. In light of the various challenges with the clinical and laboratory assessment for type 1 VWD, a recent report has suggested the utilization of a probabilistic diagnostic approach using Bayesian methodology [21]. In this analysis, the likelihood ratios based upon plasma VWF levels and family history were the most influential factors in predicting a diagnosis of type 1 VWD.

Incomplete penetrance of type 1 VWD has been noted for over 30 years. Initial estimates of penetrance suggested that approximately 60% of individuals who had inherited the mutant VWF allele would be penetrant for the phenotype [22,23]. Recent molecular genetic studies provide evidence that, not surprisingly, penetrance varies with specific type 1 VWD mutations. Thus, the most common type 1 variant, Y1584C, has a penetrance of approximately 70% while other type 1 VWD mutations, such as R1315C and R1205H, show complete penetrance in the limited studies performed to date. In addition to incomplete penetrance, there is also longstanding evidence of variable expressivity of the type 1 VWD phenotype within families [22]. There is currently insufficient information available to comment upon the occurrence of this phenomenon with specific genotypes.

While mutations of the *VWF* gene have been the most obvious candidates to cause the type 1 VWD phenotype, there has been increasing evidence that other genetic factors also play a significant role in determining plasma levels of VWF. The best characterized and, to date, the most important of these genetic modifiers is the ABO blood group.

The role of ABO blood group and type 1 VWD

The fact that ABO blood type influences the plasma level of VWF and FVIII has been known for the past 25 years [24]. Individuals with blood group O have VWF and FVIII levels that are 25–30% lower than those in individuals with other blood groups. Given these findings, it is not surprising that individuals with blood group O are over-represented in type 1 VWD populations, whereas in type 2 VWD the various ABO blood types are found with their expected frequency.

Studies of mono- and dizygotic twins have documented that approximately 30% of the genetic variance of VWF : Ag levels is a result of an effect of the ABO blood group [25].

In addition to its complex pattern of N- and O-linked glycosylation, VWF is also modified by the addition of blood group A, B, and H oligosaccharides [26]. In those with blood group O, the presence of a glycosyl transferase null phenotype leaves the H antigen structure unmodified by further glycan addition. How this glycan difference influences plasma VWF levels has now been established by work from several groups (Table 11.2). Most importantly, studies establishing elimination half-lives of endogenously released VWF in individuals with different ABO blood types have shown that the half-life of those in group O is approximately 40% of those with other blood types (10 h vs. 25 h) [27]. This finding is supported by the discovery that VWFpp to VWF : Ag ratios in individuals in group O are increased compared with individuals in other blood groups (1.6

Table 11.2 Influence of ABO blood group on von Willebrand factor (VWF).

Plasma VWF levels 25–30% lower in group O
Accelerated clearance of group O VWF
Enhanced ADAMTS13-mediated proteolysis of group O VWF

vs. 1.2). The finding of increased VWFpp ratios has recently been associated with accelerated clearance of VWF from the circulation. The final observation that might also contribute to lower levels of plasma VWF is that ABO blood type also seems to influence the susceptibility of VWF to ADAMTS13-mediated cleavage, with group O VWF being more cleavable than non-group O protein [28].

Thus, epidemiologic studies indicate that individuals in blood group O have significantly lower plasma VWF and FVIII levels, and subsequent mechanistic investigations have documented an accelerated clearance of group O VWF from plasma. How does this influence the diagnosis of type 1 VWD in individuals in group O? We have no evidence that blood group O itself is associated with an increased tendency for bleeding, and thus current opinion is that blood group O status is one of the significant genetic modifiers of VWF levels in what is now recognized as a complex quantitative trait. The results of recent molecular genetic studies of >300 individuals with type 1 VWD in Canada and Europe indicate that the blood group O influence on lowering VWF levels is most evident in milder forms of type 1 disease (VWF levels 0.30–0.50 IU/mL) [29,30]. When the VWF level is <0.30 IU/mL, individuals in blood group O are no longer over-represented. All of these considerations should remove the need to establish ABO-specific normal ranges to quantify VWF levels.

Although there is no definitive evidence of a role for other glycan modifications in the pathogenesis of human type 1 VWD, there is further support for this mechanistic paradigm from the study of a mouse model of type 1 disease. In the RIIIS/J inbred mouse strain in which plasma VWF levels are low, the pathogenetic mechanism has been characterized as the ectopic expression of the enzyme *N*-acetylgalactosaminyltransferase in vascular endothelial cells [31]. This enzyme is usually expressed exclusively in the gut epithelium. The switch of cell type-specific expression of this glycosyl transferase alters the pattern of glycan modification of plasma VWF and the half-life of the modified VWF is markedly reduced, resulting in a deficit of the protein in plasma. This observation, along with the ABO blood group association, suggests that additional genetic modifiers of plasma VWF levels may play a role in post-translational modification (particularly glycosylation) of the protein and may alter its biosynthesis, secretion, or circulation dynamics.

VWF gene mutations and type 1 VWD

Until very recently, the molecular genetic pathology responsible for type 1 VWD was unknown. However, the report of three contemporaneous studies performed in Europe, the UK, and Canada, published in 2006–2007, has now provided molecular genetic information on 305 type 1 VWD index cases [29, 30,32] and there are ongoing studies in North America and Europe that will add to this knowledge.

Fortunately, the results of the three reported type 1 VWD genetic studies are very similar and suggest that, at least in patients with European ancestry, the findings in these initial studies are likely to be widely applicable.

The major findings in these initial 305 type 1 VWD index cases and their families were as follows:

1 The type 1 VWD phenotype showed linkage to the VWF gene in approximately 50% of families.
2 Candidate VWF gene mutations were identified in approximately 65% of index cases of type 1 VWD.
3 More than 100 different candidate VWF gene mutations have been identified (Table 11.3).

Table 11.3 von Willebrand factor gene mutations in type 1 von Willebrand disease.

Mutations	Frequency (%)
Missense	~60
Promotor variants	~15
Splicing	~10
Small deletions/insertions	~5
Nonsense	Rare

4 Approximately 60% of the candidate VWF mutations were missense substitutions.
5 In 15–20% of cases, more than one candidate VWF gene mutation has been identified.
6 VWF gene mutations are more likely to be found with lower plasma VWF levels (particularly <0.30 IU/mL).

In addition to these general observations, the European Union (EU) study was also able to make a number of pathogenetic determinations based upon a standard of multimer analysis not available in the other studies. Thus, where an abnormal VWF multimer pattern was seen (usually subtle loss of the high-molecular-weight forms), candidate VWF gene mutations were seen in 95% of index cases [29]. In contrast, where the multimer pattern was normal, 55% of cases had candidate VWF mutations.

The initial evidence of genetic heterogeneity from these recent studies came from the results of linkage analysis. In the EU study, in which larger type 1 families with more affected members were recruited, 70% of pedigrees showed linkage to the VWF gene [33]. However, when cases in which qualitative VWF variants were present were excluded, the proportion of linked cases fell to 50%. In comparison, in the Canadian study, where smaller families with fewer affected members were assessed, the proportion of pedigrees in whom the type 1 phenotype was linked to the VWF gene was 41% [34]. Thus, from these two formal genetic linkage analyses there is strong evidence that genetic loci other than VWF contain mutations that produce a type 1 VWD phenotype. These results complement the finding that there is an absence of candidate VWF gene mutations in approximately 35% of type 1 VWD index cases.

There is good evidence from the EU and Canadian studies that the likelihood of finding candidate VWF gene mutations is increased with lower plasma VWF levels. In the Canadian study mutations were found in 75% of index cases with VWF levels <0.30 IU/mL compared with only 49% of cases with levels >0.30 IU/mL [30]. The EU study found that candidate VWF mutations were 20-fold more likely when VWF levels were <0.15 IU/mL [29]. Nevertheless, there are occasional cases (2% in the Canadian study) in which very low VWF levels (<0.20 IU/mL) are not explained by sequence variation in the VWF promoter, the coding region, and splice sites.

Another issue that has been clarified by these initial molecular genetic studies is that type 1 VWD is very seldom a heterozygous form of type 3 VWD. Thus, null mutations—the cause of type 3 VWD—were found only in rare patients with type 1 disease.

Recurrent type I VWD candidate mutations

A number of recurring mutations have been reported in the initial cohorts of patients with type 1 VWD.

In all three studies the Y1584C variant was the most prevalent, with a frequency ranging from 8% to 15%. This missense substitution in the VWF A2 domain changes a highly conserved amino acid and inserts a new cysteine that appears from the molecular model of A2 to be solvent exposed. In the Canadian study, this substitution was associated with a founder polymorphic haplotype [35]. The heterozygous state for Y1584C is associated with VWF levels of around 0.40 IU/mL, whereas rare homozygotes for the mutation have had levels of approximately 0.25 IU/mL. The phenotypic penetrance for Y1584C is approximately 70% and the substitution is almost always accompanied by co-inheritance of blood group O in cases manifesting type 1 VWD. Studies addressing the potential pathogenic mechanisms of the Y1584C mutation have indicated that both intracellular retention and altered susceptibility to ADAMTS13-mediated proteolysis may contribute to the low VWF levels [35,36].

The second most frequent candidate mutation found in the 305 index cases of type 1 VWD was the R1205H "Vicenza" mutation. Approximately 3% of index cases were documented with this substitution and, in the EU study, this variant was almost always associated with an abnormal multimer pattern. The VWF levels associated with heterozygosity for R1205H are always <0.15 IU/mL and penetrance of this phenotype is 100%. Recent studies have confirmed that this missense substitution is associated with an accelerated clearance phenotype and that while the initial response to DDAVP (1-deamino-8-D-arginine vasopressin) infusion is excellent (5- to 10-fold VWF increment), this benefit is short lived [37]. Further discussion of the accelerated clearance phenotype follows below.

Other recurrent mutations have included R1315C (2% of cases; always associated with abnormal multimers in the EU study), R854Q, and R924Q. All of these substitutions occur within hypermutable arginine codons (owing to spontaneous deamination of the cytosine in CpG dinucleotide sequences). The mechanism through which the R854Q and R924Q variants result in low VWF levels is unclear. In its homozygous form, R854Q produces type 2N VWD, but this phenotype is recessive in nature. Investigation of the R924Q variant has shown that the glutamine-substituted VWF cDNA (complementary DNA) product produces no phenotype in *in vitro* studies; therefore, this sequence variant may act as a marker for another, as yet unidentified, pathogenic change.

Noncoding sequence variants in type 1 VWD

During the characterization of mutations in the initial 305 index type 1 VWD cases, several nucleotide variations have been identified in the 5′ flanking region of the *VWF* gene. These have included a C to T transition at nucleotide −1046 from the transcriptional start site in 2–7% of index cases and a 13 nucleotide deletion in the proximal *VWF* promoter in a Canadian patient with mild VWF deficiency. To date, the functional significance of these variations has not been confirmed and, in addition, there may be other transcriptional control elements further out in the 5′ or 3′ region of the gene whose disruption could result in a significant reduction in VWF expression.

Type 1 VWD and accelerated clearance of VWF

While a large spectrum of candidate *VWF* gene mutations has already been assembled, the pathogenic mechanisms associated with most of these variations is unresolved. This is especially true for most of the missense mutants. However, until recently, the major pathophysiologic focus was on biosynthetic and secretion defects—mechanisms that can be evaluated through *in vitro* expression studies.

One pathogenetic theme that has emerged recently is the contribution from accelerated clearance of

VWF (Table 11.4). The R1205H "Vicenza" variant represents the prototypic example of this phenotype and this mutant has now been shown to exhibit a markedly abbreviated plasma half-life of <2 h [37]. With the information currently available, the accelerated clearance phenotype in type 1 VWD appears to be associated with the following features [19,20]:

1 levels of baseline VWF:Ag <0.30 IU/mL and often <0.15 IU/mL;

2 an elevated (more than twofold up to >10-fold) ratio of the plasma VWFpp to VWF:Ag;

3 an exaggerated initial response to DDAVP (>fourfold and often >10-fold) but subsequent rapid decline in VWF levels (by 4 h);

4 plasma VWF half-lives of <3 h;

5 subtly abnormal VWF multimer patterns (either presence of suprahigh-molecular-weight forms or reduced satellite triplet bands); and

6 missense mutations in the D3 or D4-CK domains.

To date, the following *VWF* missense substitutions have been associated with this phenotype: R1205H, C1130F/G/R, W1144G, C1149R, all in the D3 domain, and S2179F and C2671Y in the D4-CK domains. Although systematic assessments of this phenotype are awaited, it seems that accelerated clearance may be responsible for 5–15% of type 1 cases. It has been proposed that this variant be referred to as type 1C (clearance) disease.

Future priorities in type 1 VWD characterization

While an initial survey of pathogenic sequence variants now exists for type 1 VWD, there is still much to learn about the underlying mechanisms responsible for this complex trait (Figure 11.1). Ongoing studies in Europe and North America will continue to contribute to this area of knowledge. In addition to developing a better understanding of the modes of action of the recently characterized missense, noncoding, and splicing mutants, further studies are required to identify variants within introns and distant regulatory sequences that might affect VWF expression.

Of great interest will be the further search for new genetic modifiers of VWF plasma levels. The recently

Table 11.4 Characteristics of the accelerated clearance type 1 von Willebrand disease (VWD) phenotype.

VWF levels <0.30 and often <0.15 IU/dL
Elevated VWFpp/VWF:Ag ratio (>2.0)
Exaggerated early DDAVP response (four- to 10-fold increment)
VWF half-life <3 h
Subtly abnormal VWF multimers
Missense mutations in D3 and D4-CK domains
5–15% of all type 1 VWD mutations

VWF, von Willebrand factor; VWFpp, von Willebrand factor propeptide; DDAVP, 1-deamino-8-D-arginine vasopressin.

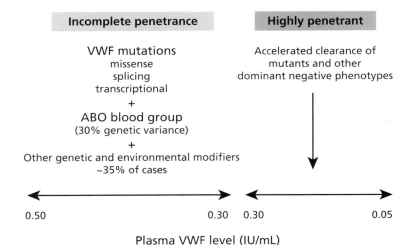

Figure 11.1 A genetic model for type 1 VWD.

derived linkage and *VWF* mutation data have confirmed that in approximately 30% of individuals with type 1, other genes are playing a major role in pathogenesis. The search for these loci has begun with plans for genome-wide association studies, but if the results of recent similar studies are applicable, these investigations will need to include very large study populations and even then may only detect loci that contribute small (1–5%) variances in the VWF level.

Reference

1 Sadler JE, Budde U, Eikenboom JC, *et al.* Update on the pathophysiology and classification of von Willebrand disease: a report of the Subcommittee on von Willebrand Factor. *J Thromb Haemost* 2006; **4**: 2103–14.

2 Rodeghiero F, Castaman G, Dini E. Epidemiological investigation of the prevalence of von Willebrand's disease. *Blood* 1987; **69**: 454–9.

3 Werner EJ, Broxson EH, Tucker EL, Giroux DS, Shults J, Abshire TC. Prevalence of von Willebrand disease in children: a multiethnic study. *J Pediatr* 1993; **123**: 893–8.

4 Castaman G, Eikenboom JC, Bertina RM, Rodeghiero F. Inconsistency of association between type 1 von Willebrand disease phenotype and genotype in families identified in an epidemiological investigation. *Thromb Haemost* 1999; **82**: 1065–70.

5 Bowman M, James PD, Godwin M, Lillicrap D. The prevalence of von Willebrand disease in the primary care setting. *Blood* 2005; **106**: 1780 (abstract).

6 Iorio A, Oliovecchio E, Morfini M, Mannucci PM. Italian Registry of Haemophilia and Allied Disorders. Objectives, methodology and data analysis. *Haemophilia* 2008; **14**: 444–53.

7 Tosetto A, Castaman G, Rodeghiero F. Assessing bleeding in von Willebrand disease with bleeding score. *Blood Rev* 2007; **21**: 89–97.

8 Rodeghiero F, Castaman G, Tosetto A, *et al.* The discriminant power of bleeding history for the diagnosis of type 1 von Willebrand disease: an international, multicenter study. *J Thromb Haemost* 2005; **3**: 2619–26.

9 Tosetto A, Rodeghiero F, Castaman G, *et al.* A quantitative analysis of bleeding symptoms in type 1 von Willebrand disease: results from a multicenter European study (MCMDM-1 VWD). *J Thromb Haemost* 2006; **4**: 766–73.

10 Sadler JE. Von Willebrand disease type 1: a diagnosis in search of a disease. *Blood* 2003; **101**: 2089–93.

11 Nichols WL, Hultin MB, James AH, *et al.* von Willebrand disease (VWD): evidence-based diagnosis and management guidelines, the National Heart, Lung, and Blood Institute (NHLBI) Expert Panel report (USA). *Haemophilia* 2008; **14**: 171–232.

12 Sadler JE, Rodeghiero F. Provisional criteria for the diagnosis of VWD type 1. *J Thromb Haemost* 2005; **3**: 775–7.

13 Abildgaard CF, Suzuki Z, Harrison J, Jefcoat K, Zimmerman TS. Serial studies in von Willebrand's disease: variability versus "variants". *Blood* 1980; **56**: 712–16.

14 Blomback M, Eneroth P, Andersson O, Anvret M. On laboratory problems in diagnosing mild von Willebrand's disease. *Am J Hematol* 1992; **40**: 117–20.

15 Miller CH, Dilley AB, Drews C, Richardson L, Evatt B. Changes in von Willebrand factor and factor VIII levels during the menstrual cycle. *Thromb Haemost* 2002; **87**: 1082–3.

16 Miller CH, Haff E, Platt SJ, *et al.* Measurement of von Willebrand factor activity: relative effects of ABO blood type and race. *J Thromb Haemost* 2003; **1**: 2191–7.

17 Tosetto A, Rodeghiero F, Castaman G, *et al.* Impact of plasma von Willebrand factor levels in the diagnosis of type 1 von Willebrand disease: results from a multicenter European study (MCMDM-1VWD). *J Thromb Haemost* 2007; **5**: 715–21.

18 Budde U, Schneppenheim R, Eikenboom J, *et al.* Detailed von Willebrand factor multimer analysis in patients with von Willebrand disease in the European study, molecular and clinical markers for the diagnosis and management of type 1 von Willebrand disease (MCMDM-1VWD). *J Thromb Haemost* 2008; **6**: 762–71.

19 Haberichter SL, Balistreri M, Christopherson P, *et al.* Assay of the von Willebrand factor (VWF) propeptide to identify patients with type 1 von Willebrand disease with decreased VWF survival. *Blood* 2006; **108**: 3344–51.

20 Haberichter SL, Castaman G, Budde U, *et al.* Identification of type 1 von Willebrand disease patients with reduced von Willebrand factor survival by assay of the VWF propeptide in the European study: molecular and clinical markers for the diagnosis and management of type 1 VWD (MCMDM-1VWD). *Blood* 2008; **111**: 4979–85.

21 Tosetto A, Castaman G, Rodeghiero F. Evidence-based diagnosis of type 1 von Willebrand disease: a Bayes theorem approach. *Blood* 2008; **111**: 3998–4003.

22 Miller CH, Graham JB, Goldin LR, Elston RC. Genetics of classic von Willebrand's disease. I. Phenotypic variation within families. *Blood* 1979; **54**: 117–36.

23 Miller CH, Graham JB, Goldin LR, Elston RC. Genetics of classic von Willebrand's disease. II. Optimal assignment of the heterozygous genotype (diagnosis) by discriminant analysis. *Blood* 1979; **54**: 137–45.

24 Gill JC, Endres-Brooks J, Bauer PJ, Marks WJ, Jr., Montgomery RR. The effect of ABO blood group on the

diagnosis of von Willebrand disease. *Blood* 1987; **69**: 1691–5.

25 Orstavik KH. Genetics of plasma concentration of von Willebrand factor. *Folia Haematol Int Mag Klin Morphol Blutforsch* 1990; **117**: 527–31.

26 Jenkins PV, O'Donnell JS. ABO blood group determines plasma von Willebrand factor levels: a biologic function after all? *Transfusion* 2006; **46**: 1836–44.

27 Gallinaro L, Cattini MG, Sztukowska M, *et al.* A shorter von Willebrand factor survival in O blood group subjects explains how ABO determinants influence plasma von Willebrand factor. *Blood* 2008; **111**: 3540–5.

28 Bowen DJ. An influence of ABO blood group on the rate of proteolysis of von Willebrand factor by ADAMTS13. *J Thromb Haemost* 2003; **1**: 33–40.

29 Goodeve A, Eikenboom J, Castaman G, *et al.* Phenotype and genotype of a cohort of families historically diagnosed with type 1 von Willebrand disease in the European study, Molecular and Clinical Markers for the Diagnosis and Management of Type 1 von Willebrand Disease (MCMDM-1VWD). *Blood* 2007; **109**: 112–21.

30 James PD, Notley C, Hegadorn C, *et al.* The mutational spectrum of type 1 von Willebrand disease: Results from a Canadian cohort study. *Blood* 2007; **109**: 145–54.

31 Mohlke KL, Purkayastha AA, Westrick RJ, *et al.* Mvwf, a dominant modifier of murine von Willebrand factor, results from altered lineage-specific expression of a glycosyltransferase. *Cell* 1999; **96**: 111–20.

32 Cumming A, Grundy P, Keeney S, *et al.* An investigation of the von Willebrand factor genotype in UK patients diagnosed to have type 1 von Willebrand disease. *Thromb Haemost* 2006; **96**: 630–41.

33 Eikenboom J, Van M, V, Putter H, *et al.* Linkage analysis in families diagnosed with type 1 von Willebrand disease in the European study, molecular and clinical markers for the diagnosis and management of type 1 VWD. *J Thromb Haemost* 2006; **4**: 774–82.

34 James PD, Paterson AD, Notley C, *et al.* Genetic linkage and association analysis in type 1 von Willebrand disease: results from the Canadian type 1 VWD study. *J Thromb Haemost* 2006; **4**: 783–92.

35 O'Brien LA, James PD, Othman M, *et al.* Founder von Willebrand factor haplotype associated with type 1 von Willebrand disease. *Blood* 2003; **102**: 549–57.

36 Davies JA, Collins PW, Hathaway LS, Bowen DJ. Effect of von Willebrand factor Y/C1584 on *in vivo* protein level and function and interaction with ABO blood group. *Blood* 2007; **109**: 2840–6.

37 Casonato A, Pontara E, Sartorello F, *et al.* Reduced von Willebrand factor survival in type Vicenza von Willebrand disease. *Blood* 2002; **99**: 180–4.

12 Clinical, laboratory, and molecular markers of type 2 von Willebrand disease

Dominique Meyer[1], Edith Fressinaud[2], and Claudine Mazurier[3]

[1]Inserm U770, Université Paris-sud, Le Kremlin-Bicêtre, Paris, France
[2]Centre National de Référence de la Maladie de Willebrand, Service d'Hématologie Biologique, Hôpital Antoine Béclère, Clamart, France
[3]Laboratoire Français du Fractionnement et des Biotechnologies, Lille, France

Introduction

Type 2 von Willebrand disease (VWD) is an inherited bleeding disorder caused by structural or functional defects of von Willebrand factor (VWF) either in mediating platelet adhesion at sites of vascular injury or in binding blood clotting factor VIII (FVIII).

Type 2 VWD is divided into four categories of variants [1], three of which induce abnormal VWF-platelet and/or VWF-connective tissue interactions [1]. In type 2A, there is decreased VWF-dependent platelet adhesion caused by a selective deficiency of high-molecular-weight (HMW) VWF multimers; in type 2B, the affinity of VWF for platelet glycoprotein Ib (GPIb) is increased; in type 2M, VWF binding to GPIb or to subendothelium is decreased despite a relatively normal distribution of VWF multimers. In the fourth type of variant, type 2N, the affinity of VWF for FVIII is markedly decreased [1].

Type 2A VWD is often further subdivided into four subtypes (IIA, IIC, IID, IIE; according to the old nomenclature) with distinct mechanisms, but today there is no recommendation to discriminate among them on a clinical basis.

The prevalence of VWD, when estimated on the basis of the number of symptomatic patients followed at hemostasis centers, ranges from 23 to 110 per million population [2], and type 2 VWD is generally reported to affect 20–45% of patients. In fact, type 2 VWD (grouping all qualitative VWF defects) may be almost as frequent as type 1 (characterized by a partial quantitative deficiency of VWF). Indeed, a recent multicenter European study, Molecular and Clinical Markers for the Diagnosis and Management of Type 1 VWD (MCMDM-1VWD), reported that one-third of patients, historically diagnosed with type 1 VWD, exhibited an abnormal VWF multimer profile with patterns previously described in patients with type 2 VWD, mostly type 2M or subtype 2A(IIE) [3]. The distribution of the different type 2 variants varies considerably among studies [4,5]. Lastly, type 2N VWD may still be misdiagnosed as hemophilia A.

Thus, depending on the classification criteria used and on the quantity and quality of specialized tests performed, it may be difficult to recognize a functionally abnormal VWF. However, identifying patients with type 2 VWD is important not only because this diagnosis predicts bleeding symptoms thought to be more severe than in patients with type 1 but also because these patients have a weaker probability of a positive response to desmopressin than those with type 1 and may therefore present specific therapeutic needs.

Discrimination among type 2 variants requires tests that are only performed in specialized hemostasis laboratories; moreover, *VWF* gene sequencing is useful in the diagnosis of type 2 VWD as the probability of detecting a *VWF* mutation is very high and because its localization on the *VWF* gene is clearly associated with a defined variant.

In this chapter we will take into account the results of a multicenter study entitled "French INSERM Network on Molecular abnormalities in VWD",

Von Willebrand Disease, 1st edition. Edited by Augusto B. Federici, Christine A. Lee, Erik E. Berntorp, David Lillicrap, Robert R. Montgomery. © 2011 Blackwell Publishing Ltd.

which was conducted between 1996 and 2003 to extensively estimate the value of phenotypic and molecular markers for the diagnosis of type 2 VWD [4,6–8].

Clinical manifestations

Bleeding symptoms in type 2 VWD are thought to be more severe than in type 1 and less severe than in type 3, but this assertion needs to be modulated between the different type 2 variants and requires further evaluation.

Clearly, patients with type 2 VWD have therapeutic needs distinct from those with type 1, as desmopressin releases dysfunctional VWF and pregnancy induces an increased production of abnormal VWF.

It is also well known that the loss of HMW VWF multimers is associated with deficient VWF–platelet or VWF–connective tissue interactions, thus exposing patients showing these characteristics to significant bleeding involving mucous membranes and skin sites. An international survey has indicated that, in contrast to patients with type 1 VWD, those with type 2 VWD are exposed to gastrointestinal bleeding caused by angiodysplasia [9].

Very few studies demonstrate the prevalence of bleeding symptoms in the different VWD types. The Italian registry reported that, apart from joint bleeding, the distribution of other types of bleeding (epistaxis, menorrhagia, postsurgical bleeding, postpartum bleeding, etc.) is similar for the different VWD types (1, 2, and 3) [10]. The frequency of bleeding events seems to vary among types: an Italian prospective study followed patients with VWD for 1 year and reported a more frequent occurrence of bleeding episodes in type 3 (57.7%) than in type 2 (18.3%) or type 1 (12.4%) VWD [10].

A quantitative evaluation of bleeding symptoms using a standardized bleeding score is required to compare the clinical expression of the different types of VWD and to evaluate the association between the bleeding score and both clinical and laboratory characteristics of patients with different types and subtypes. A bleeding questionnaire applied to a large panel of families with type 1 VWD enrolled in the MCMDM-1VWD study provided interesting findings such as a consistent increase of the bleeding risk throughout life and a clinical severity clearly related to the levels of circulating plasma VWF and FVIII [11]. Moreover, among these variants, we need to identify those associated with a high risk of bleeding and to know, for example, whether there is a correlation between bleeding score and VWF multimer pattern; patients lacking HMW multimers are predicted as having a higher bleeding score.

Using a condensed version of the MCMDM-1VWD bleeding questionnaire, a recent Canadian study evaluated the bleeding score of 42 patients (type 1 VWD, $n = 16$; type 2 VWD, $n = 14$; type 3 VWD, $n = 12$); there was a significant difference in bleeding score between the three types, with type 3 > type 2 > type 1 [12]. It would be clinically useful to evaluate the extensive MCMDM-1VWD bleeding questionnaire in large cohorts of patients with different type 2 variants. Recently, Federici et al. reported that the bleeding score was inversely correlated to the platelet count at baseline in a group of patients with type 2B VWD [13].

The clinical expression of type 2N VWD, mainly characterized by post-traumatic or surgery-related bleeding, is more comparable to that observed in moderate or minor hemophilia A than to that observed in other VWD types, except in some patients who also have a low VWF level and in whom the multimerization VWF process is modified.

Laboratory diagnosis

Initial testing

The initial tests used to detect VWD include measurements of plasma levels of VWF and FVIII. Three tests, available in most laboratories, should be performed together to estimate (i) the amount of VWF protein in plasma, i.e., VWF antigen (VWF:Ag) assay; (ii) the function of the protein, measured by its ability to interact with platelets, i.e., VWF ristocetin cofactor (VWF:RCo) assay; and (iii) the ability to carry FVIII, i.e., FVIII assay.

Results of these tests may already suggest a type 2 variant with abnormal VWF function indicated by a low VWF:RCo to VWF:Ag ratio or a low FVIII to VWF:Ag ratio.

Platelet count should be included in this initial evaluation because the discovery of thrombocytopenia is very suggestive of type 2B VWD. In our experience with the French INSERM network, 27 of 64 patients (42%), secondarily diagnosed with type 2B VWD, were initially tested with a platelet count $<150 \times 10^9$/L.

Ratio of VWF:RCo to VWF:Ag

Initially, an abnormal VWF:RCo/VWF:Ag ratio was defined as <0.7 in a relevant study of healthy controls (mean 1.0; range 0.72–1.26; SD 2) [14]. Other authors proposed a threshold of 0.6 [15] or even 0.5. What is clear is that the VWF:RCo assay has been shown to have a coefficient of variation (CV) as high as 30% in several studies, especially at low levels of VWF. The VWF:RCo/VWF:Ag ratio is thus unreliable when basal VWF:Ag levels are less than 15–20 IU/dL.

Indeed, technical limitations should be considered. Concerning the VWF:Ag assay, the old Laurell gel procedure (electro-immunodiffusion), still performed in some laboratories because of its low cost, may overestimate the level of VWF protein in some VWF variants; thus, it is replaced by the enzyme-linked immunosorbent assay (ELISA) or the latex immunoassay, the latter being less specific in the presence of rheumatoid factor [16].

The VWF:RCo assay is still the most widely accepted functional test for VWF. The binding of VWF to platelet GPIb induced by ristocetin is assessed by methods using that inducer, formalin-fixed normal platelets and dilutions of patient plasma. The platelet clumping may be evaluated by either aggregometry or visual inspection (both methods being quantitative to 6–12 IU/dL), or automated turbidometric tests (quantitative to 10–20 IU/dL) [17]. ELISA assays assessing direct binding of patient plasma VWF to platelet GPIb (glycocalicin or recombinant GPIbα) have been developed as they have a lower intra-assay variability and a higher sensitivity (measuring VWF:RCo to <1–3 IU/dL) [18,19]. Lastly, several monoclonal ELISAs that use antibodies directed to the VWF epitope containing the GPIb binding site are now available [20], but they are distinct from the VWF:RCo assay as they are not based on ristocetin-induced binding; moreover, these ELISAs can be criticized as they do not directly assess the function of the largest VWF multimers [21].

In the framework of the French INSERM network, the phenotype of 217 patients with VWD characterized with a type 2 (2A, 2B, 2M) *VWF* gene mutation has been analyzed (Table 12.1). VWF:Ag levels were clearly higher in patients with type 2A(IIA) and type 2B VWD than in those with type 2A(IIC), type 2A(IID), type 2A(IIE), and type 2M VWD. The VWF:RCo/VWF:Ag ratio was less than 0.7 in all patients with types 2A(IIA), 2A(IIC), 2A(IID), and type 2M. Among patients with type 2A(IIE) VWD, 5 of 7 (71%) showed a VWF:RCo/VWF:Ag ratio >0.7; among patients with type 2B VWD, 23 of 86 (29%) exhibited a VWF:RCo/VWF:Ag ratio >0.7. Consequently, patients with type 2A(IIE) may be frequently misclassified with type 1 VWD. A quarter of patients with type 2B may also be identified

Table 12.1 Phenotypic data for the French cohort of type 2 von Willebrand disease: all patients except those with type 2N.

Type (subtype)	FVIII:C	VWF:RCo	VWF:Ag	VWF:RCo/Ag
2A(IIA); $n = 40$	51 (39–70)	11 (8–22)	50 (35–73)	0.22 (0.20–0.39)
2A(IIC); $n = 2$	20–24	5–5	11–16	0.31–0.45
2A(IID); $n = 2$	25–33	6–8	16–15	0.38–0.53
2A(IIE); $n = 7$	31 (26–40)	12 (10–14)	18 (13–28)	0.67 (0.54–0.74)
2B; $n = 86$	46 (36–61)	22 (13–36)	46 (34–60)	0.48 (0.34–0.74)
2M; $n = 80$	40 (29–58)	10 (6–15)	26 (19–37)	0.38 (29–51)

VWF:Ag levels were evaluated using enzyme-linked immunosorbent assay (ELISA) or latex immunoassay, VWF:RCo levels using agglutination or aggregometry.
Values are arithmetic median (25th to 75th percentiles) in IU/dL.

as type 1 VWD, the thrombocytopenia being too inconsistent to help the diagnosis. Furthermore, in patients with type 2M, some with the lowest values of VWF:Ag may also be difficult to distinguish from type 1.

Thus, a VWF:RCo/VWF:Ag ratio >0.7 does not allow the exclusion of type 2 VWD, whereas when it is <0.7 it is highly in favor of type 2 VWD.

Further laboratory evaluation

Patients with an abnormal VWF:RCo/VWF:Ag ratio and patients with a normal ratio but VWF:Ag levels lower than <30 IU/dL should benefit from further evaluation, including at least VWF multimer analysis.

Ristocetin-induced platelet aggregation (RIPA) using a low concentration of ristocetin, usually <0.7 mg/mL, should also be performed in all patients whatever the VWF:RCo/VWF:Ag ratio or VWF:Ag levels, and particularly in patients with thrombocytopenia not clearly associated with decreased VWF levels.

VWF multimer study

The electrophoretic analysis of VWF multimers is the gold standard for differentiating type 2 from type 1 and for identifying the various type 2 subtypes. Methods should use low-resolution gels (0.65–1.2% agarose) to distinguish the largest multimers from the intermediate and small multimers, and medium- (1.5–1.8% agarose) or high-resolution gels (2–3% agarose) to separate each multimer band into satellite bands. These methods should include a quantitative evaluation by densitometry. The recent MCMDM-1VWD study proposed to define a decrease of the large multimers as <70% of the amount of large multimers of normal pooled plasma [3]. Specific abnormal characteristics of the migration pattern are described and discussed in the paragraph on molecular aspects of type 2 VWD.

Ristocetin-induced platelet aggregation

The interest of RIPA carried out in platelet-rich plasma is to detect most patients with type 2B using low concentrations of ristocetin, usually <0.7 mg/mL; these low doses induce VWF binding and platelet aggregation in patients with either type 2B VWD or platelet-type VWD, but not in patients with other types of VWD.

However, some patients with type 2B may not exhibit platelet aggregation with a low dose of ristocetin, whereas they might show a loss in large plasma VWF multimers. The apparent 2A phenotype of the corresponding patients may be explained by the spontaneous binding of plasma HMW and intermediate-molecular-weight multimers to platelets and by the presence in the circulation of only small multimers unable to bind to platelets. Diagnosis can then be established by gene analysis showing a mutation in the A1 domain of VWF and by expression studies confirming the type 2B mutation. In the French INSERM network, we identified 8 of 64 patients (12%) with a type 2B mutation who lacked low-dose RIPA; this characteristic was preferentially associated with some mutations (C1272R, C1272G, R1308C) [4].

At higher concentrations of ristocetin (1.1–1.3 mg/mL), RIPA may be reduced in patients with type 2A or 2M VWD; however, the test is not sufficiently sensitive to consider this result as a requirement for the diagnosis.

Plasma VWF binding to platelets

This method determines the amount of patient plasma VWF bound to normal paraformaldehyde-fixed platelets using variable concentrations of ristocetin and a radiolabeled anti-VWF antibody [22]. It is often replaced by the measurement of VWF binding to a recombinant fragment of GPIbα with an ELISA-based method [23].

Increased VWF binding at low concentrations of ristocetin (0.2–0.6 mg/mL) is characteristic of type 2B VWD and allows differentiating it from platelet-type VWD. However, like for RIPA, the enhanced affinity of 2B VWF for platelets may not be detected in some patients.

Decreased VWF binding at higher ristocetin concentrations (1.1–1.3 mg/mL) is observed in patients with type 2A (IIA, IIC, IID) and type 2M VWD.

Replacement of ristocetin by botrocetin may be informative, as these two inducers involve distinct domains of VWF. In patients with type 2A VWD, decreased binding in the presence of either ristocetin or botrocetin is linked to the loss of HMW multimers. In patients with type 2M VWD, decreased affinity of VWF for platelets, directly connected to the impaired VWF binding to GPIb sites, is observed when the binding is induced by ristocetin but not by botrocetin [4]. However, patients with type 2M exhibiting a relative loss of HMW multimers may show decreased botrocetin-induced binding to GPIb.

VWF collagen-binding assay and the VWF:CB/VWF:Ag ratio

The capacity of VWF to bind to collagen (VWF:CB) is measured by an ELISA. The primary VWF binding site to fibrillar collagen is located in the A3 domain. Like, or even more than, VWF:RCo, VWF:CB is dependent upon VWF multimeric size, with the largest multimers binding more avidly than the smaller forms. Thus, some authors propose to use the VWF:CB assay in the initial evaluation of VWD in order to determine the VWF:CB/VWF:Ag ratio and better discriminate type 2 from type 1 VWD. However, the VWF:CB assay lacks standardization, and its sensitivity to detect type 2 VWD or to discriminate among VWD variants is highly dependent on the source of collagen, a collagen mixture of 95% type I and 5% type III having been proven to be the most sensitive. Indeed, in the MCMDM-1VWD study, the VWF:CB/VWF:Ag ratio did not perform better (or was even worse) than the VWF:RCo/VWF:Ag ratio to prevent the misidentification of type 2 with type 1 VWD [3]. In particular, the VWF:CB assay is not suitable for discriminating between type 2A(IIE) and type 1 VWD.

We estimate that VWF:CB testing can neither replace VWF:RCo nor negate the need to perform multimer analysis. However, for laboratories that cannot perform VWF multimer analysis, the VWF:CB assay evaluated in patients with a decreased VWF:RCo/VWF:Ag ratio may rapidly help to discriminate between most of those with type 2A (IIA, IIC, IID) and those with type 2M.

Lastly, the VWF:CB assay is probably the only test able to identify the very rare patients with a specific collagen-binding defect associated with a mutation of VWF in the A3 domain [24].

Ratio of FVIII to VWF:Ag and binding assay of VWF to FVIII

The initial evaluation may indicate an abnormal FVIII/VWF:Ag ratio whatever the FVIII assay (one-stage or two-stage chronometric, chromogenic, or immunologic assay). This low ratio may be detected in patients with decreased VWF:Ag levels, in favor of type 2N VWD, or in patients with normal VWF:Ag levels, generally in favor of hemophilia A. Type 2N VWD is recessively inherited and patients are either homozygous (each allele bearing the same type 2N mutation) or compound heterozygous (one allele bearing a type 2N mutation and the other being a null allele, or each allele carrying a different type 2N mutation). Thus, these compound heterozygous patients may appear with decreased VWF:Ag levels. Whatever the VWF:Ag levels, in the case of a low FVIII/VWF:Ag ratio, the evaluation of the VWF binding to FVIII (VWF:FVIIIB) is mandatory in order not to miss the type 2N VWD diagnosis. Indeed, around 10% of patients with a low FVIII/VWF:Ag ratio recruited by the INSERM network exhibited a markedly decreased or absent VWF:FVIIIB, the laboratory hallmark of type 2N VWD. All 111 patients with type 2N VWD had an FVIII/VWF:Ag ratio <0.5. The FVIII level depends on the severity of the VWF:FVIIIB defect: data from the INSERM network indicated that FVIII levels were significantly lower in patients with completely absent FVIII binding function than in patients in whom this function is only markedly decreased (Table 12.2) [6]. This characteristic is clearly dependent upon the involved mutation [6].

Since the original description of the VWF:FVIIIB assay [25], several modifications have been published: in France, the capacity of plasma VWF to bind exogeneous FVIII is now measured with an ELISA test, which is easier to perform using only commercially available reagents [26]. The assay allows the easy differentiation of markedly reduced or absent VWF:FVIIIB, leading to the diagnosis of type 2N VWD, from moderately reduced VWF:FVIIIB, indicating the presence of a type 2N mutation in the heterozygous state. The latter cannot by itself account for FVIII deficiency owing to the recessive nature of

Table 12.2 FVIII levels related to VWF:FVIIIB in the French cohort of type 2N von Willebrand disease.

VWF:FVIIIB	FVIII:C (IU/dL)	FVIII/VWF:Ag
Nil (*n* = 22)	8 ± 5	0.13 ± 0.06
Markedly decreased (*n* = 45)	22 ± 9	0.31 ± 0.15

Values are mean ± 2SD; $P < 0.001$.

141

type 2N VWD. Thus, the finding of a low FVIII/VWF:Ag ratio with a moderately reduced VWF:FVIIIB should lead to the analysis of the *FVIII* gene for a coexistent hemophilic mutation.

Molecular markers

The importance of specific domains of VWF involved in its function (binding to platelet GPIb, to connective tissue, or to FVIII), its structure (multimerization and dimerization of VWF), and its proteolysis and clearance is now well known. The identification of these functional domains has guided the search for the molecular abnormalities responsible for qualitative defects of VWF so that the location of mutations in a defined VWF domain may be associated with a specific subtype of type 2 VWD (Table 12.3).

Mutations are listed on the VWF database (http://www.vwf.group.shef.ac.uk/).

In the French INSERM network on molecular abnormalities in VWD [4,6–8], 298 unrelated patients were diagnosed with a VWD variant. The gene analysis identified 102 distinct mutations, half of which were expressed and characterized. Molecular abnormalities mostly consisted of missense mutations (80%), but also insertion (2%), deletion (2%), or nonsense mutations (16%) were observed in patients with type 2N VWD who were compound heterozygotes with one copy of a null allele. Classification of patients was not only performed according to the characteristics of the VWF multimer profile but also according to results of the functional tests performed using patient plasma VWF (and using the analysis of recombinant VWF in the case of candidate mutations). The distribution of variants, shown in Figure 12.1, was roughly

Table 12.3 Localization of molecular defects, pathogenesis, and von Willebrand factor (VWF) multimer patterns in the von Willebrand disease (VWD) type 2 variants.

Localization of molecular defect on *VWF* gene	Pathogenesis	VWF multimer pattern	VWD variants
Propeptide (D1, D2)	Abnormal multimerization of VWF	Absence of large multimers Absence of outer proteolytic bands	2A(IIC)
D', D3	Decreased binding of VWF to FVIII ± abnormal multimer assembly	Normal or relative loss of large multimers and smear around central bands	2N
D3	Abnormal disulfide bonding ± intracellular retention ± decreased binding to FVIII ± increased clearance	Relative loss of large multimers Smear around central bands and lack of the outer bands	2A(IIE)
A1	Decreased binding of VWF to platelets ± abnormal folding of A1 loop and defect in multimerization	Normal Or relative loss of large multimers and smear around the central bands	2M 2M(2A-like)
A1	Increased binding of VWF to platelets	Absence of large multimers with increased outer flanking subbands or normal	2B
A2	Increased proteolysis of VWF by ADAMTS13 ± intracellular defect in multimer assembly	Absence of large and intermediate multimers Increased outer flanking subbands	2A(IIA)
A3	Decreased binding of VWF to subendothelium	Normal	2M
CK	Abnormal dimerization of VWF	Absence of large multimers Odd-numbered oligomers	2A(IID)

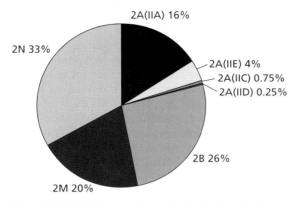

Figure 12.1 Distribution of variants in the French cohort of type 2 von Willebrand disease (VWD). 298 unrelated patients were characterized phenotypically and genetically. Phenotyping included multimer analysis and functional assays (binding to platelets, to collagen, and to FVIII).

similar between the four subtypes but with a surprising high prevalence of type 2N.

We will summarize the molecular basis of the different VWD variants by taking into account our own experience.

Type 2A VWD

Type 2A VWD includes variants with decreased VWF-dependent platelet function caused by the selective deficiency of HMW multimers. However, causative mutations and involved mechanisms are heterogeneous, as are the VWF multimeric patterns (Table 12.3).

Type 2A(IIA)

In this subtype with dominant inheritance, responsible mutations, all located in the A2 domain, cause an increased proteolysis by ADAMTS13 (group 2 mutations) and in some cases also an impaired intracellular transport, resulting in the absence of secretion of HMW multimers (group 1 mutations) [1]. Multimeric patterns show a severe loss of the large- and often intermediate-molecular-weight multimers and an increase of the intensity of the outer proteolytic flanking subbands. In the French INSERM network, we found 22 distinct mutations in 47 families. Two mutations, R1597W and I1628T (both group 2), were particularly frequent, being identified in one-third of patients.

Type 2A(IIC)

In this subtype with recessive inheritance, mutations are located in the D1 or D2 domains of the VWF propeptide (which are necessary to catalyze intermolecular bonding at the D3 domain of the mature VWF), further preventing polymerization of VWF dimers to multimers. Phenotypic data from these patients showed significantly more decreased VWF:Ag levels than in the classic subtype IIA (Table 12.1) and also a distinct multimeric profile with an increase in the protomer and absence of the outer proteolytic satellite bands. This subtype of type 2A VWD is much less frequent—in France we diagnosed only two families, each with a distinct mutation in the homozygous state (C623W and InsG625) [27].

Type 2A(IID)

With a recessive or dominant inheritance pattern, this rare form of type 2A VWD is caused by mutations located in the CK domain, often involving cysteine residues, which impair formation of disulfide-linked dimers and therefore subsequent multimerization [28]. Phenotypic data resemble those of the subtype IIC except for the multimeric pattern showing, besides the lack of the large multimers, the typical odd-numbered oligomers. In France, only one family with a recessive inheritance was diagnosed with the A2801D mutation [29].

Type 2A(IIE)

In this relatively frequent 2A subtype that shows dominant inheritance, described by Zimmerman et al. [30], causative mutations are located in the D3 domain. These mutations affect the participation of cysteine residues in the intermolecular disulfide bonding of the mature VWF subunit, which is essential for VWF multimerization. As stated by Sadler et al. [1], mutations in the D3 domain may interfere with multimer assembly, reduce VWF secretion, increase VWF clearance, and/or decrease VWF affinity for FVIII. Phenotypic data from these patients are completely different from those of patients with classic type 2A VWD (Table 12.1), but have many characteristics of patients with type 1 VWD. Only a sensitive multimeric analysis may distinguish them, with subtype IIE showing a relative loss of the largest multimers and a lack of outer satellite bands with some smear around the central bands. In the French INSERM network, we diagnosed six families with five distinct mutations (C1101R, C1101W, C1157F, C1196R, C1234W); the incidence of this subtype is, however, probably underestimated as patients showing no clear criteria of type 2 VWD were not recruited. Indeed, the first publication reporting a mutated cysteine residue in the D3 domain (C1130F) classified these patients as having type 1 VWD, as the authors found the multimer abnormality insufficient for classification as type 2 VWD [31]. Standardization will be useful as, depending on the authors, patients with the same mutation are classified either in type 2A or type 1 VWD.

Most of our patients with subtype IIE exhibited a positive response to desmopressin. This is why it is clinically useful to distinguish patients with subtype IIE from other patients with type 2A (IIA, IIC, IID).

Type 2M VWD

Type 2M VWD, with dominant inheritance, includes variants with decreased VWF-dependent platelet adhesion not caused by the absence of HMW multimers.

Type 2M *with impaired binding to GPIb*

Type 2M VWD is characterized by a defective binding of VWF to GPIb despite a relatively normal-sized distribution of VWF multimers [1]. In the INSERM network, we identified different groups of patients who fit with this definition (60 families).

In the first group, patients showed a typical phenotype with decreased binding of VWF to GPIb in the presence of ristocetin but not of botrocetin and the presence of large VWF multimers. Causative mutations (G1324A, E1359K, and K1362T) were identified in the A1 domain. These residues are localized within the GPIb binding sites in the part of the A1 domain that interacts with the β-switch of the terminus part of GPIbα [32]; thus, these mutations may directly impair GPIb binding.

In the second group, patients showed decreased VWF binding to GPIb in the presence of ristocetin and of botrocetin, and a relative decrease of the large multimers without clear abnormality of the triplet structure but often a smear around the central bands. Causative mutations (L1276P, R1315C/G, R1374C/H/L/S, and P1462A) are also localized within the GPIb binding sites, in the part of the A1 domain that interacts with the β-finger site of the GPIbα [32].

These mutations may disrupt the salt bridge network of the A1 domain and thus induce an abnormal folding of the A1 domain that indirectly impairs GPIb binding. The mutations involving cysteine residues at position 1315 and 1374 are extremely frequent and have been detected in 52% of our patients with type 2M VWD. The corresponding mutated rVWFs have been studied by our group [33,34]; whereas the structural alterations affecting the GPIb sites dramatically decreased reactivity for GPIb, HMW multimers were only minimally diminished. Patients harboring these mutations may be classified as type 2M, 2A-like, 2A, or remain as unclassified type 2 VWD. Moreover, the mutations at positions 1315 and 1374 were detected in patients studied in type 1 VWD cohorts, although harboring a low (often <0.4) VWF:RCo/VWF:Ag ratio, and reclassified as type 2M in the Canadian study [35] and as type 2A (with a smeary multimeric pattern) in the European study [3]. Clearly, standardization of the classification is needed for patients who harbor these frequent mutations.

Lastly, we also diagnosed patients with a type 2M phenotype whose responsible mutations were located in the A1 domain but were remote from GPIb binding sites (L1282R, S1285F, L1296P, D1302G, L1383R, R1399C, G1402R, L1408del, I1425F, and C1458Y). These mutations, leading to changes in the A1 structure, may disrupt the GPIb binding sites, generally without affecting multimer assembly [14,22,36].

Type 2M *with impaired binding to subendothelium*

This type has been detected in one French and two UK families in whom the affected family members showed isolated, decreased VWF:CB and a mutation in the A3 domain (S1731T) [24].

We will not discuss the "Vicenza" subtype, which is now classified among type 1 VWD [1].

Type 2B VWD

Type 2B VWD, with dominant inheritance, is caused by an increased affinity of VWF for platelet GPIb. Studies on the crystal structure of the VWF–GPIbα complex showed that the VWF A1 domain changes conformation when it binds to GPIb [32]. Mutations clustered within or near the VWF A1 domain do not impair the assembly and secretion of VWF multimers but confer a bound conformation on the A1 domain with increased accessibility to the β-finger site of GPIbα. The large multimers bind spontaneously to platelets and become cleaved by ADAMTS13; thrombocytopenia may occur with a slight increase of platelet size. In the INSERM network, we detected 79 unrelated patients with a type 2B mutation: we found 23 distinct mutations on 14 residues. Five mutations (R1306W, R1308C, V1316M, P1337L, and R1341W) were frequent, detected in 82% of patients.

There is a wide degree of heterogeneity both in the multimeric pattern and in the platelet count of patients. Molecular predictors of this heterogeneity have been reported [13].

In some patients, mutated VWF showed a remarkably high affinity for the GPIbα, which led to the loss of high- and also intermediate-molecular-weight multimers and hence to the absence of RIPA at low ristocetin concentrations, as in type 2A VWD. Nevertheless, most patients still exhibited thrombocytopenia in stress conditions. The latter characteristic was preferentially associated with some mutations: C1272R/G, R1308C, V1314F [4].

The relatively frequent P1266L mutation is associated with type 2B "Malmö/New York" VWD that shows heightened RIPA at low ristocetin concentrations but a normal set of multimers and no thrombocytopenia induced by stress conditions or desmopressin [1]. Recently, patients carrying the R1308L mutation were also described with this same phenotype [13].

Some patients presented with severe thrombocytopenia, sometimes associated with giant platelets and spontaneous platelet aggregates; the *VWF* V1316M mutation may be associated with this phenotype [37,38] and type 2B VWD must always be considered in the differential diagnosis of genetic thrombocytopenia. Indeed, the *VWF* V1316M mutation was recently detected in patients previously described with Montreal platelet syndrome [39]. Severe thrombocytopenia was also detected in patients with the R1308P mutation and clearly associated with impaired megakaryocytopoiesis [40].

Type 2N VWD

Type 2N VWD, recessively inherited, refers to variants with a markedly decreased affinity of VWF for FVIII and was originally described in French patients [25,41]. Patients are homozygous or compound het-

erozygous. Sometimes both alleles have a type 2N mutation, but often one allele has a type 2N mutation while the other allele expresses little or no VWF; in the latter, VWF levels are decreased and the FVIII/VWF:Ag ratio is abnormally decreased.

Mutations are localized in the FVIII binding site of VWF that spans the D′ domain and part of the D3 domain. In the INSERM network, we diagnosed 118 patients (100 families) with type 2N VWD. We described mutations in either the D′ domain (R763G, G785E, T791M, Y795C, C804F, R816W, R854Q, and C858F) or the D3 domain (D879N, Q1053H, C1060R, E1078K, and C1099Y) [6]. The R854Q mutation is extremely frequent, occurring on at least one allele in 90% of patients with type 2N VWD.

Expression studies consistently showed the dramatic impairment of VWF:FVIIIB [6]. Some mutations (C788Y, C788R, D879N, C858F, and C1225G), most of them involving cysteine residues, not only decrease FVIII binding but also induce a defect in expression and a decrease in the HMW multimers [6].

The plasma FVIII levels correlate with specific mutations. Thus, FVIII levels are significantly lower in mutations that induce a complete lack of FVIII binding than in mutations (R854Q and Q1053H) in which the VWF:FVIIIB is markedly decreased [6]. This distinction has clinical utility, as patients with the R854Q mutation show a therapeutically useful response to desmopressin and an improvement during pregnancy, whereas those with the other mutations do not [42]. Indeed, it is important to stress that heterozygous carriers of a type 2N mutation have a moderate decrease of VWF:FVIIIB, which cannot by itself account for an FVIII deficiency: such patients should not be considered as having type 2N VWD.

Concluding remarks

Type 2 VWD is extremely heterogeneous, and the identification of its numerous variants requires an approach based on the knowledge of the pathologic mechanisms of *VWF* gene mutations and of their impact on VWF structure and function. The refined classification of variants based on genotypic analysis should help to predict clinical expression and therefore aid in the diagnosis and management of this disease.

References

1 Sadler JE, Budde U, Eikenboom JC, *et al.* Update on the pathophysiology and classification of von Willebrand disease: a report of the Subcommittee on von Willebrand Factor. *J Thromb Haemost* 2006; **4**: 2103–14.

2 Sadler JE, Mannucci PM, Berntorp E, *et al.* Impact, diagnosis and treatment of von Willebrand disease. *Thromb Haemost* 2000; **84**: 160–74.

3 Budde U, Schneppenheim R, Eikenboom J, *et al.* Detailed von Willebrand factor multimer analysis in patients with von Willebrand disease in the European study, molecular and clinical markers for the diagnosis and management of type 1 von Willebrand disease (MCMDM-1VWD). *J Thromb Haemost* 2008; **6**: 762–71.

4 Meyer D, Fressinaud E, Gaucher C, *et al.* Gene defects in 150 unrelated French cases with type 2 von Willebrand disease: from the patient to the gene. INSERM Network on Molecular Abnormalities in von Willebrand Disease. *Thromb Haemost* 1997; **78**: 451–6.

5 Budde U, Drewke E, Mainusch K, Schneppenheim R. Laboratory diagnosis of congenital von Willebrand disease. *Semin Thromb Hemost* 2002; **28**: 173–90.

6 Meyer D, Fressinaud E, Hilbert L, Ribba AS, Lavergne JM, Mazurier C. Type 2 von Willebrand disease causing defective von Willebrand factor-dependent platelet function. *Best Pract Res Clin Haematol* 2001; **14**: 349–64.

7 Mazurier C, Goudemand J, Hilbert L, Caron C, Fressinaud E, Meyer D. Type 2N von Willebrand disease: clinical manifestations, pathophysiology, laboratory diagnosis and molecular biology. *Best Pract Res Clin Haematol* 2001; **14**: 337–47.

8 Fressinaud E, Mazurier C, Meyer D. Molecular genetics of type 2 von Willebrand disease. *Int J Hematol* 2002; **75**: 9–18.

9 Fressinaud E, Meyer D. International survey of patients with von Willebrand disease and angiodysplasia. *Thromb Haemost* 1993; **70**: 546.

10 Federici AB, Castaman G, Mannucci PM. Guidelines for the diagnosis and management of von Willebrand disease in Italy. *Haemophilia* 2002; **8**: 607–21.

11 Tosetto A, Rodeghiero F, Castaman G, *et al.* A quantitative analysis of bleeding symptoms in type 1 von Willebrand disease: results from a multicenter European study (MCMDM-1 VWD). *J Thromb Haemost* 2006; **4**: 766–73.

12 Bowman M, Mundell G, Grabell J, *et al.* Generation and validation of the Condensed MCMDM-1VWD Bleeding Questionnaire for von Willebrand disease. *J Thromb Haemost* 2008; **6**: 2062–6.

13 Federici AB, Mannucci PM, Castaman G, *et al.* Clinical and molecular predictors of thrombocytopenia and risk of bleeding in patients with von Willebrand disease type 2B: a cohort study of 67 patients. *Blood* 2009; **113**: 526–34.

14 Hillery CA, Mancuso DJ, Sadler JE, *et al.* Type 2M von Willebrand disease: F606I and I662F mutations in the glycoprotein Ib binding domain selectively impair ristocetin- but not botrocetin-mediated binding of von Willebrand factor to platelets. *Blood* 1998; **91**: 1572–81.

15 James PD, Paterson AD, Notley C, *et al.* Genetic linkage and association analysis in type 1 von Willebrand disease: results from the Canadian type 1 VWD study. *J Thromb Haemost* 2006; **4**: 783–92.

16 Veyradier A, Fressinaud E, Sigaud M, Wolf M, Meyer D. A new automated method for von Willebrand factor antigen measurement using latex particles. *Thromb Haemost* 1999; **81**: 320–1.

17 Nichols WL, Hultin MB, James AH, *et al.* von Willebrand disease (VWD): evidence-based diagnosis and management guidelines, the National Heart, Lung, and Blood Institute (NHLBI) Expert Panel report (USA). *Haemophilia* 2008; **14**: 171–232.

18 Federici AB, Canciani MT, Forza I, *et al.* A sensitive ristocetin co-factor activity assay with recombinant glycoprotein Ibalpha for the diagnosis of patients with low von Willebrand factor levels. *Haematologica* 2004; **89**: 77–85.

19 Vanhoorelbeke K, Pareyn I, Schlammadinger A, *et al.* Plasma glycocalicin as a source of GPIbalpha in the von Willebrand factor ristocetin cofactor ELISA. *Thromb Haemost* 2005; **93**: 165–71.

20 Pinol M, Sales M, Costa M, Tosetto A, Canciani MT, Federici AB. Evaluation of a new turbidimetric assay for von Willebrand factor activity useful in the general screening of von Willebrand disease. *Haematologica* 2007; **92**: 712–13.

21 Fischer BE, Thomas KB, Dorner F. von Willebrand factor: measuring its antigen or function? Correlation between the level of antigen, activity, and multimer size using various detection systems. *Thromb Res* 1998; **91**: 39–43.

22 Stepanian A, Ribba AS, Lavergne JM, *et al.* A new mutation, S1285F, within the A1 loop of von Willebrand factor induces a conformational change in A1 loop with abnormal binding to platelet GPIb and botrocetin causing type 2M von Willebrand disease. *Br J Haematol* 2003; **120**: 643–51.

23 Caron C, Hilbert L, Vanhoorelbeke K, Deckmyn H, Goudemand J, Mazurier C. Measurement of von Willebrand factor binding to a recombinant fragment of glycoprotein Ibalpha in an enzyme-linked immunosorbent assay-based method: performances in patients with type 2B von Willebrand disease. *Br J Haematol* 2006; **133**: 655–63.

24 Ribba AS, Loisel I, Lavergne JM, *et al.* Ser968Thr mutation within the A3 domain of von Willebrand factor (VWF) in two related patients leads to a defective binding of VWF to collagen. *Thromb Haemost* 2001; **86**: 848–54.

25 Nishino M, Girma JP, Rothschild C, Fressinaud E, Meyer D. New variant of von Willebrand disease with defective binding to factor VIII. *Blood* 1989; **74**: 1591–9.

26 Caron C, Mazurier C, Goudemand J. Large experience with a factor VIII binding assay of plasma von Willebrand factor using commercial reagents. *Br J Haematol* 2002; **117**: 716–18.

27 Gaucher C, Dieval J, Mazurier C. Characterization of von Willebrand factor gene defects in two unrelated patients with type IIC von Willebrand disease. *Blood* 1994; **84**: 1024–30.

28 Katsumi A, Tuley EA, Bodo I, Sadler JE. Localization of disulfide bonds in the cystine knot domain of human von Willebrand factor. *J Biol Chem* 2000; **275**: 25585–94.

29 Hommais A, Stepanian A, Fressinaud E, *et al.* Impaired dimerization of von Willebrand factor subunit due to mutation A2801D in the CK domain results in a recessive type 2A subtype IID von Willebrand disease. *Thromb Haemost* 2006; **95**: 776–81.

30 Zimmerman TS, Dent JA, Ruggeri ZM, Nannini LH. Subunit composition of plasma von Willebrand factor. Cleavage is present in normal individuals, increased in IIA and IIB von Willebrand disease, but minimal in variants with aberrant structure of individual oligomers (types IIC, IID, and IIE). *J Clin Invest* 1986; **77**: 947–51.

31 Eikenboom JC, Matsushita T, Reitsma PH, *et al.* Dominant type 1 von Willebrand disease caused by mutated cysteine residues in the D3 domain of von Willebrand factor. *Blood* 1996; **88**: 2433–41.

32 Huizinga EG, Tsuji S, Romijn RA, *et al.* Structures of glycoprotein Ibalpha and its complex with von Willebrand factor A1 domain. *Science* 2002; **297**: 1176–9.

33 Hilbert L, Gaucher C, Mazurier C. Identification of two mutations (Arg611Cys and Arg611His) in the A1 loop of von Willebrand factor (vWF) responsible for type 2 von Willebrand disease with decreased platelet-dependent function of vWF. *Blood* 1995; **86**: 1010–18.

34 Ribba AN, Hilbert L, Lavergne JM, *et al.* The arginine-552-cysteine (R1315C) mutation within the A1 loop of von Willebrand factor induces an abnormal folding with a loss of function resulting in type 2A-like phenotype of von Willebrand disease: study of 10 patients and mutated recombinant von Willebrand factor. *Blood* 2001; **97**: 952–9.

35 James PD, Notley C, Hegadorn C, *et al.* Challenges in defining type 2M von Willebrand disease: results from a Canadian cohort study. *J Thromb Haemost* 2007; **5**: 1914–22.

36 Hilbert L, Jenkins PV, Gaucher C, *et al.* Type 2M vWD resulting from a lysine deletion within a four lysine residue repeat in the A1 loop of von Willebrand factor. *Thromb Haemost* 2000; **84**: 188–94.

37 Nurden P, Chretien F, Poujol C, Winckler J, Borel-Derlon A, Nurden A. Platelet ultrastructural abnormalities in three patients with type 2B von Willebrand disease. *Br J Haematol* 2000; **110**: 704–14.

38 Loffredo G, Baronciani L, Noris P, Menna F, Federici AB, Balduini CL. von Willebrand disease type 2B must be always considered in the differential diagnosis of genetic thrombocytopenias with giant platelets. *Platelets* 2006; **17**: 149–52.

39 Jackson SC, Sinclair GD, Cloutier S, Duan Z, Rand ML, Poon MC. The Montreal platelet syndrome kindred has type 2B von Willebrand disease with the VWF V1316M mutation. *Blood* 2008; **113**: 3348–51.

40 Nurden P, Debili N, Vainchenker W, *et al.* Impaired megakaryocytopoiesis in type 2B von Willebrand disease with severe thrombocytopenia. *Blood* 2006; **108**: 2587–95.

41 Mazurier C, Dieval J, Jorieux S, Delobel J, Goudemand M. A new von Willebrand factor (vWF) defect in a patient with factor VIII (FVIII) deficiency but with normal levels and multimeric patterns of both plasma and platelet vWF. Characterization of abnormal vWF/FVIII interaction. *Blood* 1990; **75**: 20–6.

42 Nishino M, Nishino S, Sugimoto M, Shibata M, Tsuji S, Yoshioka A. Changes in factor VIII binding capacity of von Willebrand factor and factor VIII coagulant activity in two patients with type 2N von Willebrand disease after hemostatic treatment and during pregnancy. *Int J Hematol* 1996; **64**: 127–34.

13 Clinical, laboratory, and molecular markers of type 3 von Willebrand disease

Luciano Baronciani[1], Augusto B. Federici[2,3], and Jeroen C.J. Eikenboom[4]

[1]Angelo Bianchi Bonomi Haemophilia and Thrombosis Centre, Department of Medicine and Medical Specialties, IRCCS Maggiore Policlinico Hospital, Mangiagalli and Regina Elena Foundation, University of Milan, Milan, Italy

[2]Division of Hematology and Transfusion Medicine, L. Sacco University Hospital, Milan, Italy

[3]Department of Internal Medicine, University of Milan, Milan, Italy

[4]Department of Thrombosis and Hemostasis, Leiden University Medical Center, Leiden, the Netherlands

General definition, history, and epidemiology

General definitions

Type 3 von Willebrand disease (VWD) is due to a virtually complete deficiency of von Willebrand factor (VWF). Type 3 VWD is inherited as an autosomal recessive trait and heterozygous relatives have mild or no bleeding symptoms. Most patients with type 3 VWD are characterized by undetectable levels of VWF antigen (VWF:Ag) and by reduced concentrations (<10 IU/dL) of factor VIII (FVIII); for this reason, type 3 VWD also has been described as "severe VWD." However, the term "severe VWD" can be misleading as it has sometimes been used to describe symptomatic patients with type 1 VWD who have very low levels of VWF. However, those with type 1 VWD can be easily distinguished from those with type 3 VWD because patients with type 1 are characterized by an autosomal dominant inheritance pattern and measurable baseline levels of VWF that can increase after desmopressin [1,2].

History

The first description of a family with type 3 VWD was originally reported by Erik A. von Willebrand, an internist at the Deaconess Hospital in Helsinki, Finland. In April 1924, a 5-year-old girl from Föglö on the islands of Åland in the Gulf of Bothnia (between Finland and Sweden) was admitted to the hospital for investigation of severe bleeding from her nose and gums. Her parents were cousins and there was a bleeding history within the family: 11 siblings had a bleeding history and three had died from gastrointestinal bleeds or menorrhagia. Erik von Willebrand described this novel bleeding disorder in 1926 and, in his original publication, he provided an impressive comprehensive description of its clinical and genetic features [3,4]. In contrast to hemophilia, the epitome of inherited bleeding disorders, both sexes were affected and mucosal bleeding was the predominant symptom. A prolonged bleeding time with a normal platelet count was the most important laboratory abnormality, and a functional disorder of the platelets associated with a systemic lesion of the vessel wall was suggested as a possible cause of the disease. von Willebrand called this novel clinical disorder "hereditary pseudo-haemophilia" [3,4]. In the 1950s, when preliminary methods to measure the antihemophilic factor (AHF), later called factor VIII (FVIII), were available, several clinicians described patients of both sexes with a prolonged bleeding time

Von Willebrand Disease, 1st edition. Edited by Augusto B. Federici, Christine A. Lee, Erik E. Berntorp, David Lillicrap, Robert R. Montgomery. © 2011 Blackwell Publishing Ltd.

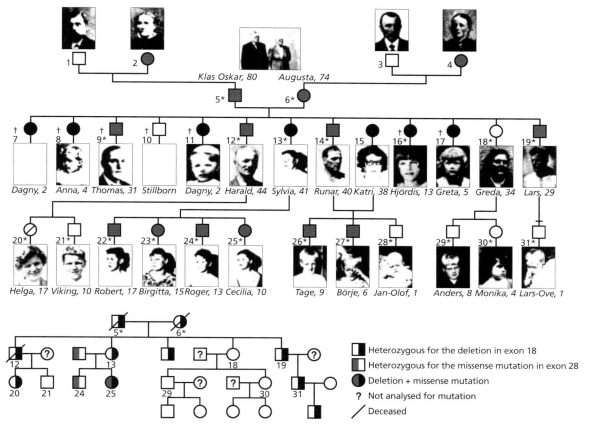

Figure 13.1 Pedigree of family S of Föglö (Historical picture adapted from Blombäk [101]).

associated with reduced FVIII. In 1957, Inga-Marie Nilsson and coworkers revisited the Åland islands and studied 15 patients belonging to the original family (Figure 13.1) and confirmed that these patients had the same clinical and laboratory features as those observed in Sweden [5].

Epidemiology

The prevalence of type 3 VWD is very low, ranging from 0.1 to 5.3 per million population [6–8] and differing considerably between countries (Table 13.1). The highest rate is found in Arabs and the lowest in southern Europeans. However, the actual prevalence of type 3 VWD is still unknown in most countries owing to the lack of retrospective or prospective studies. In Italy, the data of the national registry collected by 48 hemophilia centers have been recently

Table 13.1 Prevalence of type 3 von Willebrand disease (VWD).

Nationality	Prevalence per million population	Reference
Arabic	5.30	Berliner *et al.* [8]
Scandinavian	2.40–3.12	Mannucci *et al.* [6]
Other western European	0.11–0.55	Mannucci *et al.* [6]
Israeli	1.60	Mannucci *et al.* [6]
North American and Canadian	1.38	Weiss *et al.* [7]
European (+ Israeli and Iranian)	1.51	Weiss *et al.* [7]

Table 13.2 Prevalence (%) of bleeding symptoms in patients with von Willebrand disease (VWD) from different cohorts and in normal individuals (adapted from Federici *et al.* [13]; Silwer [11]; Lak *et al.* [12]).

VWD symptoms	Ethnicity					
	Iranian	Italian			Scandinavian	
	Type 3 VWD (*n* = 348)	Type 1 VWD (*n* = 671)	Type 2 VWD (*n* = 497)	Type 3 VWD (*n* = 66)	VWD (*n* = 264)	Normal (*n* = 500)
Epistaxis	77	61	63	66	62	5
Menorrhagia	69	32	32	56	60	25
Post-extraction bleeding	70	31	39	53	51	5
Hematomas	n.r.	13	14	33	49	12
Bleeding from minor wounds	n.r.	36	40	50	36	0.2
Gum bleeding	n.r.	31	35	56	35	7
Postsurgical bleeding	41	20	23	41	28	1
Postpartum bleeding	15	17	18	26	23	19
Gastrointestinal bleeding	20	5	8	20	14	1
Joint bleeding	37	3	4	45	8	0
Hematuria	1	2	5	12	7	1
CNS bleeding	n.r.	1	2	9	n.r.	0

CNS, central nervous system; n.r., not reported.

published [9]: 96 patients with type 3 VWD (5.8%) were identified among the 1650 cases included in the registry with a prevalence of 1.6 per million of population [9].

Clinical markers of type 3 VWD

Because of the severity of VWF defects, patients with type 3 VWD usually meet the three main criteria required for correct diagnoses of VWD: (i) positive bleeding history since childhood; (ii) reduced VWF activity in plasma; and (iii) history of bleeding in a family with autosomal recessive inheritance [10]. Clinical manifestations are excessive mucocutaneous bleeding and prolonged oozing after surgical procedures. In women, menorrhagia is a very frequent clinical manifestation. In contrast with other VWD types, soft tissue and joint bleeding can occur in most patients with type 3 VWD because FVIII is always reduced. To date, only a few detailed descriptions of symptoms are available [11–13]. Following the original description by Silwer [11], the frequency of symptoms has been evaluated specifically in Iranian and Italian patients with type 3 VWD: the most frequent

symptoms in these two cohorts of patients are epistaxis, menorrhagia, and bleeding after dental extractions, but hematoma and joint bleeding are found in 33–45% of the patients (Table 13.2). Several attempts have been made to evaluate the sensitivity and specificity of bleeding symptoms in VWD. In a multicenter study carried out in obligatory carriers of type 1 VWD, menorrhagia and epistaxis were poor predictors of the disease while cutaneous bleeding and bleeding after dental extractions were more sensitive symptoms for diagnosis [14]. A bleeding severity score (BSS) has been calculated using a detailed questionnaire devoted to collecting information on 12 bleeding symptoms in affected and nonaffected members of 154 families enrolled in a large European study, as well as in 200 normal individuals [15]. Despite the fact that this BSS was investigated prospectively in patients with type 1 VWD, this approach seems useful in all types, including type 3 VWD, as recently found in a large cohort of 814 Italian patients with VWD. Preliminary results of this prospective study in all patients with VWD suggest that the BSS can be a useful parameter to predict bleeding risk in VWD. In particular, 52 patients with type 3 VWD, enrolled by six Italian hemophilia centers, were

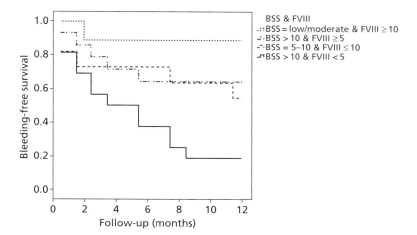

Figure 13.2 Bleeding-free survival curves calculated according to bleeding severity score (BSS) and levels of FVIII in 56 Italian patients with type 3 VWD.

exposed at enrollment to the detailed questionnaire to calculate the BSS and observed prospectively during the following 12 months for bleeding episodes. In the calculation of bleeding incidence, only the first bleeding episode after the start of follow-up was considered. As expected, in patients with type 3 VWD who showed a BSS higher than 10, the incidence of bleeding measured as percent/year (95% confidence interval [CI]) was 73.3 (44.5–102), much higher that that shown in all the other VWD types. However, four different patterns were observed in the Kaplan–Meier curves of bleeding-free survival, suggesting a high degree of heterogeneity in our cohort of patients with type 3 VWD (Figure 13.2). By multivariate model including all variables, values of BSS >10 were the most significant (hazard ratio = 5.5 [2.8–10.89]) determinant of bleeding [16].

Laboratory markers of type 3 VWD

Unlike the other VWD types, where diagnosis may often require several laboratory tests to be repeated on different occasions, patients with type 3 VWD can be identified quite easily owing to the severity of VWF and FVIII defects. Additionally, screening tests for hemostasis can be abnormal and suggest a possible diagnosis of type 3 VWD. Partial thromboplastin time (PTT) is usually prolonged because of the low concentrations of FVIII (<10 IU/dL) and the platelet count is normal but always associated with prolonged bleeding time, the original hallmark of type 3 VWD.

Bleeding time can be sometimes very prolonged (>35 min), this is due to undetectable levels of VWF in both plasma and platelets. Evaluation of closure time with the platelet function analyzer PFA-100 gives a rapid and simple measure of VWF-dependent platelet function at high shear stress: it can be performed in whole blood and therefore can be employed instead of the bleeding time in children or when the bleeding time is not feasible. This system is sensitive and reproducible for type 3 VWD screening, but the closure time is not corrected after the administration of VWF/FVIII concentrates [17]. In patients with a normal platelet count, very prolonged bleeding time, and an abnormal PTT with reduced levels of FVIII, the diagnosis of type 3 VWD should be always confirmed by measuring plasma levels of VWF:Ag. Different methods of VWF:Ag are available, but the ELISA (enzyme-linked immunosorbent assay) tests are the most sensitive. By definition, VWF:Ag levels should be undetectable with concentrations <1 IU/dL. However, there is still some debate about also considering individuals with very reduced but measurable levels of VWF:Ag as having type 3 VWD. Platelet VWF also should be undetectable in type 3 VWD, while VWF contents in platelet and plasma were found to be heterogeneous in the heterozygous carriers of type 3 VWD [18]. Owing to the very low or undetectable levels of VWF:Ag, measurements of VWF activities such as ristocetin cofactor (VWF:RCo) and collagen-binding assay (VWF:CB) are of limited use. Multimeric analyses of VWF in the plasma and platelets of patients with type 3 VWD might show

151

only VWF monomers without any organization into dimers or tetramers: all these assays can be of interest for confirming the complete deficiency of VWF in type 3 VWD.

Alloantibodies against VWF are a rare complication of replacement therapy in transfused patients with inherited type 3 VWD. An incidence of 7.5–9.5% was found in an international survey based on the 150 individuals tested [19]. No general consensus has been reached for measuring anti-VWF antibodies in patients with type 3 VWD. The assays are currently available in only a few specialized labs and they mimic the Bethesda assays for hemophilia inhibitors by performing VWF and FVIII activities in patient-normal pool plasma mixtures after 2 h incubation at 37°C. The titer of anti-VWF inhibitor is calculated by the current dilution of VWD plasma inhibiting 50% of normal plasma pool diluted 1:2 compared with control mixture. Several authors have used ristocetin-induced platelet agglutination (RIPA) in normal platelet-rich plasma (PRP) to measure anti-VWF inhibitors [19]. However, all VWF parameters should be performed, such as anti-VWF:Ag, anti-VWF:RCo, anti-VWF:CB, and anti-FVIII. Owing to the relatively low frequency of type 3 VWD, the costs and difficulties of its molecular diagnosis, the difficulty of identifying anti-VWF antibodies, and the current worldwide prevalence, clinical–molecular diagnosis and management of this rare complication are not available. We have recently proposed an investigator-driven study entitled "Prevalence and clinical–molecular markers of alloantibodies in type 3 VWD patients" [20].

Molecular markers of type 3 VWD

Inheritance pattern

Type 3 VWD is inherited with an autosomal recessive pattern; therefore, unaffected parents, who are heterozygous for a defective *VWF* gene (carriers), have a 25% possibility of having an affected child. Evidence of this autosomal recessive transmission had already been reported by Veltkamp and van Tilburg [21] in 1973 through the observation of severely affected patients and their symptomless parents. The advent of molecular biology techniques allowed the identification of VWF gene defects. Often, patients with type 3 VWD are homozygous for a mutation owing to the consanguinity of their parents.

Large gene deletions

In the late 1980s, the first molecular defects in patients with type 3 VWD were identified using the Southern blot technique. Complete homozygous VWF gene deletions were identified in two out of 19 patients with type 3 VWD by Shelton-Inloes et al. [22], and complete homozygous and heterozygous deletions were found among six patients with type 3 VWD by Ngo et al. [23]. In the 1990s, Schneppenheim et al. [24] identified one complete homozygous and one partial heterozygous deletion among 28 German patients with type 3 VWD, whereas one complete heterozygous VWF gene deletion was identified among five Italian patients with type 3 VWD [25]. Recently, Schneppenheim et al. [26] identified the exact extent of the deletion in patients who shared the same defect, with a deletion of 253,246 bp (Δ253 kb). The identification of an identical break-point in these patients led the authors to hypothesize a common genetic background for these German and Italian patients. To date, seven partial homozygous VWF gene deletions including exons 1–3, 6–16, 42, 33–38, 22–43, 23–52, and 17–18 have been described [27–32]. Among these alterations, only the Alu-mediated deletion of exons 1–3 was found in several patients, which was the most common defect in Hungarian patients with type 3 VWD [31].

Nonsense mutations

Since the first studies into the disorder [22,23], it was clear that the majority of patients with type 3 VWD would not have large gene deletions, but more subtle mutations (i.e., single nucleotide substitutions or small deletions and insertions). The first attempts of several groups to identify these defects was done by analysis of the 11 CGA arginine codons present in the VWF coding region. These codons contain the CpG dinucleotide considered to be the primary site of eukaryotic DNA methylation, which results in a mutation product TpG [33]. Therefore, at codon CGA the substitution C to T introduces a translational stop codon (TGA). The screening of these 11 arginine codons allowed the identification of four nonsense mutations (R365X, R1659X, R1853X, and

R2535X) [34–37]. Only the use of screening techniques such as single-strand confirmation polymorphism analysis, conformation-sensitive gel electrophoresis, and chemical cleavage mismatch analysis, in association with direct DNA sequencing, has now allowed the complete characterization of many type 3 VWD mutations. To date, over 30 different nonsense mutations have been identified (see Table 13.3). Of these, seven are at the 11 CGA codons. The R1659X and R2535X were the most frequently described, with R2535X reported in patients of Swedish [34,38], Dutch [35], German [24], Italian [25], and Turkish [30] origin and R1659X reported in patients from Finland [34,38], Japan [39], Iran [29], and India [40]. Also, mutation Q1311X (c.3831C→T), first reported by Casana *et al.* [41], has been reported in several patients from different countries [40,42–44]. In all cases but one [41], mutation c.3831C>T was found always with one or more nearby nucleotide substitutions as a result of gene conversion between the *VWF* gene and its pseudogene [57].

Small deletions and insertions

More than 30 small deletions or insertions [24,25,29–31,38,40,43,45–49] have so far been reported in patients with type 3 VWD (see Table 13.3). As would be expected in patients with type 3 VWD, all these defects but two (c.8241del9 and c.788del24) cause a frameshift resulting in a premature termination codon. Deletions and insertions do not occur randomly with respect to the surrounding DNA sequence; they are known to be strongly influenced by the presence of direct repeats, inverted repeats, and symmetric elements in the immediate vicinity of the lesion [58]. Ten of these deletions occurred within a run of the same nucleotide (AA, TT, TTT, GGG, GGGG, GGGGG, TTTTT, CCCCCC) and three occurred within a stretch of a dinucleotide (ACACAC, GTGTGTGT, and CTCTCTCTCT). Six insertions of a single base were identified in a string of the same nucleotide (GG, TTT, CCC, CCCC, CCCCC, CCCCCC, and CCCCCCC). The deletions of 9 and 24 nucleotides were found to be surrounded by a repetitive sequence (CCA, CTGGAGT) that is probably responsible for a slipped strand mispairing at the replication fork, as has been reported by Efstratiadis *et al.* [59].

Only a few mutations have been reported more than once, with the exception of the c.2435delC (c.2680delC when numbered from the transcription initiation) [45]. This single cytosine deletion in exon 18 was first reported as the most common mutation in Swedish patients with type 3 VWD, in whom it was identified in about 50% of the mutant alleles [45]. This mutation was also identified [60] in the first ever patient with type 3 VWD studied by Erik von Willebrand. The c.2435delC was found with a high prevalence in Germany [24], Poland [48], Hungary [31], and rarely in Italy [25,43,47], whereas it was not found among patients with type 3 VWD from the USA [61], Turkey [30], Iran [43], India [40,43], and Greece [40]. The high prevalence of c.2435delC in northern Europe favors a founder effect rather than a recurrent mutation at a mutational hot spot. Apparently, linkage studies support a possible common origin of c.2435delC mutation in the Swedish population [38] but not in the German and Polish populations, where most cases were linked to different haplotypes [24,48]. However, the different polymorphic haplotypes may be a result of the recombination or an instability of repeats [62]. The mutation c.7130insC, first reported [25] in the Italian population, was found in three unrelated Indian patients [29,43], but with different haplotypes (VNTR1–VNTR2: Italy 8–3 vs. India 12–7), supporting the independent origin of the insertion.

Also, deletions c.2016del4 [43,47] and c.6182delT [29,47] have been found more than once, but always among the same population, and therefore it is likely that the patients shared a common ancestor.

Splice site mutations

More than 15 splice site mutations have so far been identified (see Table 13.3). However, the majority of these nucleotide substitutions have not been confirmed at the mRNA level. Therefore, in contrast to nonsense and frameshift mutations, these nucleotide substitutions should only be considered as putative mutations. Nevertheless, half of these substitutions affect the guanine at position +1 or −1 and so are very likely to alter normal splicing. Only two of these mutations have been evaluated at the mRNA level, mutation c.1534–3C>A [25] (or IVS13–3C>A according to the human gene Nomenclature Working Group [63]) and mutation c.8155+3G>T [50] (IVS50+3G>T).

Table 13.3 Molecular genetic defects in type 3 von Willebrand disease (VWD).

Type of defect	Nucleotide change	Amino acid change	Exon	References
Large gene deletions	Complete VWF gene deletion		1–52	Shelton-Inloes et al. [22]; Ngo et al. [23]; Schneppenheim et al. [24]; Eikenboom et al. [25]; Schneppenheim et al. [26]
	Large partial VWF gene deletion		1–3	Mohl et al. [31]
	Large partial VWF gene deletion		6–16	Xie et al. [32]
	Large partial VWF gene deletion		17–18	Abuzenadah et al. [30]
	Large partial VWF gene deletion		22–43	Mancuso et al. [28]
	Large partial VWF gene deletion		23–52	Baronciani et al. [29]
	Large partial VWF gene deletion		33–38	Mancuso et al. [28]
	Large partial VWF gene deletion		42	Peake et al. [27]
	Large partial VWF gene deletion		Unspecified	Schneppenheim et al. [24]
mRNA expression defects	No VWF mRNA detectable		n.a.	Eikenboom et al. [35]; Nichols et al. [98]
Nonsense mutations	c.171C>A	C57X	3	Abuzenadah et al. [30]
	c.229C>T	Q77X	4	Castaman et al. [47]
	c.592C>T	Q198X	6	Castaman et al. [47]
	c.652C>T	Q218X	6	Baronciani et al. [29]
	c.666G>A	W222X	7	Baronciani et al. [29]
	c.970C>T	R324X	8	Schneppenheim et al. [24]; Gupta et al. [40]
	c.1093C>T	R365X	9	Baronciani et al. [29]; Bahnak et al. [36]; Baronciani et al. [43]; Castaman et al. [47]
	c.1117C>T	R373X	10	Baronciani et al. [29]; Gupta et al. [40]
	n.r.	W553X	14	Gupta et al. [40]
	c.1693C>T	Q565X	14	Gupta et al. [40]
	c.1830C>A	Y610X	15	Baronciani et al. [43]
	c.1858G>T	E620X	15	Zhang et al. [38]
	c.1926G>A	W642X	15	Baronciani et al. [43]
	c.1930G>T	E644X	15	Baronciani et al. [29]
	c.2116C>T	Q706X	16	Baronciani et al. [29]
	c.2848G>T	E950X	22	Titapiwatanakun et al. [53]

c.3427G>T	E1143X	27	Wetzstein et al. [49]
c.3800T>A	L1267X	28	Gupta et al. [40]
c.3931C>T	Q1311X	28	Gupta et al. [40]; Casan et al. [41]; Surdhar et al. [42]; Baronciani et al. [43]; Gupta et al. [44]; Castaman et al. [47]
c.4013C>G	S1338X	28	Baronciani et al. [29]
c.4036C>T	Q1346X	28	Baronciani et al. [29]
c.4368C>A	Y1456X	28	Xie et al. [46]
c.4626C>G	Y1542X	28	Baronciani et al. [29]
c.4975C>T	R1659X	28	Baronciani et al. [29]; Zhang et al. [34]; Zhang et al. [37]; Zhang et al. [38]; Hagiwara et al. [39]; Gupta et al. [40]
c.5557C>T	R1853X	32	Zhang et al. [34]; Zhang et al. [38]
c.5692C>T	Q1898X	34	Mohl et al. [31]
c.5941G>T	E1981X	35	Baronciani et al. [43]
c.6385G>T	E2129X	37	Baronciani et al. [29]
n.r.	Y2392X	42	Abuzenadah et al. [30]
c.7300C>T	R2434X	43	Baronciani et al. [43]
c.7603C>T	R2535X	45	Schneppenheim et al. [24]; Eikenboom et al. [25]; Abuzenadah et al. [30]; Zhang et al. [34]; Eikenboom et al. [35]; Zhang et al. [38]; Enayat et al. [56]
c.7630C>T	Q2544X	45	Baronciani et al. [43]
Small insertions			
c.276insT	Frameshift	4	Enayat et al. [56]
c.893insG	Frameshift	8	Xie et al. [46]
c.1657insT	Frameshift	14	Zhang et al. [38]
c.2734insT	Frameshift	21	Abuzenadah et al. [30]
c.3259insT	Frameshift	25	Gupta et al. [40]
c.3737insCC	Frameshift	28	Gupta et al. [40]
c.4331ins8	Frameshift	28	Gupta et al. [40]
c.4414insC	Frameshift	28	Baronciani et al. [43]
c.4415insG	Frameshift	28	Abuzenadah et al. [30]; Baronciani et al. [43]
c.4975insC	Frameshift	28	Zhang et al. [38]
c.7130insC	Frameshift	42	Eikenboom et al. [25]; Baronciani et al. [29]; Baronciani et al. [43]
c.7139insT	Frameshift	42	Baronciani et al. [43]
c.7173insT	Frameshift	42	Gupta et al. [40]
c.7449insA	Frameshift	44	Abuzenadah et al. [30]
c.7674insC	Frameshift	45	Baronciani et al. [29]

(Continued)

Table 13.3 (*Continued*)

Type of defect	Nucleotide change	Amino acid change	Exon	References
Small deletions	c.191delG	Frameshift	3	Baronciani et al. [29]
	c.276delT	Frameshift	4	Baronciani et al. [43]
	c.410del13	Frameshift	5	Enayat et al. [56]
	c.788del24	263del8	7	Baronciani et al. [43]
	c.1384delG	Frameshift	12	Gupta et al. [40]
	c.1930del20	Frameshift	15	Zhang et al. [38]
	c.2016del4	Frameshift	16	Baronciani et al. [43]; Castaman et al. [47]
	c.2157delA	Frameshift	16	Baronciani et al. [43]
	c.2269delCT	Frameshift	17	Baronciani et al. [43]
	c.2435delC	Frameshift	18	Schneppenheim [24]; Baronciani et al. [29]; Mohl et al. [31]; Zhang et al. [38]; Zhang et al. [45]; Gazda et al. [48]; Wetzstein et al. [49]
	c.2516delG	Frameshift	19	Enayat et al. [56]
	c.2641delC	Frameshift	20	Abuzenadah et al. [30]
	c.3385delAG	Frameshift	26	Abuzenadah et al. [30]
	c.3622delT	Frameshift	27	Mohl et al. [31]
	c.3938delG	Frameshift	28	Gupta et al. [40]
	c.4092delAC	Frameshift	28	Baronciani et al. [43]
	c.4449delG	Frameshift	28	Eikenboom et al. [25]
	c.4635delG	Frameshift	28	Schneppenheim et al. [24]
	c.6182delT	Frameshift	36	Baronciani et al. [29]; Castaman et al. [47]
	c.7294delGT	Frameshift	43	Baronciani et al. [43]
	c.7683delT	Frameshift	45	Baronciani et al. [43]
	c.8241del9	2748del3	51	Baronciani et al. [29]
Splice site mutations	c.658-3C>A	n.a.	7	Enayat et al. [56]
	c.874+1G>A	n.a.	7	Gadisseur et al. [99]
	c.1110-1G>A	n.a.	10	Baronciani et al. [29]
	c.1534-3C>A	n.a.	14	Eikenboom et al. [25]; Castaman et al. [47]
	c.1946-4C>T	n.a.	16	Baronciani et al. [43]
	c.2453-1G>C	n.a.	19	Castaman et al. [47]
	c.3108+5G>A	n.a.	23	Baronciani et al. [43]
	c.3379+1G>A	n.a.	25	Baronciani et al. [43]
	c.5053+1G>T	n.a.	28	Abuzenadah et al. [30]
	c.5053+1G>A	n.a.	28	Baronciani et al. [43]
	c.5170+10C>T	n.a.	29	Baronciani et al. [29]

	Nucleotide change	Exon	Amino acid change	Reference
	c.6977-1G>C	41	n.a.	Baronciani et al. [29]
	c.7437G>A	43	n.a.	Zhang et al. [38]
	c.7729+7C>T	45	n.a.	Baronciani et al. [43]
	c.7770+1G>T	46	n.a.	Castaman et al. [47]
	c.8155+3G>T	50	n.a.	Mertes et al. [50]
Missense mutations	c.100C>G	3	R34G	Abuzenadah et al. [30]
	c.139G>C	3	D47H	Baronciani et al. [43]
	c.253T>C	4	S85P	Baronciani et al. [43]
	c.257T>A	4	V86E	Gupta et al. [40]; Gupta et al. [44]
	c.421G>T	5	D141Y	Baronciani et al. [43]
	c.421G>A	5	D141N	Baronciani et al. [43]
	c.449T>A	5	L150Q	Zhang et al. [38]; Zhang et al. [51]
	c.817C>T	7	R273W	Gupta et al. [40]; Allen et al. [52]
	c.823T>A	7	C275S	Baronciani et al. [29]
	n.r.	8	N318K	Gupta et al. [40]
	c.1131G>T	10	W377C	Schneppenheim et al. [24]
	c.1152T>G	10	C384T	Enayat et al. [56]
	c.1280T>A	11	I427N	VWF database[a]
	n.r.	20	R854Y	Castaman et al. [47]
	c.3212G>T	24	C1071F	Baronciani et al. [43]
	Gene conversion	28		Eikenboom et al. [25]
	c.3943C>T	28	R1315C	Zhang et al. [38]; Zhang et al. [51]
	c.4027A>G	28	I1343V	Castaman et al. [47]
	c.5191T>A	30	S1731T	Castaman et al. [47]
	c.5380A>G	31	K1794E	Gupta et al. [40]
	c.6187C>T	36	P2063S	Abuzenadah et al. [30]
	c.6520T>G	37	C2174G	Baronciani et al. [29]
	c.6965A>T	40	E2322V	Titapiwatanakun et al. [53]
	c.7085G>T	42	C2362F	Eikenboom et al. [25]
	c.7433G>A	43	R2478Q	Titapiwatanakun et al. [53]
Missense mutations, dimerization region	c.8012G>A	49	C2671Y	Eikenboom et al. [25]
	c.8216G>A	51	C2739Y	Zhang et al. [38]
	c.8262T>G	52	C2754W	Schneppenheim et al. [55]
	c.8411G>A	52	C2804Y	Baronciani et al. [29]
	c.8416T>C	52	C2806R	Montogmery et al. [54]

Nucleotides are numbered from the A of the initiator ATG as +1; amino acids are numbered from 1 to 2813 starting at the translation initiation codon(Goodeve et al. [100]).

VWF, von Willebrand factor; n.a., not applicable; n.r., not reported.

[a]VWF Online Database. International Society on Thrombosis and Haemostasis Scientific and Standardization Committee VWF information homepage; Available from: http://www.vwf.group.shef.ac.uk/ [accessed on 19 October 2010].

Both result in a premature termination codon, one at the acceptor splice site (IVS13–3C>A) by causing the skipping of exon 14, and one at the donor splice site (IVS50+3G>T) by causing the skipping of exon 50. No apparent common defect was found among these splice defects—only the c.1534–3C>A mutation was found in more than one study—but in all cases the patients were from the same country [25,47].

Missense mutation

We would not expect to frequently find missense mutations in patients with type 3 VWD. In contrast to large deletions, nonsense mutations, and frameshift mutations, missense mutations can only be considered putative disease-producing mutations, as a cause and effect relationship between the amino acid substitution and the low VWF level is not certain. In addition, how these missense mutations cause a quantitative VWF defect is often not easily understood. Nevertheless, about 30 candidate missense mutations have been reported in patients with type 3 VWD [24,25,29, 30,38,40,43,47,51–56]. In a subgroup of patients with autosomal recessive severe VWD characterized by a significant increase in FVIII:C after desmopressin infusion [64], a missense mutation was identified predicting the loss of the cysteine residue C2362F [25]. The probands were either homozygous for the C2362F mutation or compound heterozygous, the second allele being a null allele (splice defect, nonsense mutation or frameshift). Because of the null allele, the compound heterozygotes are phenotypically similar to the homozygotes [25]. *In vitro* transient expression of the full-length mutant VWF-C2362F protein showed impaired secretion and intracellular retention of the mutant protein [65]. Although the proteolysis of VWF C2362F was shown to be increased [66], the transfection experiments showed that this could not be explained by increased susceptibility of recombinant VWF-C2362F to ADAMTS13 [65]. Almost half of the missense mutations identified in type 3 VWD are located in the propeptide of VWF. Only three of these mutations (D141Y, R273W, and C275S) have been expressed in COS-7 cells. *In vitro* studies showed that the mutations strongly impaired the VWF multimerization process and that recombinant mutant VWF was retained intracellularly [52,67].

The missense mutations in type 3 VWD are heterogeneous, but there may be subgroups of mutations that cause VWF deficiency through a common mechanism. One subgroup could be mutated cysteine residues in the C terminal region of VWF, a region responsible for the dimerization of the pro-VWF subunits [68]. Six mutations resulting in the loss of a cysteine in the C terminus have been described: C2671Y [25], C2739Y [38], HYC2748–2750del [29], C2754W [55], C2804Y [29], and C2806R [54]. Expression studies of C2754W [55] and C2806R [54] showed a failure of C terminal dimerization.

Prenatal and molecular diagnosis of type 3 VWD

Compared with hemophilia, most patients with VWD show relatively mild bleeding symptoms. Therefore, prenatal diagnosis is required mainly in cases where parents are already known to be carriers of type 3 VWD, with gene defects identified in their first affected child. Neonatal diagnosis can be performed in cases of children from parents with VWF defects already characterized, but phenotypic diagnosis of VWD should be always confirmed later on in the child and compared with the other affected members within the same family. In the past, prenatal diagnoses were performed by polymerase chain reaction (PCR) amplification of variable number tandem repeat region of *VWF* gene [69]. Nowadays, prenatal diagnosis can be performed by using PCR amplification of the region of the *VWF* gene where mutations or deletions could be found in the propositus. As young children with type 3 VWD might carry deletions of the *VWF* gene that predispose them to developing alloantibodies to VWF, searching for deletions could be considered in a new child with type 3 VWD before starting extensive therapy with exogenous VWF concentrates. New methods for screening large deletions are now available [70].

Treatment and prevention of bleeding in type 3 VWD

The goal of treatment is to correct the dual defects of hemostasis, that is, abnormal platelet adhesion owing to low or defective VWF and abnormal intrinsic coagulation due to low FVIII [71]. Two main therapeutic approaches are available: (i) desmopressin (DDAVP, 1-deamino-8-D-arginine vasopressin), which releases endogenous VWF from endothelial cells; and (ii) exogenous VWF contained in VWF/FVIII concentrates.

As the response to DDAVP depends on the endogenous synthesis of VWF, patients with type 3 VWD are unresponsive to desmopressin [72,73]. Therefore, there is no place for DDAVP in the treatment of patients with type 3 VWD. Recently, however, a subgroup of patients with autosomal recessive severe VWD has been described, in whom the FVIII:C increased to near-normal levels (49–70 IU/dL) after DDAVP infusion [64]. These patients were characterized by a very low but measurable concentration of VWF:Ag (0.5–3.5 IU/dL) that increased after DDAVP infusion to 8–9 IU/dL. One of those patients even underwent an uncomplicated dental extraction using desmopressin. Thus, this response to desmopressin represents a unique phenotype, and the DDAVP infusion data should not be generalized to other patients with type 3 VWD. Moreover, DDAVP could act as an adjuvant to replacement therapy as it has been shown in patients treated with cryoprecipitate that the addition of DDAVP shortens the bleeding time independent of the release of endogenous VWF [74].

VWF/FVIII concentrates are the treatment of choice for patients with type 3 VWD. The minimal requirements for plasma-derived VWF/FVIII concentrates in VWD management are as follows: (i) they must contain biologically active VWF that could correct the primary hemostasis defect and stabilize the endogenous FVIII molecule (the latter objective can be achieved independently of the content in exogenous FVIII); (ii) they should be treated by virucidal methods; and (iii) before clinical use, they should be tested for pharmacokinetics and efficacy in retrospective or prospective clinical trials in relatively large numbers of patients with VWD [71]. Among many VWF/FVIII concentrates available in the market, only a few can meet these requirements (Table 13.4). VWF/FVIII concentrates can be given to stop bleeding episodes when they occur (treatment on demand), to prevent bleeding during surgery (prophylaxis for surgery), and to prevent recurrent bleeding at specific sites (secondary long-term prophylaxis). The pharmacokinetics and clinical efficacy results of the first prospective study in VWD were published in 2002 [75]. This study included 53 patients receiving treatment with a doubly virus-inactivated VWF/FVIII concentrate (Alphanate; Grifols Biologicals Inc., Los Angeles, CA, USA) for 87 bleeding episodes and 39 patients receiving treatment for 71 surgical or invasive diagnostic procedures. A good clinical response with this VWF/

FVIII concentrate was observed in 86% of the spontaneous bleeding episodes and in 71% of surgical or invasive procedures [75]. Two retrospective studies and one prospective study have also been performed using Fanhdi (Instituto Grifols, S.A. Barcelona, Spain), a concentrate manufactured using a process very similar to that of Alphanate [76–78].

Haemate-P/Humate-P, an intermediate-purity VWF/FVIII concentrate, has been widely used in VWD. This product was introduced into clinical practice in Europe (Haemate-P; CSL Behring, Marburg, Germany) in 1984 and into the USA (Humate-P; CSL Behring, Marburg, Germany) in 1999. The first pharmacokinetics study of Haemate-P, published in 1998, was a single-center evaluation involving six patients with type 3 VWD [79]. Results of a large retrospective study organized by the Canadian Hemophilia Centers were published in 2002 [80]. Other published studies include two retrospective analyses of Haemate-P/Humate-P efficacy and safety in Italian patients with VWD [81,82], as well as two prospective multicenter open-label, nonrandomized studies conducted in the USA on Haemate-P/Humate-P used in urgent bleeding and urgent surgical events [83,84]. The results of another prospective study in elective surgery with Haemate-P/Humate-P with dosing based on pharmacokinetics have been recently published [85].

The use of Wilate (Octapharma, Vienna, Austria) in VWD management has been reported in Germany since 2005 [86], and the results of efficacy and safety in acute bleeding episodes, in surgical interventions and in secondary long-term prophylaxis, will be published within a few months. Data on the pharmacokinetics and clinical efficacy of Biostate (CSL Behring, Marburg, Germany), a VWF/FVIII concentrate available in Australia and Asia, have also been reported [87,88]. A distinct plasma-derived VWF concentrate with low FVIII levels was introduced in France in 1992, and the first pharmacokinetics study in type 3 VWD was published in 1996 [89]. An improved version of this concentrate (Wilfactin; LFB, Lille, France), which is almost devoid of FVIII, was evaluated in two large French and European studies, and data on pharmacokinetics have been already published [90]. Results in type 3 VWD show no major differences in VWF:RCo and VWF:Ag for the concentrates that did or did not contain FVIII, the only difference was an approximate 6-h delay in FVIII increase with the concentrate devoid of FVIII.

Table 13.4 Plasma-derived concentrates containing von Willebrand factor (VWF).

Concentrate	Purification procedures	Virucidal Rx	VWF:RCo/Ag[a]	VWF:RCo/FVIII[a]	Available in	Manufacturer
A. Concentrates with published activity in patients with VWD						
Alphanate[b]	Heparin ligand CT	SD; dry heat	0.6	1.2	Germany, Italy, United Kingdom, USA	Grifols (USA)
Biostate[c]	Precipitation/heparin ligand CT	SD; dry heat	0.8	2.0	Australia, Asia	CSL Behring
Fanhdi[d]	Precipitation, heparin ligand CT	SD; dry heat	0.6	1.6	Spain, Italy	Grifols (Spain)
Haemate-P[e,c]	Polyelectrolyte precipitations	Pasteurization	0.8	2.5	Asia, Europe, USA	CSL Behring
Wilate[f]	Affinity CT, size exclusion	SD; dry heat	0.7	0.8	Germany	Octapharma
Wilfactin[g]	Ion-exchange, affinity CTs	SD; NF; dry heat	0.7	60	France	LFB (Lille)
B. Concentrates with limited activity or no published studies in patients with VWD						
Emoclot[h]	Ion-exchange CT	SD; dry heat	0.5	1.2	Brazil, Italy	Kedrion
Immunate[i]	Ion-exchange CT	SD; vapor heat	0.2	0.2	Europe	Baxter
Innobrand[g]	Ion-exchange CT	SD	0.7	2.5	France	LFB (Lille)
Koate DVI[j]	Precipitations, size exclusion	SD; dry heat	0.5	1.2	USA	Talecris
8Y[k]	Heparin/glycine precipitations	Dry heat	0.3	0.8	United Kingdom	BioProducts

VWD, von Willebrand disease; CT, chromatography; SD, solvent-detergent (t-N-butyl-PO$_4$ with polysorbate, Tween, or otoxynol, Triton); NF, nanofiltration.

[a] Ratio of ristocetin cofactor activity (VWF:RCo) to VWF:Ag or FVIII activity expressed as IU/dL (or percent of a normal pool).
[b] Grifols Biologicals Inc., Los Angeles, CA, USA.
[c] CSL Behring, Marburg, Germany.
[d] Instituto Grifols, S.A. Barcelona, Spain.
[e] Humate-P in USA.
[f] Octapharma, Vienna, Austria.
[g] LFB, Lille, France.
[h] Kedrion S.p.A. Castelvecchio P. (LU), Italy.
[i] Baxter Bioscience, Vienna, Austria.
[j] Talecris Biotherapeutics Inc., Research Triangle Park, NC, USA.
[k] Bio Products Laboratory, Elstree, UK.

Therefore, administration of exogenous FVIII is recommended in type 3 VWD episodes of acute life-threatening bleeding or emergency surgeries [90]. Clinical efficacy results of the French and European studies have been recently reported [91].

On the whole, there is no evidence from retrospective or prospective clinical studies that the six VWF/FVIII concentrates (Alphanate, Biostate, Fanhdi, Haemate-P/Humate-P, Wilate, and Wilfactin) reported in Table 13.4 differ with regards to efficacy, because no head-to-head clinical study was carried out. Therefore all these VWF/FVIII concentrates can be effective in the management or prevention of bleeding in patients with VWD.

Treatment of patients with alloantibodies to VWF

For the rare patients with type 3 VWD who develop anti-VWF alloantibodies after multiple transfusions, the use of VWF/FVIII concentrates is not only ineffective, but may even cause postinfusion anaphylaxis as a result of the formation of immune complexes [92]. These reactions may be life threatening. To overcome this drawback, a patient undergoing emergency abdominal surgery was treated with recombinant FVIII, because this product, which contains no VWF, could not cause anaphylactic reactions. In view of the very short half-life of FVIII without its VWF carrier, recombinant FVIII had to be administered by continuous intravenous infusion at very large doses to keep FVIII levels above 50 IU/dL for 10 days after surgery [92]. Another possible therapeutic approach is recombinant activated factor VII (rFVIIa), which can be used in VWD with alloantibodies according to the same dosage and regimen as for patients with hemophilia A with inhibitors [93,94].

Secondary long-term prophylaxis

Patients with severe forms of VWD may have frequent hemarthroses, especially when FVIII levels are below 10 IU/dL, so that some of them develop target joints like patients with moderate hemophilia A. Some patients have recurrent gastrointestinal bleeding, often without lesions in the gastrointestinal tract, and need treatment every day or every other day. Finally, there are children who have epistaxis frequently and severely enough to cause anemia. In these frequent and severe bleeders, the optimal therapy may be regular prophylaxis with VWF concentrates rather than on-demand treatment on the occasion of bleeding episodes. The largest experience with secondary prophylaxis in VWD has been collected in Sweden in 35 patients with severe forms of VWD [95]. Secondary prophylaxis was also implemented in a cohort of Italian patients with VWD [96]. These two retrospective studies suggest that cost-effectiveness of these prophylaxis regimens versus on-demand therapy should be further evaluated in larger prospective studies.

Future perspectives

On the whole, treatments currently available for VWD are quite satisfactory. For patients with type 3 VWD, VWF/FVIII concentrates are the only form of available treatment. The fact that they are fractionated from plasma is of concern for some, even if more than one viral inactivation method is used for most concentrates in the manufacturing process. Haemate-P/Humate-P is the only concentrate that uses only one viral inactivation method (pasteurization), but the safety record of this product is impeccable. This favorable situation notwithstanding, there are advanced plans to develop a therapeutic preparation of recombinant VWF. This product, containing only VWF, will require the concomitant administration of FVIII for the control of acute bleeding episodes and for the prevention of excessive bleeding at the time of major surgery. Attempts to partially correct VWD through gene replacement therapy are also in progress [97].

Acknowledgements

We acknowledge the work of Dr. Luigi Flaminio Ghilardini, who prepared the figures reported in this manuscript.

References

1 Eikenboom JC. Congenital von Willebrand disease type 3: clinical manifestations, pathophysiology and molecular biology. *Best Pract Res Clin Haematol* 2001; **14**: 365–79.

2 Sadler JE, Budde U, Eikenboom JC, *et al.* Update on the pathophysiology and classification of von Willebrand disease: a report of the Subcommittee on von Willebrand Factor. *J Thromb Haemost* 2006; **4**: 2103–14.

3 von Willebrand EA. Hereditär pseudohemofili. *Finska Läkaresällskapets Handlingar* 1926; **68**: 87–112.

4 Nilsson IM. Commentary to Erik von Willebrand's original paper from 1926 "Hereditar pseudohemofili". *Haemophilia* 1999; **5**: 220–1.

5 Nilsson IM, Blomback M, Blomback B. von Willebrand's disease in Sweden. Its pathogenesis and treatment. *Acta Med Scand* 1959; **164**: 263–78.

6 Mannucci PM, Bloom AL, Larrieu MJ, *et al.* Atherosclerosis and von Willebrand factor. I. Prevalence of severe von Willebrand's disease in western Europe and Israel. *Br J Haematol* 1984; **57**: 163–9.

7 Weiss HJ, Ball AP, Mannucci PM. Incidence of severe von Willebrand's disease (letter). *N Engl J Med* 1982; **307**: 127.

8 Berliner SA, Seligsohn U, Zivelin A, *et al.* A relatively high frequency of severe (type III) von Willebrand's disease in Israel. *Br J Haematol* 1986; **62**: 535–43.

9 Iorio A, Oliovecchio E, Morfini M, *et al.* Italian Registry of Haemophilia and Allied Disorders. Objectives, methodology and data analysis. *Haemophilia* 2008; **14**: 444–53.

10 Federici AB, Mannucci PM. Management of inherited von Willebrand disease in 2007. *Ann Med* 2007; **39**: 346–58.

11 Silwer J. von Willebrand's disease in Sweden. *Acta Paediatr Scand Suppl* 1973; **238**: 1–159.

12 Lak M, Peyvandi F, Mannucci PM. Clinical manifestations and complications of childbirth and replacement therapy in 385 Iranian patients with type 3 von Willebrand disease. *Br J Haematol* 2000; **111**: 1236–9.

13 Federici AB, Castaman G, Mannucci PM. Guidelines for the diagnosis and management of von Willebrand disease in Italy. *Haemophilia* 2002; **8**: 607–21.

14 Rodeghiero F, Castaman G, Tosetto A, *et al.* The discriminant power of bleeding history for the diagnosis of type 1 von Willebrand disease: an international, multicenter study. *J Thromb Haemost* 2005; **3**: 2619–26.

15 Tosetto A, Rodeghiero F, Castaman G, *et al.* A quantitative analysis of bleeding symptoms in type 1 von Willebrand disease: results from a multicenter European study (MCMDM-1 VWD). *J Thromb Haemost* 2006; **4**: 766–73.

16 Federici AB, Bucciarelli P, Castaman G, *et al.* Incidence and determinants of bleeding in different types of von Willebrand disease: results of the first prospective multicenter study on 814 Italian patients *Blood* 2007; **110**: 713.

17 Cattaneo M, Federici AB, Lecchi A, *et al.* Evaluation of the PFA-100 system in the diagnosis and therapeutic monitoring of patients with von Willebrand disease. *Thromb Haemost* 1999; **82**: 35–9.

18 Mannucci PM, Lattuada A, Castaman G, *et al.* Heterogeneous phenotypes of platelet and plasma von Willebrand factor in obligatory heterozygotes for severe von Willebrand disease. *Blood* 1989; **74**: 2433–6.

19 Mannucci PM, Federici AB. Antibodies to von Willebrand factor in von Willebrand disease. *Adv Exp Med Biol* 1995; **386**: 87–92.

20 Federici AB. Clinical and molecular markers of inherited von Willebrand disease type 3: are deletions of the VWF gene associated with alloantibodies to VWF? *J Thromb Haemost* 2008; **6**: 1726–8.

21 Veltkamp JJ, van Tilburg NH. Detection of heterozygotes for recessive von Willebrand's disease by the assay of antihemophilic-factor-like antigen. *N Engl J Med* 1973; **289**: 882–5.

22 Shelton-Inloes BB, Chehab FF, Mannucci PM, *et al.* Gene deletions correlate with the development of alloantibodies in von Willebrand disease. *J Clin Invest* 1987; **79**: 1459–65.

23 Ngo KY, Glotz VT, Koziol JA, *et al.* Homozygous and heterozygous deletions of the von Willebrand factor gene in patients and carriers of severe von Willebrand disease. *Proc Natl Acad Sci USA* 1988; **85**: 2753–7.

24 Schneppenheim R, Krey S, Bergmann F, *et al.* Genetic heterogeneity of severe von Willebrand disease type III in the German population. *Hum Genet* 1994; **94**: 640–52.

25 Eikenboom JCJ, Castaman G, Vos HL, *et al.* Characterization of the genetic defects in recessive type 1 and type 3 von Willebrand disease patients of Italian origin. *Thromb Haemost* 1998; **79**: 709–17.

26 Schneppenheim R, Castaman G, Federici AB, *et al.* A common 253-kb deletion involving VWF and TMEM16B in German and Italian patients with severe von Willebrand disease type 3. *J Thromb Haemost* 2007; **5**: 722–8.

27 Peake IR, Liddell MB, Moodie P, *et al.* Severe type III von Willebrand's disease caused by deletion of exon 42 of the von Willebrand factor gene: Family studies that identify carriers of the condition and a compound heterozygous individual. *Blood* 1990; **75**: 654–61.

28 Mancuso DJ, Tuley EA, Castillo R, *et al.* Characterization of partial gene deletions in type III von Willebrand disease with alloantibody inhibitors. *Thromb Haemost* 1994; **72**: 180–5.

29 Baronciani L, Cozzi G, Canciani MT, *et al.* Molecular characterization of a multiethnic group of 21 patients with type-3 von Willebrand disease. *Thromb Haemost* 2000; **84**: 536–40.

30 Abuzenadah AM, Gursel T, Ingerslev J, *et al.* Mutational analysis of the von Willebrand factor gene in 27 families from Turkey with von Willebrand disease *Thromb Haemost* 1999; **82**: 283.

31 Mohl A, Marschalek R, Masszi T, *et al.* An Alu-mediated novel large deletion is the most frequent cause of type 3 von Willebrand disease in Hungary. *J Thromb Haemost* 2008; **6**: 1729–35.

32 Xie F, Wang X, Cooper DN, *et al.* A novel Alu-mediated 61-kb deletion of the von Willebrand factor (VWF) gene whose breakpoints co-locate with putative matrix attachment regions. *Blood Cells Mol Dis* 2006; **36**: 385–91.

33 Cooper DN, Krawczak M. The mutational spectrum of single base-pair substitutions causing human genetic disease: patterns and predictions. *Hum Genet* 1990; **85**: 55–74.

34 Zhang ZP, Lindstedt M, Falk G, *et al.* Nonsense mutations of the von Willebrand factor gene in patients with von Willebrand disease type III and type I. *Am J Hum Genet* 1992; **51**: 850–8.

35 Eikenboom JCJ, Ploos van Amstel HK, Reitsma PH, *et al.* Mutations in severe type III von Willebrand's disease in the Dutch population: candidate missense and nonsense mutations associated with reduced levels of von Willebrand factor messenger RNA. *Thromb Haemost* 1992; **68**: 448–54.

36 Bahnak BR, Lavergne JM, Rothschild C, *et al.* A stop codon in a patient with severe type III von Willebrand disease. *Blood* 1991; **78**: 1148–9.

37 Zhang ZP, Falk G, Blombäck M, *et al.* Identification of a new nonsense mutation in the von Willebrand factor gene in patients with von Willebrand disease type III. *Hum Mol Genet* 1992; **1**: 61–2.

38 Zhang ZP, Blombäck M, Egberg N, *et al.* Characterization of the von Willebrand factor gene (vWF) in von Willebrand disease type III patients from 24 families of Swedish and Finnish origin. *Genomics* 1994; **21**: 188–93.

39 Hagiwara T, Inaba H, Yoshida S, *et al.* A novel mutation Gly 1672->Arg in type 2A and a homozygous mutation in type 2B von Willebrand disease. *Thromb Haemost* 1996; **76**: 253–7.

40 Gupta PK, Saxena R, Adamtziki E, *et al.* Genetic defects in von Willebrand disease type 3 in Indian and Greek patients. *Blood Cells Mol Dis* 2008; **41**: 219–22.

41 Casana P, Martinez F, Haya S, *et al.* Q1311X: a novel nonsense mutation of putative ancient origin in the von Willebrand factor gene. *Br J Haematol* 2000; **111**: 552–5.

42 Surdhar GK, Enayat MS, Lawson S, *et al.* Homozygous gene conversion in von Willebrand factor gene as a cause of type 3 von Willebrand disease and predisposition to inhibitor development. *Blood* 2001; **98**: 248–50.

43 Baronciani L, Cozzi G, Canciani MT, *et al.* Molecular defects in type 3 von Willebrand disease: updated results from 40 multiethnic patients. *Blood Cells Mol Dis* 2003; **30**: 264–70.

44 Gupta PK, Adamtziki E, Budde U, *et al.* Gene conversions are a common cause of von Willebrand disease. *Br J Haematol* 2005; **130**: 752–8.

45 Zhang ZP, Falk G, Blombäck M, *et al.* A single cytosine deletion in exon 18 of the von Willebrand factor gene is the most common mutation in Swedish von Willebrand disease type III patients. *Hum Mol Genet* 1992; **1**: 767–8.

46 Xie F, Wang X, Cooper DN, *et al.* Compound heterozygosity for two novel mutations (1203insG/Y1456X) in the von Willebrand factor gene causing type 3 von Willebrand disease. *Haemophilia* 2007; **13**: 645–8.

47 Castaman G, Giacomelli SH, Coppola A, *et al.* Molecular bases of type 3 von Willebrand disease in Italy: report on 12 families. *Blood Transfus* 2008; (Suppl. 3): S44.

48 Gazda H, Budde U, Krey S, *et al.* Delta C in exon 18 of the von Willebrand factor gene is the most common mutation in patients with severe von Willebrand disease type 3 in Poland. *Blood* 1997; **90** (Suppl. 1): 94b.

49 Wetzstein V, Budde U, Oyen F, *et al.* Intracranial hemorrhage in a term newborn with severe von Willebrand disease type 3 associated with sinus venous thrombosis. *Haematologica* 2006; **91**: 163–5.

50 Mertes G, Ludwig M, Finkelnburg B, *et al.* A G+3-to-T donor splice site mutation leads to skipping of exon 50 in von Willebrand factor mRNA. *Genomics* 1994; **24**: 190–1.

51 Zhang ZP, Lindstedt M, Blombäck M, *et al.* Effects of the mutant von Willebrand factor gene in von Willebrand disease. *Hum Genet* 1995; **96**: 388–94.

52 Allen S, Abuzenadah AM, Hinks J, *et al.* A novel von Willebrand disease-causing mutation (Arg273Trp) in the von Willebrand factor propeptide that results in defective multimerization and secretion. *Blood* 2000; **96**: 560–8.

53 Titapiwatanakun R, Guenther JC, Asmann YW, *et al.* Novel mutations in types 2 & 3 von Willebrand disease and correlation with von Willebrand factor multimer patterns. *Blood* 2007; **110**: 2136.

54 Montgomery RR, Jozwiak MA, Hutter JJ, *et al.* A homozygous variant of the von Willebrand factor (VWF) that fails to c-terminal dimerize resulting in loss of VWF multimers larger than dimer. *Blood* 1999; **94** (Suppl. 1): 443a.

55 Schneppenheim R, Budde U, Drewke E, *et al.* Cysteine mutations of von Willebrand factor correlate with different types of von Willebrand disease. *Thromb Haemost* Suppl 1999; **82**: 283.

163

56 Enayat MS, Guilliatt AM, Surdhar GK, *et al*. Identification of five novel mutations in families with type 3 von Willebrand's disease. *Thromb Haemost* Suppl 2001; **86**: P1810.

57 Eikenboom JCJ, Vink T, Briët E, *et al*. Multiple substitutions in the von Willebrand factor gene that mimic the pseudogene sequence. *Proc Natl Acad Sci USA* 1994; **91**: 2221–4.

58 Krawczak M, Cooper DN. Gene deletions causing human genetic disease: mechanisms of mutagenesis and the role of the local DNA sequence environment. *Hum Genet* 1991; **86**: 425–41.

59 Efstratiadis A, Posakony JW, Maniatis T, *et al*. The structure and evolution of the human beta-globin gene family. *Cell* 1980; **21**: 653–68.

60 Zhang ZP, Blombäck M, Nyman D, *et al*. Mutations of von Willebrand factor gene in families with von Willebrand disease in the Aland Islands. *Proc Natl Acad Sci USA* 1993; **90**: 7937–40.

61 Mohlke KL, Nichols WC, Rehemtulla A, *et al*. A common frameshift mutation in von Willebrand factor does not alter mRNA stability but interferes with normal propeptide processing. *Br J Haematol* 1996; **95**: 184–91.

62 Eikenboom JCJ, Reitsma PH, van der Velden PA, *et al*. Instability of repeats of the von Willebrand factor gene variable number tandem repeat sequence in intron 40. *Br J Haematol* 1993; **84**: 533–5.

63 Antonarakis SE. Recommendations for a nomenclature system for human gene mutations. Nomenclature Working Group. *Hum Mutat* 1998; **11**: 1–3.

64 Castaman G, Lattuada A, Mannucci PM, *et al*. Factor VIII: C increases after desmopressin in a subgroup of patients with autosomal recessive severe von Willebrand disease. *Br J Haematol* 1995; **89**: 147–51.

65 Tjernberg P, Castaman G, Vos HL, *et al*. Homozygous C2362F von Willebrand factor induces intracellular retention of mutant von Willebrand factor resulting in autosomal recessive severe von Willebrand disease. *Br J Haematol* 2006; **133**: 409–18.

66 Castaman G, Eikenboom JC, Lattuada A, *et al*. Heightened proteolysis of the von Willebrand factor subunit in patients with von Willebrand disease hemizygous or homozygous for the C2362F mutation. *Br J Haematol* 2000; **108**: 188–90.

67 Baronciani L, Federici AB, Cozzi G, *et al*. Expression studies of missense mutations p.D141Y, p.C275S located in the propeptide of von Willebrand factor in patients with type 3 von Willebrand disease. *Haemophilia* 2008; **14**: 549–55.

68 Voorberg J, Fontijn R, Calafat J, *et al*. Assembly and routing of von Willebrand factor variants: the requirements for disulfide-linked dimerization reside within the carboxy-terminal 151 amino acids. *J Cell Biol* 1991; **113**: 195–205.

69 Peake IR, Bowen D, Bignell P, *et al*. Family studies and prenatal diagnosis in severe von Willebrand disease by polymerase chain reaction amplification of a variable number tandem repeat region of the von Willebrand factor gene. *Blood* 1990; **76**: 555–61.

70 Acquila M, Bottini F, DI Duca M, Vijzelaar R, Molinari AC, Bicocchi MP. Multiplex ligation-dependent probe amplification to detect a large deletion within the von Willebrand gene. *Haemophilia* 2009; **15**: 1346–8.

71 Mannucci PM. Treatment of von Willebrand's Disease. *N Engl J Med* 2004; **351**: 683–94.

72 Federici AB, Mazurier C, Berntorp E, *et al*. Biologic response to desmopressin in patients with severe type 1 and type 2 von Willebrand disease: results of a multicenter European study. *Blood* 2004; **103**: 2032–8.

73 Castaman G, Lethagen S, Federici AB, *et al*. Response to desmopressin is influenced by the genotype and phenotype in type 1 von Willebrand disease (VWD): results from the European Study MCMDM-1VWD. *Blood* 2008; **111**: 3531–9.

74 Cattaneo M, Moia M, Della Valle P, *et al*. DDAVP shortens the prolonged bleeding times of patients with severe von Willebrand disease treated with cryoprecipitate. Evidence for a mechanism of action independent of released von Willebrand factor. *Blood* 1989; **74**: 1972–5.

75 Mannucci PM, Chediak J, Hanna W, *et al*. Treatment of von Willebrand disease with a high-purity factor VIII/von Willebrand factor concentrate: a prospective, multicenter study. *Blood* 2002; **99**: 450–6.

76 Federici AB, Baudo F, Caracciolo C, *et al*. Clinical efficacy of highly purified, doubly virus-inactivated factor VIII/von Willebrand factor concentrate (Fanhdi) in the treatment of von Willebrand disease: a retrospective clinical study. *Haemophilia* 2002; **8**: 761–7.

77 Bello IF, Yuste VJ, Molina MQ, *et al*. Fanhdi, efficacy and safety in von Willebrand's disease: prospective international study results. *Haemophilia* 2007; **13** (Suppl. 5): 25–32.

78 Federici AB, Barillari G, Zanon E, *et al*. Efficacy and safety of highly-purified, doubly virus-inactivated VWF/FVIII concentrates in patients with von Willebrand disease: an Italian retrospective study on 120 cases. *Haemophilia* 2010; **16**: 101–10.

79 Dobrkovska A, Krzensk U, Chediak JR. Pharmacokinetics, efficacy and safety of Humate-P in von Willebrand disease. *Haemophilia* 1998; **4** (Suppl. 3): 33–9.

80 Lillicrap D, Poon MC, Walker I, *et al*. Efficacy and safety of the factor VIII/von Willebrand factor concentrate, haemate-P/humate-P: ristocetin cofactor unit

dosing in patients with von Willebrand disease. *Thromb Haemost* 2002; **87**: 224–30.

81 Franchini M, Rossetti G, Tagliaferri A, *et al*. Efficacy and safety of factor VIII/von Willebrand's factor concentrate (Haemate-P) in preventing bleeding during surgery or invasive procedures in patients with von Willebrand disease. *Haematologica* 2003; **88**: 1279–83.

82 Federici AB, Castaman G, Franchini M, *et al*. Clinical use of Haemate P in inherited von Willebrand's disease: a cohort study on 100 Italian patients. *Haematologica* 2007; **92**: 944–51.

83 Gill JC, Ewenstein BM, Thompson AR, *et al*. Successful treatment of urgent bleeding in von Willebrand disease with factor VIII/VWF concentrate (Humate-P): use of the ristocetin cofactor assay (VWF:RCo) to measure potency and to guide therapy. *Haemophilia* 2003; **9**: 688–95.

84 Thompson AR, Gill JC, Ewenstein BM, *et al*. Successful treatment for patients with von Willebrand disease undergoing urgent surgery using factor VIII/VWF concentrate (Humate-P). *Haemophilia* 2004; **10**: 42–51.

85 Lethagen S, Kyrle PA, Castaman G, *et al*. von Willebrand factor/factor VIII concentrate (Haemate P) dosing based on pharmacokinetics: a prospective multicenter trial in elective surgery. *J Thromb Haemost* 2007; **5**: 1420–30.

86 Stadler M, Gruber G, Kannicht C, *et al*. Characterisation of a novel high-purity, double virus inactivated von Willebrand Factor and Factor VIII concentrate (Wilate). *Biologicals* 2006; **34**: 281–8.

87 Favaloro EJ, Lloyd J, Rowell J, *et al*. Comparison of the pharmacokinetics of two von Willebrand factor concentrates [Biostate and AHF (High Purity)] in people with von Willebrand disorder. A randomised cross-over, multi-centre study. *Thromb Haemost* 2007; **97**: 922–30.

88 Shortt J, Dunkley S, Rickard K, *et al*. Efficacy and safety of a high purity, double virus inactivated factor VIII/von Willebrand factor concentrate (Biostate) in patients with von Willebrand disorder requiring invasive or surgical procedures. *Haemophilia* 2007; **13**: 144–8.

89 Menache D, Aronson DL, Darr F, *et al*. Pharmacokinetics of von Willebrand factor and factor VIIIC in patients with severe von Willebrand disease (type 3 VWD): estimation of the rate of factor VIIIC synthesis. Cooperative Study Groups. *Br J Haematol* 1996; **94**: 740–5.

90 Goudemand J, Scharrer I, Berntorp E, *et al*. Pharmacokinetic studies on Wilfactin, a von Willebrand factor concentrate with a low factor VIII content treated with three virus-inactivation/removal methods. *J Thromb Haemost* 2005; **3**: 2219–27.

91 Borel-Derlon A, Federici AB, Roussel-Robert V, *et al*. Treatment of severe von Willebrand disease with a high-purity von Willebrand factor concentrate (Wilfactin): a prospective study of 50 patients. *J Thromb Haemost* 2007; **5**: 1115–24.

92 Bergamaschini L, Mannucci PM, Federici AB, *et al*. Postransfusion anaphylactic reaction in a patient with severe von Willebrand disease: role of complement and alloantibodies to von Willebrand factor. *J Lab Clin Med* 1995; **125**: 348–55.

93 Ciavarella N, Schiavoni M, Valenzano E, *et al*. Use of recombinant factor VIIa (NovoSeven) in the treatment of two patients with type III von Willebrand's disease and an inhibitor against von Willebrand factor. *Haemostasis* 1996; **26** (Suppl. 1): 150–4.

94 Boyer-Neumann C, Dreyfus M, Wolf M, *et al*. Multi-therapeutic approach to manage delivery in an alloimmunized patient with type 3 von Willebrand disease. *J Thromb Haemost* 2003; **1**: 190–2.

95 Berntorp E, Petrini P. Long-term prophylaxis in von Willebrand disease. *Blood Coagul Fibrinolysis* 2005; **16** (Suppl. 1): S23–S26.

96 Federici AB, Gianniello F, Canciani MT, *et al*. Secondary long-term prophylaxis in severe patients with von Willebrand disease: an Italian cohort study. *Blood* 2005; **106**: 507a.

97 De Meyer SF, Vanhoorelbeke K, Chuah MK, *et al*. Phenotypic correction of von Willebrand disease type 3 blood-derived endothelial cells with lentiviral vectors expressing von Willebrand factor. *Blood* 2006; **107**: 4728–36.

98 Nichols WC, Lyons SE, Harrison JS, *et al*. Severe von Willebrand disease due to a defect at the level of von Willebrand factor mRNA expression: detection by exonic PCR-restriction fragment length polymorphism analysis. *Proc Natl Acad Sci USA* 1991; **88**: 3857–61.

99 Gadisseur AP, Vrelust I, Vangenechten I, *et al*. Identification of a novel candidate splice site mutation (0874 + 1G > A) in a type 3 von Willebrand disease patient. *Thromb Haemost* 2007; **98**: 464–6.

100 Goodeve AC, Eikenboom JC, Ginsburg D, *et al*. A standard nomenclature for von Willebrand factor gene mutations and polymorphisms. On behalf of the ISTH SSC Subcommittee on von Willebrand factor. *Thromb Haemost* 2001; **85**: 929–31.

101 Blombäck M. Scientific visits to the Åland Islands. *Haemophilia* 1999; **5**(Suppl. 2): 12–8.

14 Pediatric aspects of von Willebrand disease

Jorge Di Paola[1] and Thomas Abshire[2]
[1]Department of Pediatrics, University of Colorado School of Medicine, Denver, CO, USA
[2]BloodCenter of Wisconsin, Milwaukee, WI, USA

Introduction

Erik von Willebrand held an academic position in the Department of Internal Medicine of the Deaconess Institute in Helsinki. However, as was common in those days, he was asked to see a pediatric patient from the Åland Islands, a 5-year-old girl named Hjördis, who suffered from severe epistaxis [1]. Hjördis was the ninth of 11 children from a family in which four of the children had died at an early age from uncontrolled hemorrhages. Eventually, Dr. von Willebrand proceeded to investigate this family and Hjördis would become the index case for this Åland Island pedigree with "hereditary pseudohemophilia" (now known as von Willebrand disease [VWD]). Unfortunately, Hjördis died of bleeding during a menstrual period in her teenage years. This case underscores some of the unique aspects of this disorder among children and adolescents.

Although the clinical signs and symptoms of VWD are almost indistinguishable between children and adults, there are specific aspects regarding diagnosis and treatment that are almost exclusive to the pediatric population (defined here as birth to 18 years). This chapter will attempt to briefly describe those aspects and explore the distinctive characteristics of pediatric VWD.

Diagnosis of VWD in childhood

Clinical presentation and screening tests

Many patients with VWD are diagnosed in childhood. The majority of children with VWD have their first encounter with a pediatric hematologist owing to a family practitioner's or pediatrician's concerns regarding either excessive mucocutaneous bleeding or a family history of bleeding. In most cases, the referring physician will have already performed several screening tests including a complete blood count, a prothrombin time, an activated partial thromboplastin time (PTT), and the fibrinogen level to exclude other causes of bleeding. Sometimes additional testing may have been performed such as the bleeding time or the platelet function analyzer (PFA-100). Therefore, an initial evaluation by the pediatric hematologist will include a review of the personal and family history, a physical examination, and careful evaluation of the blood smear, in addition to a review of already obtained laboratory testing.

The bleeding associated with VWD primarily involves the skin and mucous membranes. Spontaneous joint or deep muscle bleeding are relatively uncommon in children with this disorder. Bleeding manifestations within the skin can be characterized by their size, elevation, and distribution. These comprise petechiae, purpura, and hematomas. Petechiae can occur in VWD but are much more common in disorders of platelet number or function. Purpura are usually smaller in size (1–3 cm) than those in disorders such as hemophilia and often may appear only in a "normal" distribution on the lower extremities among toddlers or on bony surfaces in children. In these cases, the number of small purpuric lesions (four to five) may be indicative of a platelet-vessel bleeding disorder such as VWD. Hematomas may also be present in VWD, but are more likely a characteristic of factor deficiency bleeding. Close attention should also be given to the distribution and elevation of the lesions as this can be helpful in distinguishing VWD-related bleeding from other causes such as vasculitic disease or nonaccidental injury. For example, the lesions associated with Henoch–Schönlein purpura, a vasculitic childhood disease, are raised and often appear in a classic distribution involving dependent surfaces and the lower extremities [2]. Unusual or regular patterns of skin lesions (handprint, linear distribution, etc.) may suggest the possibility of nonaccidental injury.

Platelet disorders and VWD are also associated with mucosal surface bleeding including epistaxis, bleeding within the oral cavity, upper and lower gastrointestinal hemorrhage, hematuria, and menorrhagia. Epistaxis may appear to be more common among children without an underlying bleeding disorder but careful questioning can distinguish "normal" or prominent nasal vessel-related epistaxis from that associated with VWD and platelet disorders. VWD-related epistaxis is usually from both nostrils, lasts longer than 10–15 min, does not stop spontaneously (without appropriate pressure), and is not seasonal. These individuals have often sought medical attention to alleviate the epistaxis. Menorrhagia is a common presenting complaint in young women and it is estimated that up to 15% of women with menorrhagia will have platelet dysfunction or VWD [3,4]. This bleeding manifestation will be described more fully in the section on adolescents. VWD should also be suspected in the presence of increased bleeding following dental extraction (including wisdom teeth), tonsillectomy, and other surgical procedures.

Screening methods have been utilized in an attempt to identify individuals with a high likelihood of having VWD or a platelet disorder. A rapid assay with high sensitivity would be expected to lower the need for further, more costly, invasive testing. The bleeding time was the first of these methods to be widely used, but its clinical utility is questionable owing to difficulties with standardization, reproducibility, and lack of sensitivity and specificity [5]. It has been suggested that the recently introduced PFA-100 could have a role in the screening of individuals with suspected VWD.

Initial studies focused on the efficacy of the PFA-100 in the evaluation of individuals with known VWD and severe platelet disorders such as Glanzmann thrombasthenia and Bernard–Soulier syndrome. In these patient populations with VWD and VWF levels <25 IU/dL or severe platelet disorders, both the sensitivity and specificity of the PFA-100 approach 90%. These results suggested that the PFA-100 could have utility as an initial diagnostic tool in the evaluation of children with suspected VWD or a platelet-related bleeding disorder [6–9]. Recently, however, the initial enthusiasm for the usefulness of the PFA-100 as a screening tool has diminished because of the low sensitivity (24–41%) of the device reported in individuals with VWD and VWF levels >25 IU/dL, mild platelet secretion defects, and storage pool disorders, especially in the preoperative setting [10–13].

In summary, the existing screening laboratory methods available to pediatric hematologists have very limited value. Therefore, in clinical practice, if the personal history of mucocutaneous bleeding is significant, specific laboratory assays for VWD should be ordered. In Figure 14.1 we propose a simple algorithm for the diagnosis of VWD in children.

Diagnosis of type 1 VWD versus low VWF levels as a risk factor for bleeding

Over the last decade the definition of mild (type 1) VWD has been contested. It is becoming clearer that borderline normal plasma VWF levels represent a continuous variable and may be one of many risk factors for bleeding. The presence of plasma VWF levels between 30 (0.3 kIU/L) and 40 IU/dL (0.4 kIU/L) does not automatically assign an individual to the disease group [14]. For practicing pediatric hematologists, this conceptual dilemma becomes a critical issue when they have to categorize patients and identify their risk for bleeding before conducting surgery. Presurgical evaluation to rule out VWD is not an uncommon reason for consultation. We have previously stated that screening tests are not always useful for diagnosing VWD. So what tools are available for practicing hematologists to aid the diagnosis of VWD and to adequately predict bleeding?

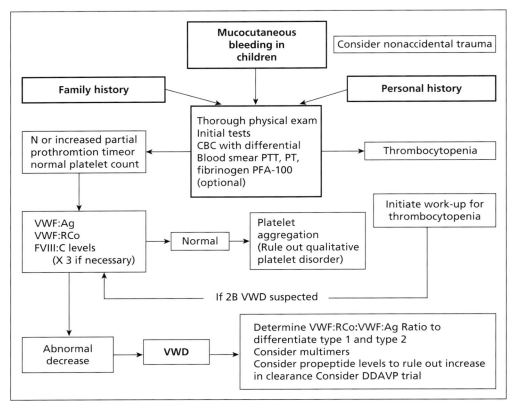

Figure 14.1 Proposed algorithm for diagnosis of von Willebrand disease (VWD) in children who present with mucotaneous bleeding. Some aspects are omitted for didactic purposes. PTT, partial thromboplastin time; DDAVP, 1-deamino-8-D-arginine vasopressin.

It is well known that clinical bleeding in patients with VWD does not always correlate with VWF levels. On the other hand, mild bleeding and bruising may be common in the general population without an identifiable bleeding disorder, and some symptoms may overlap between bleeders and healthy controls. Type 1 VWD is very heterogeneous, and in clinical practice more than two-thirds of the individuals with low levels of VWF are asymptomatic or have minimal bleeding symptoms that are most of the time indistinguishable from those in the general "healthy" population. Therefore, the issue of prevalence is intimately related to the accurate characterization of the bleeding phenotype and ultimately to how type 1 VWD is defined. Two epidemiologic studies among schoolchildren have reported a prevalence of 0.8% and 1.3% in northern Italy and the USA, respectively [15,16]. The criteria for diagnosis in these studies were based on personal and family history of bleeding plus low VWF levels. Interestingly, investigators from the Italian study followed the children diagnosed with type 1 VWD within the cohort for 13 years and although the VWF:ristocetin cofactor (VWF:RCo) levels were consistently replicated, only one child had a positive bleeding history. Moreover, a study by Biron et al. [17] demonstrated the lack of predictive power of modestly low VWF levels on serious postoperative bleeding.

This diagnostic problem is confounded by difficulties in the accurate quantification of bleeding. Recently the European Union (EU) VWD study developed a questionnaire for the determination of a bleeding phenotype. The final bleeding score that results from this questionnaire is based upon quantitative and qualitative bleeding criteria. A recent report by Rodeghiero *et al.* [18] using this tool demonstrated that exhibiting a score of 3 in males and a score of 5 in females was highly specific (98.6%) and moderately sensitive (69.1%) in diagnosing type 1 VWD. This questionnaire represents a significant advance in the phenotypic characterization of the disease; however, children (<12 years of age) were not represented. Utilizing a standardized, adult-oriented bleeding history in children is difficult as they may not have been exposed to the hemostatic challenges that are a prominent feature of the EU bleeding score. New pediatric-oriented questionnaires are being evaluated and will hopefully provide pediatric hematologists with grading tools to contribute to accurate diagnosis and assessment of bleeding risk.

VWD in neonates

Unless an infant has a significant family history of the disease, VWD is rarely diagnosed in the neonatal period. Prenatal diagnosis is recommended only for known carriers of type 3 VWD. Some newborns with type 3 disease may have large deletions of *VWF*, which could potentially predispose them to the development of alloantibodies upon replacement with exogenous VWF-containing concentrates. Genetic testing then may be warranted for the detection of such deletions before replacement therapy as the calculated prevalence of antibody development in these patients ranges from 2.6% to 9.5%. These antibodies can also cause severe anaphylactic reactions [19].

It is well known that there is a marked increase of several coagulation factors in women during gestation including the VWF and factor VIII:C [20]. However, VWF, a very large multimeric protein, does not cross the placenta and thus the maternal elevation of this protein has little impact on VWF levels in newborns. Despite a few isolated reports, serious VWD-related bleeding in the fetal and neonatal period is rare, even in severe cases [21–24]. Postcircumcision bleeding has been reported in males with type 3 VWD who did not receive prophylactic replacement, but it is otherwise rare in other types of VWD. Special consideration should be given to the

diagnosis of type 2B VWD in neonates with persistent thrombocytopenia and giant platelets, as this may mimic other platelet disorders [25].

Acquired VWD in childhood

Acquired VWD is a relatively rare bleeding disorder, which in adults has been associated with several conditions including, but not limited to, myeloproliferative disorders, autoimmune disease, and monoclonal gammopathies [26–29].

In children there are essentially three acquired conditions that have been associated with low VWF levels and bleeding: congenital or acquired hypothyroidism, congenital heart disease, and Wilms tumor. These associations are based upon a mechanistic rationale, but also, and more importantly, on the fact that when patients were treated for their disease, VWF levels increased to the normal range and bleeding disappeared [30]. For example, when patients with hypothyroidism are treated with thyroid hormone replacement their VWF levels normalize as soon as they become euthyroid [31]. It appears that hypothyroidism is associated with decreased synthesis of VWF [30].

Some children with congenital heart disease, such as ventricular septal defect [32] and pulmonary hypertension [33], have been reported to have decreased VWF levels, mainly due to acquired loss of high-molecular-weight VWF multimers. This is similar to the acquired VWD observed in adults with aortic stenosis, and similarly to those cases levels will normalize after surgical intervention [34]. The mechanism for VWF decrease is not known, but it appears that the high shear stress characteristic of these anatomical defects has an impact on the VWF multimeric molecule which makes it more susceptible to cleavage by the VWF protease ADAMTS13 [35].

Finally, Wilms tumor, a kidney neoplasm almost exclusively seen in childhood, has been reported to be associated with acquired VWD. The mechanism for this disease is not completely understood, but it has been reported that the secretion of hyaluronic acid by the tumor may cause concomitant decrease of VWF levels [36,37].

In any of these cases of acquired VWD the treatment of acute bleeding is similar to the treatment of bleeding

169

in patients with type 1 VWD, either by the administration of DDAVP (1-deamino-8-D-arginine vasopressin) or by utilizing a VWF-containing concentrate.

VWD in adolescents

The diagnosis of VWD during adolescence is more common in females because of menstrual bleeding. While excessive menstrual bleeding (menorrhagia) in older women is mostly related to anatomical causes, anovulatory cycles are a frequent cause of menorrhagia in adolescents. However, over the last decade there has been an increasing recognition of the high prevalence of mild bleeding disorders in women with menorrhagia [3,38,39] but only a few articles specifically address the issue of menorrhagia during the teenage years. Mikhail *et al.* [40] reported a retrospective study in which they thoroughly evaluated 61 adolescent patients between the ages of 11 and 19 years who were referred to the Hemophilia Treatment Center for evaluation of menorrhagia. Overall, they identified a disorder of hemostasis in 41% of the patients. Low VWF levels (<40%) were found in 36% of the patients. One-third of these patients exhibited menorrhagia within the first few periods.

The treatment for menorrhagia in adolescents with VWD follows the same principles utilized for treating menorrhagia in adult women. However, some interventions, such as the use of oral contraceptive pills in young girls, may have underscored family and cultural concerns that warrant attention. Also, surgical options such as endometrial ablation or hysterectomy cannot be reasonably entertained. (A detailed description of the diagnosis and treatment of menorrhagia in patients with VWD is offered in Chapter 15.) The diagnosis of VWD in males during adolescence is rare and most likely limited to post-trauma or postsurgical procedural bleeding.

Treatment strategies in children

General principles

The fundamentals of treating VWD are very similar between children and adults. Patients with type 1 VWD who display moderately low protein levels and functional activity are likely to receive DDAVP for most bleeding episodes and VWF-containing concentrates for some major surgery or life-threatening bleeds. Similarly, some patients with type 2 VWD (dysfunctional molecules) may receive DDAVP for some bleeding episodes but are more likely to receive VWF-containing concentrates. Similar to their adult counterparts, children with type 3 VWD are treated with VWF-containing products. Ancillary therapy is also successfully used in children with VWD. Aminocaproic acid is widely utilized for mucosal bleeding and surgical procedures such as tonsillectomy and wisdom teeth extraction. Aspirin and nonsteroidal anti-inflammatory drugs should be avoided in children with VWD owing to their effect on platelet function.

DDAVP

DDAVP is a synthetic analog of the antidiuretic hormone vasopressin that has been used extensively over the last three decades for the treatment of bleeding episodes in mild to moderate hemorrhagic disorders. Chapter 16 includes a detailed description of the use of DDAVP in VWD. In this chapter we present some aspects that are relevant to the pediatric population.

As in the adult population, a therapeutic trial of DDAVP is highly recommended to determine the child's responsiveness to the drug and its use in future therapeutic interventions. The dose of DDAVP is 0.3 μg/kg of body weight administered intravenously in 25–50 mL of saline over a period of 20–30 min. The same dose has proven effective via the subcutaneous route [41]. The drug can also be administered in an intranasal form (Stimate; CSL Behring, King of Prussia, PA, USA) with a concentration of 1.5 mg/mL [42,43].

The dose of intranasal DDAVP in teenagers and adults (weighing >50 kg) is 300 μg (150 μg or one puff in each nostril). For children weighing <50 kg, the recommended dose is 150 μg (one puff). It is difficult to utilize this nasal form in preschool children. Also, severe rhinorrhea could jeopardize absorption. A more diluted (100 μg/mL) form of DDAVP is available on the market for patients with diabetes insipidus and enuresis. It is important for clinicians to know that this particular form is ineffective for the treatment of VWD.

Administration of DDAVP causes fluid retention, and appropriate precautions regarding fluid restriction must be given to avoid possible serious electrolyte imbalance. Because of this complication its use in children under two years of age should be approached with caution. Several case series indicate that the use of either intranasal or intravenous DDAVP in children has been associated with severe hyponathremia and seizures. In most of these cases, this was exacerbated by concomitant use of hypotonic solutions or the lack of fluid restriction [44,45]. If DDAVP is absolutely required in young children, close monitoring with serial electrolyte measurements, fluid restriction, and avoidance of hypotonic solutions in the first 24 h after the administration of the drug are highly recommended [45]. Tachyphylaxis to DDAVP will most likely develop if multiple daily doses of DDAVP are given [46].

Replacement therapy

Replacement therapy with VWF-containing concentrates in children is usually recommended for bleeding episodes that are unresponsive to DDAVP or for episodes that are severe enough to require more aggressive management. This usually applies to significant bleeding episodes and surgery. Most of the VWF-containing concentrates available contain factor VIII as well as VWF. Although most data for VWF replacement have originated from clinical trials focusing mostly on adults, the historical use of these concentrates supports their use for bleeding episodes and surgical procedures in children [47–49]. Prophylactic treatment for severe forms of VWD has been utilized with a significant decrease in the number of bleeding episodes in patients with intractable epistaxis, oral bleeding, and menorrhagia unresponsive to other treatment options as well as the prevention of arthropathy in children with type 3 VWD [50,51]. A new international study is under way to systematically explore this treatment concept for this group of patients [52].

Conclusions

von Willebrand disease is a common bleeding disorder often diagnosed in childhood. This diagnosis could have a significant impact on the lifestyle and medical care of the affected child and family. Accordingly, it is essential to understand those aspects of the disorder that are characteristic in childhood.

This approach will likely assure correct diagnosis and management of VWD as well as a successful transition to adult care.

References

1 Berntorp E. Erik von Willebrand. *Thromb Res* 2007; **120** (Suppl. 1): S3–4.

2 Chen KR, Carlson JA. Clinical approach to cutaneous vasculitis. *Am J Clin Dermatol* 2008; **9**: 71–92.

3 Kadir RA, Economides DL, Sabin CA, Owens D, Lee CA. Frequency of inherited bleeding disorders in women with menorrhagia. *Lancet* 1998; **351**: 485–9.

4 Bevan JA, Maloney KW, Hillery CA, Gill JC, Montgomery RR, Scott JP. Bleeding disorders: A common cause of menorrhagia in adolescents. *J Pediatr* 2001; **138**: 856–61.

5 Peterson P, Hayes TE, Arkin CF, *et al.* The preoperative bleeding time test lacks clinical benefit: College of American Pathologists' and American Society of Clinical Pathologists' position article. *Arch Surg* 1998; **133**: 134–9.

6 Cariappa R, Wilhite TR, Parvin CA, Luchtman-Jones L. Comparison of PFA-100 and bleeding time testing in pediatric patients with suspected hemorrhagic problems. *J Pediatr Hematol Oncol* 2003; **25**: 474–9.

7 Cattaneo M, Federici AB, Lecchi A, *et al.* Evaluation of the PFA-100 system in the diagnosis and therapeutic monitoring of patients with von Willebrand disease. *Thromb Haemost* 1999; **82**: 35–9.

8 Harrison P, Robinson MS, Mackie IJ, *et al.* Performance of the platelet function analyser PFA-100 in testing abnormalities of primary haemostasis. *Blood Coagul Fibrinolysis* 1999; **10**: 25–31.

9 Harrison P. The role of PFA-100 testing in the investigation and management of haemostatic defects in children and adults. *Br J Haematol* 2005; **130**: 3–10.

10 Quiroga T, Goycoolea M, Munoz B, *et al.* Template bleeding time and PFA-100 have low sensitivity to screen patients with hereditary mucocutaneous hemorrhages: comparative study in 148 patients. *J Thromb Haemost* 2004;. **2**: 892–8.

11 Harrison C, Khair K, Baxter B, Russell-Eggitt I, Hann I, Liesner R. Hermansky-Pudlak syndrome: infrequent bleeding and first report of Turkish and Pakistani kindreds. *Arch Dis Child* 2002; **86**: 297–301.

12 Cattaneo M, Lecchi A, Agati B, Lombardi R, Zighetti ML. Evaluation of platelet function with the PFA-100 system in patients with congenital defects of platelet secretion. *Thromb Res* 1999; **96**: 213–17.

13 Roschitz B, Thaller S, Koestenberger M, *et al.* PFA-100 closure times in preoperative screening in 500 pediatric patients. *Thromb Haemost* 2007; **98**: 243–7.

14 Sadler JE. Von Willebrand disease type 1: a diagnosis in search of a disease. *Blood* 2003; **101**: 2089–93.

15 Rodeghiero F, Castaman G, Dini E. Epidemiological investigation of the prevalence of von Willebrand's disease. *Blood* 1987; **69**: 454–9.

16 Werner EJ, Broxson EH, Tucker EL, Giroux DS, Shults J, Abshire TC. Prevalence of von Willebrand disease in children: a multiethnic study. *J Pediatr* 1993; **123**: 893–8.

17 Biron C, Mahieu B, Rochette A, *et al*. Preoperative screening for von Willebrand disease type 1: low yield and limited ability to predict bleeding. *J Lab Clin Med* 1999; **134**: 605–9.

18 Rodeghiero F, Castaman G, Tosetto A, *et al*. The discriminant power of bleeding history for the diagnosis of type 1 von Willebrand disease: an international, multicenter study. *J Thromb Haemost* 2005; **3**: 2619–26.

19 Federici AB. Diagnosis of inherited von Willebrand disease: a clinical perspective. *Semin Thromb Hemost* 2006; **32**: 555–65.

20 Brenner B. Haemostatic changes in pregnancy. *Thromb Res* 2004; **114**: 409–14.

21 Mullaart RA, Van Dongen P, Gabreels FJ, van Oostrom C. Fetal periventricular hemorrhage in von Willebrand's disease: short review and first case presentation. *Am J Perinatol* 1991; **8**: 190–2.

22 Silwer J. von Willebrand's disease in Sweden. *Acta Paediatr Scand Suppl* 1973; **238**: 1–159.

23 Lak M, Peyvandi F, Mannucci PM. Clinical manifestations and complications of childbirth and replacement therapy in 385 Iranian patients with type 3 von Willebrand disease. *Br J Haematol* 2000; **111**: 1236–9.

24 Wetzstein V, Budde U, Oyen F, *et al*. Intracranial hemorrhage in a term newborn with severe von Willebrand disease type 3 associated with sinus venous thrombosis. *Haematologica* 2006; **91** (Suppl. 12): ECR60.

25 Loffredo G, Baronciani L, Noris P, Menna F, Federici AB, Balduini CL. von Willebrand disease type 2B must be always considered in the differential diagnosis of genetic thrombocytopenias with giant platelets. *Platelets* 2006; **17**: 149–52.

26 Michiels JJ, Berneman Z, Gadisseur A, *et al*. Immune-mediated etiology of acquired von Willebrand syndrome in systemic lupus erythematosus and in benign monoclonal gammopathy: therapeutic implications. *Semin Thromb Hemost* 2006; **32**: 577–88.

27 Niiya M, Niiya K, Takazawa Y, *et al*. Acquired type 3-like von Willebrand syndrome preceded full-blown systemic lupus erythematosus. *Blood Coagul Fibrinolysis* 2002; **13**: 361–5.

28 Michiels JJ, Schroyens W, van der Planken M, Berneman Z. Acquired von Willebrand syndrome in systemic lupus erythematodes. *Clin Appl Thromb Hemost* 2001; **7**: 106–12.

29 Federici AB. Acquired von Willebrand syndrome: an underdiagnosed and misdiagnosed bleeding complication in patients with lymphoproliferative and myeloproliferative disorders. *Semin Hematol* 2006; **43** (Suppl. 1): S48–58.

30 Galli-Tsinopoulou A, Stylianou C, Papaioannou G, Nousia-Arvanitakis S. Acquired von Willebrand's syndrome resulting from untreated hypothyroidism in two prepubertal girls. *Haemophilia* 2006; **12**: 687–9.

31 Dalton RG, Dewar MS, Savidge GF, *et al*. Hypothyroidism as a cause of acquired von Willebrand's disease. *Lancet* 1987; **1**: 1007–9.

32 Gill JC, Wilson AD, Endres-Brooks J, Montgomery RR. Loss of the largest von Willebrand factor multimers from the plasma of patients with congenital cardiac defects. *Blood* 1986; **67**: 758–61.

33 Lopes AA, Maeda NY, Aiello VD, Ebaid M, Bydlowski SP. Abnormal multimeric and oligomeric composition is associated with enhanced endothelial expression of von Willebrand factor in pulmonary hypertension. *Chest* 1993; **104**: 1455–60.

34 Vincentelli A, Susen S, Le Tourneau T, *et al*. Acquired von Willebrand syndrome in aortic stenosis. *N Engl J Med* 2003; **349**: 343–9.

35 Sadler JE. Aortic stenosis, von Willebrand factor, and bleeding. *N Engl J Med* 2003; **349**: 323–5.

36 Scott JP, Montgomery RR, Tubergen DG, Hays T. Acquired von Willebrand's disease in association with Wilm's tumor: regression following treatment. *Blood* 1981; **58**: 665–9.

37 Bracey AW, Wu AH, Aceves J, Chow T, Carlile S, Hoots WK. Platelet dysfunction associated with Wilms tumor and hyaluronic acid. *Am J Hematol* 1987 **24**: 247–57.

38 Philipp CS, Dilley A, Miller CH, *et al*. Platelet functional defects in women with unexplained menorrhagia. *J Thromb Haemost* 2003; **1**: 477–84.

39 Dilley A, Drews C, Miller C, *et al*. von Willebrand disease and other inherited bleeding disorders in women with diagnosed menorrhagia. *Obstet Gynecol* 2001; **97**: 630–6.

40 Mikhail S, Varadarajan R, Kouides P. The prevalence of disorders of haemostasis in adolescents with menorrhagia referred to a haemophilia treatment centre. *Haemophilia* 2007; **13**: 627–32.

41 Rodeghiero F, Castaman G, Mannucci PM. Prospective multicenter study on subcutaneous concentrated desmopressin for home treatment of patients with von Willebrand disease and mild or moderate hemophilia A. *Thromb Haemost* 1996; **76**: 692–6.

42 Kohler M, Hellstern P, Miyashita C, von Blohn G, Wenzel E. Comparative study of intranasal, subcutaneous and intravenous administration of desamino-D-ar-

ginine vasopressin (DDAVP). *Thromb Haemost* 1986; **55**: 108–11.

43 Leissinger C, Becton D, Cornell C Jr., Cox Gill J. High-dose DDAVP intranasal spray (Stimate) for the prevention and treatment of bleeding in patients with mild haemophilia A, mild or moderate type 1 von Willebrand disease and symptomatic carriers of haemophilia A. *Haemophilia* 2001; **7**: 258–66.

44 Koskimies O, Pylkkanen J, Vilska J. Water intoxication in infants caused by the urine concentration test with vasopressin analogue (DDAVP). *Acta Paediatr Scand* 1984; **73**: 131–2.

45 Das P, Carcao M, Hitzler J. DDAVP-induced hyponatremia in young children. *J Pediatr Hematol Oncol* 2005; **27**: 330–2.

46 Canavese C, Salomone M, Pacitti A, Mangiarotti G, Calitri V. Reduced response of uraemic bleeding time to repeated doses of desmopressin. *Lancet* 1985; **1**: 867–8.

47 Lillicrap D, Poon MC, Walker I, Xie F, Schwartz BA; Association of Hemophilia Clinic Directors of Canada. Efficacy and safety of the factor VIII/von Willebrand factor concentrate, haemate-P/humate-P: ristocetin cofactor unit dosing in patients with von Willebrand disease. *Thromb Haemost* 2002; **87**: 224–30.

48 Thompson AR, Gill JC, Ewenstein BM, Mueller-Velten G, Schwartz BA; Humate-P Study Group. Successful treatment for patients with von Willebrand disease undergoing urgent surgery using factor VIII/VWF concentrate (Humate-P). *Haemophilia* 2004; **10**: 42–51.

49 Gill JC, Ewenstein BM, Thompson AR, Mueller-Velten G, Schwartz BA; Humate-P Study Group. Successful treatment of urgent bleeding in von Willebrand disease with factor VIII/VWF concentrate (Humate-P): use of the ristocetin cofactor assay (VWF:RCo) to measure potency and to guide therapy. *Haemophilia* 2003; **9**: 688–95.

50 Berntorp E. Prophylaxis in von Willebrand disease. *Haemophilia* 2008; **14** (Suppl. 5): 47–53.

51 Federici AB. Prophylaxis of bleeding episodes in patients with von Willebrand's disease. *Blood Transfus* 2008; **6** (Suppl. 2): s26–32.

52 Berntorp E, Abshire T. The von Willebrand disease prophylaxis network: exploring a treatment concept. *J Thromb Haemost* 2006; **4**: 2511–12.

15 Women with von Willebrand disease

Christine A. Lee[1], Rezan A. Kadir[2], and Peter A. Kouides[3]
[1]University of London, London, UK
[2]Royal Free Hospital, London, UK
[3]Rochester General Hospital, Rochester, NY, USA

When Erik von Willebrand first described the bleeder family in Åland in 1926, he noted that whereas 16 of 35 women had the trait, it was found in only seven of 31 men. Thus, von Willebrand made the observation that "the trait seemed especially to be seen among the women ... in the female bleeders, the diathesis becomes manifest both in a milder and a graver form, whereas males only show a mild form. Among the female members five deaths have occurred." Hjördis, the index case, presented with epistaxis but died during her fourth menstrual period. Although her mother, Mrs. S, had frequent and persistent nosebleeding during her entire youth and her menstruation was described as "copious," she delivered 12 children without heavy bleeding. In contrast her maternal grandmother, Mrs. Augusta S, had bled to death in childbirth. Thus, in his paper von Willebrand stated that for women "genital hemorrhage" in connection with menstruation and delivery was the second most common cause of bleeding. However, he also pointed out that menstruation and delivery might be completely normal [1].

Epidemiology of VWD in women

Menorrhagia is defined as heavy regular menstrual bleeding [2]. Normal menstrual blood loss (MBL) is on average 40 mL per month [3]. The most accepted definition of the upper limit of normal MBL is 80 mL, which was established by studying how much an otherwise healthy woman could bleed every month without becoming iron deficient or anemic [4]. More recent recommendations suggest that the upper limits of normal MBL ranges from 60 to 120 mL [5].

The prevalence of objectively verified menorrhagia is around 10% [6]. A study by the Royal College of General Practitioners in the UK in 1981–82 showed that 5% of women aged 30–49 years consulted their physician for menorrhagia [7]. Furthermore, in 1992, 12% of gynecologic referrals in the UK were for menorrhagia [8]. However, although menorrhagia is a common complaint, it is difficult to define—patient history alone is a poor indicator of true menorrhagia.

A comparison using the Pictorial Blood Assessment Chart (PBAC) and the alkaline hematin method to assess MBL showed that a score over 100 was equivalent to >80 mL blood loss and could therefore be used as an objective measure of MBL. The PBAC is shown in Figure 15.1—the scores assigned were 1 for each lightly stained tampon, 5 if moderately soiled, and 10 if completely saturated with blood. Towels were given ascending scores of 1, 5, and 20, and small and large clots scored 1 and 5, respectively [9]. Using this methodology, it was possible to assess the frequency of von Willebrand disease (VWD) among patients attending a gynecology clinic for menorrhagia in London [10]. All patients with a history of heavy, regular bleeding gave a menstrual and bleeding history and completed the PBAC. The 150 sequential patients who scored over 100 were further evaluated and it was found that 15 had mild VWD and three

Von Willebrand Disease, 1st edition. Edited by Augusto B. Federici, Christine A. Lee, Erik E. Berntorp, David Lillicrap, Robert R. Montgomery. © 2011 Blackwell Publishing Ltd.

Pictorial blood assessment chart

Start date: Score:

Towel	1	2	3	4	5	6	7	8
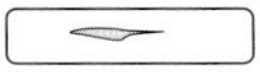 (lightly stained)	//	/	/		/	/		
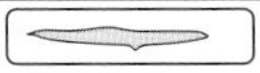 (moderately soiled)			///	//				
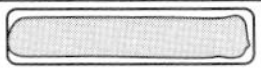 (saturated)		//	//					
Clots/Flooding		50p × 1	1p × 3					

Tampon	1	2	3	4	5	6	7	8
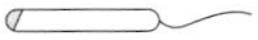 (lightly stained)		/			//	/		
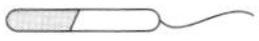 (moderately soiled)		//	///	//				
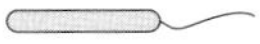 (saturated)		/	////					
Clots/Flooding								

Towels

1 point	For each lightly stained towel
5 point	For each moderately soiled towel
20 point	If the towel is completely saturated with blood

Tampons

1 point	For each lightly stained tampon
5 point	For each moderately soiled tampon
20 point	If the tampon is completely saturated with blood

1 point	For small clots (size of 1p coin)
5 point	For large clots (size of 50p coin)

Figure 15.1 The pictorial bleeding assessment chart, from Higham [9]. (a) An example of a completed chart. (b) Scoring system.

had moderate VWD, a prevalence of 13%. Menorrhagia from the menarche and a history of bleeding after tooth extraction, surgery, or parturition were highly predictive of VWD (Table 15.1).

A systematic review has summarized the overall prevalence of the laboratory diagnosis of VWD in women presenting with menorrhagia to be 13% (confidence interval 11–15.6%) of a total 988 women in 11 studies [11]. Further studies from India and Taiwan have reported a similar prevalence [12,13] (Figure 15.2).

The diagnosis of VWD in women

There is a variation of von Willebrand factor (VWF) during the menstrual cycle, however, because of the wide inter- and intra-individual variation in these factor levels, for example significantly higher levels of VWF have been found in black women [14,15].

Real differences between the different phases of the menstrual cycle may be missed unless large groups of women are studied using approaches that take account of the large variation between individuals. In

175

Table 15.1 (a) Demographic features and details of menstrual history.

	All patients (n = 150)	No bleeding disorders (n = 123)	von Willebrand disease (n = 20)	P
Median age in years (range)	39 (15–50)	39 (15–50)	40 (27–50)	0.83
Hemoglobin <110 g/L (%)	22 (14.7)	19 (15.5)	2 (10.0)	0.74
Blood group				
A (%)	58 (38.7)	49 (39.8)	6 (30.0)	0.40
O (%)	62 (41.3)	48 (39.0)	11 (55.0)	
Others (%)	30 (20.0)	26 (21.1)	3 (15.0)	
Family history of bleeding disorder (%)	4 (2.7)	2 (1.6)	1 (5.0)	0.37
History of blood transfusion (%)	17 (11.3)	10 (8.1)	3 (15.0)	0.39
Duration of menorrhagia				
<24 months (%)	61 (40.7)	57 (46.3)	3 (15.0)	0.001
>24 months (%)	62 (41.3)	55 (44.7)	4 (20.0)	
Since menarche (%)	27 (18.0)	11 (8.9)	13 (65.0)	
Duration of menstruation				
Median in days (range)	6.5 (3–13)	6.5 (3–13)	6.5 (5–12)	0.36
Passage of clots (%)	131 (87.9)	107 (87.7)	17 (85.0)	0.72
Episodes of flooding (%)	106 (70.7)	84 (63.8)	16 (80.0)	0.43
Median PBAC score (range)	184 (100–1036)	172 (100–667)	297 (122–800)	<0.001

PBAC, Pictorial Blood Assessment Chart.

Table 15.1 (b) Other bleeding symptoms and bleeding score from Kadir [10].

	Total (n = 150)	No bleeding disorders (n = 123)	von Willebrand disease (n = 20)	P
Bleeding symptoms				
Bruising (%)	88 (58.7)	66 (53.7)	16 (80)	0.05
Nosebleeding (%)	22 (14.7)	17 (13.8)	5 (25.0)	0.20
Gum bleeding (%)	54 (36)	41 (33.3)	9 (45.0)	0.45
Bleeding after tooth extraction[a] (%)	13/98 (13.3)	6/81 (7.4)	6/13 (46.2)	0.001
Postoperative bleeding[a] (%)	18/109 (16.5)	7/90 (7.8)	8/13 (61.5)	<0.001
Postpartum bleeding[a] (%)	29/27 (29.9)	17/80 (21.3)	8/13 (61.5)	0.005
Symptom score				
0 (%)	40 (26.7)	39 (31.7)	0	
1–2 (%)	78 (52.0)	65 (52.9)	11 (55.0)	
3–4 (%)	28 (18.7)	17 (13.8)	7 (35.5)	
5–6 (%)	4 (2.7)	2 (1.6)	2 (10.0)	<0.001
Median (range)	1 (0–5)	1 (0–5)	2 (1–5)	<0.001

[a] Expressed as a percentage of women who had the event or procedure.

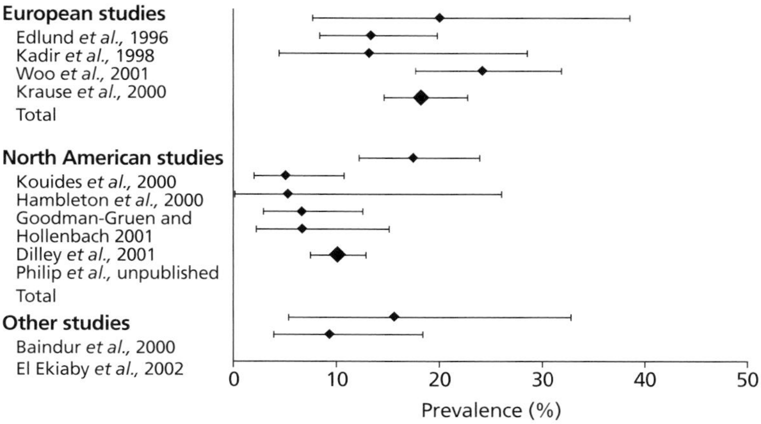

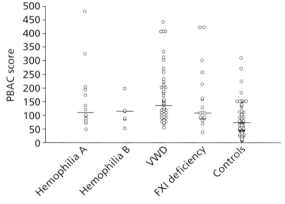

Figure 15.2 Prevalence rates with confidence intervals for von Willebrand disease. Adapted from Shankar et al. [11].

a cross-sectional study of 123 women using multilevel modeling methods it was shown that blood sampling is best in the early follicular phase, no later than day 7 of the cycle [14]—this is supported by a more recent cross-sectional analysis [16]. It is possible that the failure to find a decrease in levels during the menses in a further study was because sampling was not performed early enough in the menstrual cycle [17].

Historically, it was considered that oral contraceptive use could obscure the diagnosis of VWD because estrogens can raise the VWF level [18]. However, there is currently a lack of evidence to show a definite effect with current combination oral contraceptives that have a lower dose potency than previous preparations. In a recent study the use of oral contraceptives actually dampened the VWF levels [14].

It is recommended that, as a significant proportion of women with idiopathic menorrhagia have an underlying bleeding disorder, the most common being VWD, testing for this disorder should be considered [19]. This requires the expertise of a specialized laboratory capable of measuring both VWF:AC and VWF:Ag—the activated partial thromboplastin time (APTT) can be normal in the face of a low VWF level and therefore is inadequate as a screening test.

Clinical aspects of menorrhagia in women with VWD

The prevalence of menorrhagia, primarily in type 1 VWD, has been reported as being between 78% and

Figure 15.3 Pictorial Blood Assessment Chart (PBAC) scores in women with inherited bleeding disorders including von Willebrand disease (VWD). Reproduced from Kadir et al. [20].

97% [20–22]. Using the PBAC, 78% of women with VWD were found to have menorrhagia [20] (Figure 15.3). Women with VWD use more tampons and pads than menstruating women without VWD and have frequent staining of underclothes [22] as well as a higher prevalence of anemia [22–24]. These women also have a much higher frequency of mucocutaneous bleeding than women without VWD [10,22,23].

A relatively high rate of hysterectomy, 8–26%, has been reported in patients with type 1 VWD even though there is only a mild depression of VWF levels [20–24]. In a case–control study in 102 women with

VWD, 26% had undergone hysterectomy compared with 8% of controls [24]. Underlying uterine pathology was found in the hysterectomy specimen in two studies that demonstrated how mild VWD may "unmask" a uterine fibroid [20,22]. A statistically higher rate of fibroids compared with age-matched controls, 32% versus 17%, was noted [24]. A higher prevalence of endometriosis, 30% versus 10%; endometrial hyperplasia, 10% versus 1%; and endometrial polyps, 8% versus 1%, were also found in women with VWD compared with controls [24]. It has been suggested that VWD may exacerbate the retrograde menstrual flow implicated in the pathophysiology of endometriosis, whereas the higher prevalence of endometrial hyperplasia and polyps in women with VWD can be explained in terms of "unmasking" these lesions [25].

There are fewer studies specifically in women with type 2 and type 3 VWD, but one study has reported a high incidence of menorraghia with a quarter of those involved requiring hysterectomy [26].

Adolescent menorrhagia and VWD

Menstrual periods in adolescents are often irregular because of frequent anovulation, and the condition "adolescent menorrhagia" is quite often menometrorrhagia—heavy with at least some irregular bleeding [2]. A significant proportion of adolescent girls with menorrhagia have an underlying bleeding disorder; in a retrospective study of 106 adolescents with menorrhagia, 11 (10.4%) were found to have an underlying bleeding disorder. A positive family history of bleeding symptoms was a significant predictor of a bleeding disorder in this study [27], as well as acute adolescent menorrhagia requiring hospital admission [28]. In a further study of adolescents requiring hospitalization, 15 (33%) of 46 had an underlying hematologic disease, with VWD accounting for five (11%) cases [29]. In a study of 61 adolescents referred for hemostasis evaluation, a prevalence of VWD of 36% (22 of 61) was found [30].

Menstruation is likely to be the first hemostatic challenge faced by girls with VWD and the menorrhagia is usually very severe with an acute presentation. This can be explained by the correlation of VWF levels increasing with age [14,31]. Thus, adolescents who present with acute menorrhagia should be investigated for a bleeding disorder, particularly VWD. For prepubertal girls known to have VWD, or where there is a positive history of VWD, plans should be made in anticipation of the possibility of acute menorrhagia at the onset of menarche [19].

Medical treatment of menorrhagia

Tranexamic acid

Tranexamic acid is an antifibrinolytic agent that has been shown to reduce mean MBL in a dose of 1 g every 6–8 h in women without a bleeding disorder [32]. It is recommended as a first-line treatment for menorrhagia [33]. Tranexamic acid has been widely used in women with VWD, orally, intravenously, topically, alone, or as adjuvant therapy, in the prevention and management of oral cavity bleeding, epistaxis, gastrointestinal bleeding, and menorrhagia. However, there are no specific data on the efficacy in the reduction of menstrual blood loss in VWD. The recommended oral dose of tranexamic acid is 0.5–1 g four times a day for 3–4 days and it is helpful to start the medication before the onset of bleeding. There has been a report of successful use of a single high dose (4 g daily) in three patients with types 2A and 2B VWD, but this regime can be associated with severe nausea and vomiting [34]. There is an ongoing study of a new sustained release formulation of tranexamic acid (XP12B), which is currently being investigated in the USA [35].

DDAVP

Desmopressin (1-desamino-8-D-arginine vasopressin, DDAVP) has been reported in nonrandomized cohort studies. Approximately two-thirds of patients with either subcutaneous [36] or intranasal [37] DDAVP (IN-DDAVP) reported by self-assessment that the treatment was "effective"/"very effective." However, in 30 women with VWD and menorrhagia using the PBAC in a randomized control crossover study, there was no difference with DDAVP compared with a placebo [38]. Regardless of whether the first treatment period was with a placebo or with IN-DDAVP, there was a reduction in the PBAC score that was statistically significant ($P = 0.01$). Similar results were obtained in 20 women with menorrhagia and a prolonged bleeding time comparing 300 μg of IN-DDAVP with a placebo. In this study, the MBL was measured spectrometrically by the alkaline hematin method and there was no statistical difference between the decrease in blood loss using DDAVP compared with tranexamic acid. However, there was a significant reduction in MBL when DDAVP was combined with tranexamic acid [39]. In a multicenter US trial of women with abnormal hemostasis including VWD, crossover comparison of IN-DDAVP and tranexamic acid using the PBAC to assess MBL showed tranexamic acid to be more effective [40]. Since DDAVP induces increased fibrinolytic activity (t-PA) and tranexamic acid counteracts this, it is likely that the optimum treatment in women with VWD and menorrhagia is a combination of both drugs.

Combined oral contraceptives

There is some evidence that combined oral contraceptives (COCs) significantly reduce MBL in women [41,42]. However, the efficacy of COCs in reducing MBL in women with VWD is unknown. A survey of women with type 2 and type 3 VWD, who were unresponsive to DDAVP, showed that COCs were an effective treatment for menorrhagia in 88% of women [43]. However, in type 1 VWD a standard dose and a higher dose COC were effective in only 24% and 37% cases, respectively. Traditionally, COCs are administered daily for 21 days, followed by a pill-free week during which uterine bleeding occurs [44]. In recent years, the continuous administration of a COC (>28 days active pills) has been reported as a successful regimen in the treatment of endometriosis, dysmenorrhea, and other menstruation-associated symptoms [45,46]. Cyst rupture and the resulting hemoperitoneum is a rare but potentially life-threatening event in women with VWD and therefore it has been recommended that COCs should be used as first-line therapy for the adult or adolescent who does not desire pregnancy but may desire future childbearing [47,48].

Clotting factor concentrate

Approximately 10–15% women with VWD will not respond to DDAVP because they have severe type 1, type 2, or type 3 VWD. In these women, who may also be refractory to treatment with antifibrinolytic therapy, a plasma-derived VWF-containing concentrate may be required [49]. This can be self-administered by intravenous injection as monthly prophylaxis [50]. An international prophylaxis study is ongoing for women with type 2 and type 3 VWD-related menorrhagia [51].

It is interesting that the first use of a clotting factor containing VWF (factor 1-O) was in a woman with VWD who was bleeding uncontrollably from menorrhagia [52].

Surgical treatment

Mirena (LNG IUS)

The levonorgestrel (LNG) intrauterine system (IUS), Mirena (Schering, Germany), is an IUS with a T-shaped plastic frame that is 32 mm long with a reservoir on the vertical stem containing 52 mg of LNG. It releases 20 μg of LNG every 24 h over a recommended duration of use of 5 years. It suppresses endometrial growth, causing the glands of the endometrium to become atrophic and the epithelium inactive [53]. The use of the LNG-IUS in women with inherited bleeding disorders has been evaluated in 16 women (13 with VWD, two with an FXI deficiency, and one with Hermansky–Pudlak syndrome) with menorrhagia who were nonresponsive to medical treatment. After 9 months, the PBAC score had decreased significantly from a median of 213 (range 98–386) to a median of 47 (range 24–75) and the hemoglobin concentration had increased from a median of 12.1 g/dL (range 8.0–13.2 g/dL) to 13.1 g/dL (range 12.3–14 g/dL); $P = 0.0001$. Before insertion of the LNG-IUS, all women had at least 1 day per month when their life was detrimentally affected by their periods and six women reported that 3 days were affected. However, 9 months after the insertion of the LNG-IUS none of the women had any days of the month when menstruation detrimentally affected their life [54]. Long-term follow-up at a median of 53 (range 24–60) months has shown persistent benefit [55], although a recent case report in a patient with VWD described prolonged spotting after insertion which may require removal of the device [56].

Women with VWD could be at risk of bleeding at the time of insertion, and therefore hemostatic cover may be required [19].

Hysterectomy

An underlying bleeding disorder may be the reason for failure of medical treatment and a hysterectomy may be required [57]. Surgical intervention in women with VWD requires adequate hemostasis and the use of surgical drains should be considered.

In the UK, a large cohort study evaluated 37,298 hysterectomies between 1994 and 1995 which found that the mortality rate was 0.38% per 1000 population, the overall complication rate was 3.5% (3% severe), and the postoperative complication rate was 9% (severe 1%) [58,59]. Thus, the less invasive method of endometrial ablation has been developed for treating menorrhagia [60].

Endometrial ablation

First-generation techniques—resection, laser, and rollerball—were introduced in the 1980s and are performed under direct vision with the requirement of specialized surgical skills. Second-generation techniques are designed to ablate the full thickness of the endometrium by the controlled application of heat, cold, microwave, or other forms of energy. They require sophisticated equipment and are mostly performed blindly [19]. One study evaluated thermal balloon ablation in 70 women with severe menorrhagia and severe systematic disease, including 25 with "coagulopathy." The procedure was performed under local anesthesia and the success rate was over 90% at 3-year follow-up [61]. The findings of a smaller retrospective study, which assessed the efficacy of endometrial ablation in seven women with VWD-related menorrhagia, were less favorable. Four women experienced recurrence of menorrhagia at a median of 8 months postablation, and three women eventually underwent hysterectomy at a median of 11 months postablation [62].

Hemorrhagic ovarian cyst

Women with bleeding disorders are most likely to bleed from ruptured ovarian follicles [19]. During ovulation the ovum is expelled from the ovarian follicle into the peritoneal cavity and bleeding can result in the formation of a hemorrhagic cyst in the residual follicle or corpus luteum, or bleeding into the broad ligament can result in a retroperitoneal hematoma. In a recent review, 15 case reports and case series were identified [63]. In one study of women with VWD, nine of 136 women had experienced hemorrhagic ovarian cysts [64]. In a survey of 81 menstruating women with type 1 VWD, 60 reported midcycle Mittelschmerz pain at a median intensity of 4 on a scale of 1–10, which was similar to the pain of their menstrual cycle [44] There is ultrasonically demonstrated pelvic fluid in two-thirds of midcycle pain [65]. This suggests that Mittelscherz is associated with bleeding at the time of ovulation, which explains why it is common in women with VWD. Clotting factor therapy has been used successfully to control Mittelscherz and in some cases it may be necessary for surgical intervention [66]. Recurrences of hemorrhagic cysts are common in women with VWD, and COCs, which inhibit ovulation, have been used effectively [67–69].

Pregnancy

Counseling before pregnancy

VWD is inherited as an autosomal condition with variable penetrance. For types 1 and 2 VWD there is a 50% risk of a mother transmitting the condition to her child. Type 3 VWD is an autosomal recessive disorder and affected individuals are either homozygotes or compound heterozygotes. Where a child with type 3 has already been born in the family, the risk of a subsequent child being affected is 25%—this is common where there is marriage between first cousins. Antenatal diagnosis is not usually requested in types 1 and 2 VWD because the bleeding is relatively mild. However, if the fetus is at risk of type 3 (severe) VWD, parents may request antenatal diagnosis. Ideally, this should be planned in advance to allow the causative mutation to be identified [19].

Antenatal management

In type 1 VWD there is usually a progressive rise in FVIII coagulant activity (FVIII:Co), VWF:Ag, and VWF:AC [70]. Most women with type 1 VWD achieve VWF levels in the nonpregnant range by the third trimester [71]. However, some women severely affected with type 1 VWD fail to achieve normal VWF levels by this time [72]. In a series of 24 pregnancies in 24 women with VWD studied retrospectively, it was noted that FVIIIC and VWF:Ag rose above baseline levels by 1.5 times in most cases. A baseline VWF:AC of <15 IU/dL (four of 14 cases were predictive of a third trimester VWF level of <50 IU/dL [72].

In type 2 VWD, FVIII and VWF:Ag levels increase but there is minimal or no increase of VWF:AC levels [71,72]. In type 2N VWD, the FVIII level remains low because of impaired binding by VWF [73]. In type 2B VWD, thrombocytopenia may worsen in pregnancy because the increase in abnormal intermediate multimers induces platelet aggregation [74]. There is little or no increase of VWF in type 3 VWD [70,75].

Regular monitoring of VWF:Ag and VWF:AC together with FVIII:C is recommended during pregnancy because of the variability of hemostatic response [19]. The platelet count should also be monitored in those with type 2B VWD [74]. If the VWF:AC does not reach 50 IU/dL by the third trimester, consideration should be made for prophylactic treatment with a clotting factor concentrate containing VWF [19,76].

Miscarriage

The normal spontaneous miscarriage rate has been reported as 15% [77]. In a review of 84 pregnancies from 1980 to 1996 in women with all types of VWD, 33% reported vaginal bleeding during the first trimester with an overall spontaneous miscarriage rate of 21% [70]. In another study, the rate of miscarriage in women with VWD was reported as 22% [26]. Thus, it would seem that, although there is a higher rate of vaginal bleeding in the first trimester, women with VWD do not have an increase in miscarriage rate.

However, there is an increased risk of bleeding complications in association with spontaneous miscarriage or elective termination [26,70,74]. In one study, 10% of spontaneous or elective abortions were complicated by excessive bleeding requiring transfusion, and in 30% of cases intermittent bleeding occurred 2 weeks after the miscarriages [70]. Most miscarriages occur in the first or second trimester before the VWF:AC level has increased substantially [72]. Thus, women with VWD who present with spontaneous miscarriages or who opt for termination of pregnancy should have their VWF:AC level measured, and prophylactic treatment should be offered if it is <50 IU/dL [19].

Treatment

DDAVP

The use of DDAVP in pregnancy is controversial. The concerns include a vasoconstrictive effect leading to decreased placental blood flow, the risk of premature labor because of the weak V2 receptor activity, and the risk of neonatal hyponatremia [78]. In one survey, 50% and 30% of hematologists reported using intravenous and intranasal DDAVP, respectively, for postpartum hemorrhage in type 1 VWD and only 31% considered pregnancy as a contraindication [79]. DDAVP has been used in 31 women with VWD who underwent chorionic villus sampling or amniocentesis in the second trimester and there were no adverse events [80]. A study of peripartum use of DDAVP showed no adverse events when this was administered to cover 52 deliveries in women with a low third trimester VWF level and 20 deliveries by cesarean section. In the same report, DDAVP was given successfully to 54 women postpartum [81]. DDAVP has been successfully administered to mothers with VWD at the time of delivery and after cutting the cord [82]. Thus, the evidence suggests that DDAVP is not contraindicated in an uncomplicated pregnancy.

Clotting factor concentrate containing VWF

Virally inactivated concentrates containing VWF are the treatment of choice for women with VWD who are unresponsive to DDAVP. If the FVIIIC and/or VWF:AC is <50 IU/dL, prophylactic infusion should start at the onset of labor with the aim of maintaining a level of VWF:AC >50 IU/dL, which should be maintained for at least 3 days post delivery and 5 days post caesarean section [19]. DDAVP should be generally avoided in those with type 2B VWD because it can precipitate thrombocytopenia, and platelet transfusions have been administered when the platelet count is <20 × 10 L [83,74]. Recombinant FVIII has been used successfully in type 2N VWD [84]. In type 3 VWD, concentrate is always required to cover delivery because the VWF level does not increase in pregnancy.

Epidural anesthesia

Guidelines recommend that epidural anesthesia is safe if the VWF levels have normalized (>50 IU/dL) by the third trimester either physiologically or with treatment [19,48]. These guidelines have an evidence base of four institutional studies including approximately 100 deliveries [81,85–87].

Postpartum management

Women with VWD are at increased risk from primary (>500 mL of blood loss in the first 24 h) and secondary (500 mL of blood loss 24 h to 6 weeks post partum) postpartum hemorrhage (PPH) because of the fall in VWF and FVIIIC postnatally. In three series comprising 51 women and 92 deliveries, the primary PPH rate was 16–29% and the secondary PPH rate was 20–29% [70,72,88]. The VWF level should be checked post delivery particularly in those with a low predelivery baseline. The risk of PPH is higher in types 2 and 3 VWD, and in these women the VWF level should be maintained at >50 IU/dL for at least 3 days post delivery or 5 days after a cesarean section. There is a variable fall in VWF levels post delivery and there are anecdotal reports of a decrease from 41 to 9 IU/dL over the course of a week [72], and in another case there was a fall to half values within 24 h of delivery [89]. The presentation of PPH in women with VWD was found to be 16 days [90] and therefore there may be a need for observation and prophylaxis for several weeks post partum. Prolonged and/or intermittent secondary PPHs have been reported in women with VWD [70,72]. Comprehensive guidelines have been published on the management of PPH in women with VWD [19,48,76].

Neonates

Neonates with severe VWD are at risk of head bleeding, scalp hematoma, and intracerebral hemorrhage during labor and delivery. Thus, the use of invasive monitoring techniques such as fetal scalp electrodes, fetal blood sampling, instrumental deliveries, vacuum extraction, and midcavity/rotational forceps should be avoided where the fetus could have type 2, 3, or moderately affected type 1 VWD. It is, however, pos-

sible that some neonates with VWD could be protected by the increase of VWF and FVIII induced by the stress of labor [91].

Conclusion

It is now recognized that VWD is an important cause of menorrhagia. The World Health Organization have estimated that 18 million women worldwide have menorrhagia and therefore it is important that the diagnosis of VWD is considered. Conversely, individuals with diagnosed VWD should be assessed and treated for menorrhagia. Pregnancy may also be a problem in those women who have a baseline VWF level of <15 IU/dL. Early diagnosis and possible therapy with hemostatic agents means that the deaths in childbirth and from menorrhagia, reported in the kindred that Erik von Willebrand described in 1926, are confined to history. Morbidity from VWD can now be avoided, resulting in an improved quality of life for women with this condition.

References

1 Von Willebrand EA. Hereditar pseudohemofili. *Finska Lakarsallskapets Handl* 1926; **67**: 7–112.
2 Edland M. Physiology of menstruation and menorrhagia. in: Lee CA, Kadir R, Kouides P (eds.). *Inherited Bleeding Disorders in Women*. Wiley-Blackwell: Oxford, 2009.
3 Hallberg L, Hogdahl AM, Nilsson L, Rybo G. Menstrual blood loss: a population study. *Acta Obstet Gynecol Scand* 1966; **45**: 25–56.
4 Rybo G. Clinical and experimental studies on menstrual blood loss. *Acta Obstet Gynecol Reprod Gynecol Scand* 1966; **45**: 1–23.
5 Janssen CA, Scholten PC, Heintz AP. Reconsidering menorrhagia in gynaecological practice. Is a 30-year old definition still valid? *Eur J Obstet Gynecol Reprod Biol* 1998; **78**: 69–72.
6 Van Eijkeren MA, Christiaens GH, Scholten PC, Sixma JJ. Menorrhagia. Current drug treatment concepts. *Drugs* 1992; **43**: 201–9.
7 Royal College of General Practitioners, Office of Population Censuses and Surveys, Department of Health and Social Security. Morbidity statistics from general practice. Third national study 1981–2. Series MBS no 1. London, UK: HMSO, 1986.
8 Bradlow J, Coulter A, Brooks P. *Patterns of Referral*. Oxford: Health Services. Research Unit, 1992.

9 Highham JM, O'Brien PMS, Shaw RW. Assessment of menstrual blood loss using a pictorial chart. *Br J Obstet Gynaecol* 1990; **97**: 734–9.

10 Kadir RA, Economides DL, Sabin CA, Owens D, Lee CA. Frequency of inherited bleeding disorders in women with menorrhagia. *Lancet* 1998; **351**: 485–9.

11 Shankar M, Lee CA, Sabin CA, Economides DL, Kadir RA. von Willebrand disease in women with menorrhagia: a systematic review. *BJOG* 2004; **111**: 734–40.

12 Trasi S, Pathare AV, Shetty S, Ghosh K, Salvi V, Mohanty D. The spectrum of bleeding disorders in women with menorrhagia; a report from Western India. *Ann Haematol* 2005; **84**: 339–42.

13 Chen YC, Chao TY, Cheng SN, Hu SH, Liu JY. Prevalence of von Willebrand disease in women with iron deficiency anaemia and menorrhagia in Taiwan. *Haemophilia* 2008; **14**: 768–74.

14 Kadir RA, Economides DL, Sabin CA, Owens D, Lee CA. Variations in coagulation factors in women: effects of age, ethnicity, menstrual cycle and combined oral contraceptive. *Thromb Haemost* 1999; **82**: 1456–61.

15 Miller CH, Haff E, Platt SJ, *et al*. Measurement of von Willebrand factor activity: relative effects of ABO blood type and race. *J Thromb Haemost* 2003; **1**: 2191–7.

16 Miller CH, Dilley A, Drews C, Richardson L, Evatt B. Changes in von Willebrand factor and factor VIII levels during the menstrual cycle. *Thromb Haemost* 2002; **87**: 1082–3.

17 Onundarson PT, Gumundsdottir BR, Arnfinnsdottir AV, Kjeld M, Olafsson O. Von Willebrand factor does not vary during the normal menstrual cycle. *Thromb Haemost* 2001; **85**: 183–4.

18 Alperin JB. Estrogens and surgery in women with von Willebrand's disease. *Am J Med* 1982; **73**: 367–71.

19 Lee CA, Chi C, Pavord SR, *et al*. The obstetric and gynaecological management of women with inherited bleeding disorders—review with guidelines produced by a taskforce of UK Haemophilia Centre Doctors' Organisation. *Haemophilia* 2006; **12**: 301–36.

20 Kadir RA, Economides DL, Sabin CA, Pollard D, Lee CA. Assessment of menstrual blood loss and gynaecological problems in patients with inherited bleeding disorders. *Haemophilia* 1999; **5**: 40–8.

21 Ragni MV, Bontempo FA, Cortese Hassett A. von Willebrand disease and bleeding in women. *Haemophilia* 1999; **5**: 313–17.

22 Kouides PA, Burkhart P, Phatak P, *et al*. Gynecological and obstetrical morbidity in women with type 1 von Willebrand disease: results of a patient survey. *Haemophilia* 2000; **6**: 643–8.

23 Kadir RA, Sabin CA, Pollard D, Lee CA, Economides DL. Quality of life during menstruation in patients with inherited bleeding disorders. *Haemophilia* 1998; **4**: 836–41.

24 Kirtava A, Drews C, Lally C, Dilley A, Evatt B. Medical, reproductive and psychosocial experiences of women diagnosed with von Willebrand's disease receiving care in haemophilia treatment centres: a case-control study. *Haemophilia* 2003; **9**: 292–7.

25 James AH. More than menorrhagia: a review of the obstetric and gynaecological manifestations of bleeding disorders. *Haemophilia* 2005; **11**: 295–307.

26 Foster PA. The reproductive health of women with von Willebrand disease unresponsive to DDAVP: results of an international survey. On behalf of the Subcommittee on VWF of the SSC of the ISTH. *Thromb Haemost* 1995; **74**: 784–90.

27 Bevan JA, Maloney KW, Hillery CA, Gill JC, Montgomery RR, Scott JP. Bleeding disorders: a common cause of menorrhagia in adolescents. *J Pediatr* 2001; **138**: 856–61.

28 Claessons EA, Cowell CA. Acute adolescent menorrhagia. *Am J Obstet Gynecol* 1981; **139**: 277–80.

29 Smith YR, Quint EH, Hertzberg RB. Menorrhagia in adolescents requiring hospitalisation. *J Pediatr Adolesc Gynecol* 1998; **11**: 13–15.

30 Mikhail S, Vadadarajan R, Kouides PA. The prevalence of disorders of haemostasis in adolescents with menorrhagia referred to a haemophilia treatment centre. *Haemophilia* 2007; **13**: 627–32.

31 Conlan MG, Folsom AR, Finch A, *et al*. Associations of FVIII and von Willebrand factor with age, race, sex, and risk factors for atherosclerosis. The Atherosclerosis Risk Communities (ARIC) Study. *Thromb Haemost* 1993; **70**: 380–5.

32 Bonnar J, Sheppard BL. Treatment of menorrhagia during menstruation: Randomised controlled trial of ethamsylate, mefenamic acid, and tranexamic acid. *BMJ* 1996; **313**: 579–82.

33 Royal College of Obstetricians and Gynaecologists. *The Initial Management of Menorrhagia—National Evidence-based Clinical Guidelines*. London: RCOG, 1998.

34 Ong YL, Hull DR, Mayne EE. Menorrhagia in von Willebrand disease successfully treated with a single dose of tranexamic acid. *Haemophilia* 1998; **4**: 63–5.

35 Clinical Trials.gov. Efficacy and Safety Study of XP12B in Women with Menorrhagia. http://clinicaltrials.gov/ct/show/NCT00386308 [accessed on 1 November 2010]

36 Rodeghiero F, Castaman G, Mannucci PM. Prospective multicentre study on subcutaneous concentrated desmopressin for the home treatment of patients with von Willebrand disease and mild or moderate haemophilia A. *Thromb Haemost* 1996; **76**: 692–6.

37 Leissinger C, Becton D, Cornell C, Gill JC. High dose DDAVP intranasal spray (Stimate) for the prevention and treatment of bleeding in patients with mild haemophilia A, mild or moderate type 1 von Willebrand disease and symptomatic carriers of haemophilia A. *Haemophilia* 2001; **7**: 258–66.

38 Kadir RA, Lee CA, Sabin CA, Pollard D, Economides DL. DDAVP nasal spray for the treatment of menorrhagia in women with inherited bleeding disorders: a randomised cross over study. *Haemophilia* 2002; **8**: 87–93.

39 Edlund M, Blomback M, Fried G. Desmopressin in the treatment of menorrhagia in women with no common coagulation deficiency but with prolonged bleeding time. *Blood Coagul Fibrinolysis* 2002; **13**: 225–31.

40 Kouides PA, Byams VR, Philipp CS, *et al.* Multisite management study of menorrhagia with abnormal haemostasis: A prospective crossover study of intranasal DDAVP and oral tranexamic acid. *Br J Haematol* 2009; **145**: 212–20.

41 Callard GV, Litofsky FS, DeMerre LJ. Menstruation in women with normal or artificially controlled cycles. *Fertil Steril* 1966; **17**: 684–8.

42 Ramcharan S, Pellegrin FA, Ray RM, Hsu JP. The Walnut Creek Contraceptive Drug Study of the side effects of oral contraceptives. Volume III, an interim report: a comparison of disease occurrence leading to hospitalisation or death in users and nonusers of oral contraceptives. *J Reprod Med* 1980; **25**: 345–72.

43 Foster PA. The reproductive health of women with von Willebrand Disease unresponsive to DDAVP: results of an international survey. On behalf of the Subcommittee on von Willebrand Factor of the Scientific and Standardisation Committee of the ISTH. *Thromb Haemost* 1995; **74**: 784–90.

44 Kouides PA, Phatak PD, Burkart P, *et al.* Gynaecological and obstetrical morbidity in women with type 1 von Willebrand disease: results of a patient survey. *Haemophilia* 2000; **6**: 643–8.

45 Vercellini P, Giorgi O, Mosconi P, Stellato G, Vicentini S, Crosignani PG. Cyproterone acetate versus a continuous monophasic oral contraceptive in the treatment of recurrent pelvic pain after conservative surgery for symptomatic endometriosis. *Fertil Steril* 2002; **77**: 52–61.

46 Kwiecien M, Edelman A, Nichols MD, Jensen JT. Bleeding patterns and patient acceptability of standard or continuous dosing regimens of a low dose oral contraceptive: a randomised trial. *Contraception* 2003; **67**: 9–13.

47 Jarvis RR, Olsen ME. Type 1 von Willebrand's disease presenting as recurrent corpus haemorrhagicum. *Obstet Gynaecol* 2002; **99**: 1–8.

48 Nichols WL, Hultin MB, James AH, *et al.* von Willebrand Disease (VWD): evidence-based diagnosis and management guidelines, the National Heart, Lung, and Blood Institute (NHLBI) Expert Panel report (USA) 1. *Haemophilia* 2008; **14**: 171–232.

49 Michiels JJ, van Vliet HH, Berneman Z, *et al.* Intravenous DDAVP and factor VIII von Willebrand factor concentrate for the treatment and prophylaxis of bleedings in patients with von Willebrand disease type 1,2 and 3. *Clin Appl Thromb Hemost* 2007; **13**: 14–34.

50 Berntorp E, Petrini P. Long term prophylaxis in von Willebrand disease. *Blood Coagul Fibrinolysis* 2005; **16** (Suppl. 1): S23–6.

51 Berntorp E, Abshire T. The von Willebrand disease prophylaxis network: exploring a treatment concept. *J Thromb Haemost* 2006; **4**: 2511–12.

52 Nilsson IM, Blomback M, Blomback B. von Willebrand's disease in Sweden. Its pathogenesis and treatment. *Acta Med Scand* 1959; **164**: 263–78.

53 Silverberg SG, Haukkamaa M, Arko H, Nilsson CG, Luukkainen T. Endometrial morphology during long-term use of levonorgesterel-releasing intrauterine devices. *Int J Gynecol Pathol* 1986; **5**: 235–41.

54 Kingman CEC, Kadir RA, Lee CA, Economides DL. The use of the Levonorgesterel-releasing intrauterine system for the treatment of menorrhagia in women with inherited bleeding disorders. *BJOG* 2004; **111**: 1425–8.

55 Chi C, Chase A, Kadir RA. Levonorgestrel-releasing intrauterine system for the management of menorrhagia in women with inherited bleeding disorders: Long term follow-up. *Thromb Res* 2007; **119** (Suppl.): S101 (Abstract).

56 Lukes AS, Perry S, Ortel TL. von Willebrand's disease diagnosed after menorrhagia worsened from Levonorgestrel Intrauterine System. *Obstet Gynecol* 2005; **105**: 1223–6.

57 Lukes AS, Kouides PA. Hysterectomy versus expanded medical treatment for abnormal uterine bleeding: clinical outcomes in the medicine or surgery trial. *Obstet Gynecol* 2004; **104**: 864–5.

58 Maresh MJ, Metcalfe MA, McPherson K, *et al.* The VALUE national hysterectomy study: description of patients and their surgery. *BJOG* 2002; **109**: 302–12.

59 McPherson K, Metcalfe MA, Herbert A, *et al.* Severe complications of hysterectomy: the VALUE study. *BJOG* 2004; **111**: 688–94.

60 Lethaby A, Sheppard S, Cooke I, Farquar C. Endometrial resection and ablation versus hysterectomy for heavy menstrual bleeding. *Cochrane Database Syst Rev* 2000; CD000329.

61 Toth D, Gervaise A, Kuzel D, Fernandez H. Thermal balloon ablation in patients with multiple morbidity: 3-year follow-up. *J Am Assoc Gynecol Laparosc* 2004; **11**: 236–9.

62 Rubin G, Wortman M, Kouides PA. Endometrial ablation for von Willebrand disease-related menorrhagia—experience with seven cases. *Haemophilia* 2004; **10**: 477–82.

63 James AH. More than menorrhagia: a review of the obstetric and gynaecological manifestations of bleeding disorders. *Haemophilia* 2005; **11**: 295–307.

64 Silwer J. von Willebrand's disease in Sweden. *Acta Paediatr Scand Suppl* 1973; **238**: 1–159.

65 Hann LE, Hall DA, Black EB, Ferruci JT. Mittelschmerz. Sonographic demonstration. *JAMA* 1979; **241**: 2731–2.

66 O'Brien PM, DiMichele DM, Walterhouse DO. Management of an acute hemorrhagic cyst in a female patient with haemophilia A. *J Pediatr Hematol Oncol* 1996; **18**: 233–6.

67 Jarvis RR, Olsen ME. Type 1 von Willebrand's disease presenting as recurrent corpus hemorrhagicum. *Obstet Gynecol* 2002; **99**: 887–8.

68 Bottini E, Pareti FI, Mari D, Mannucci PM, Mugiasca ML, Conti M. Prevention of hemoperitoneum during ovulation by oral contraceptives in women with type III von Willebrand disease and afibrinogenemia. Case reports. *Haematologica* 1991; **76**: 431–3.

69 Ghosh K, Mohanty D, Pathare AV, Jijina F. Recurrent haemoperitoneum in a female patient with type III von Willebrand's disease responded to administration of oral contraceptive. *Haemophilia* 1998; **4**: 767–8.

70 Kadir RA, Lee CA, Sabin CA, Pollard D, Economides DL. Pregnancy in women with von Willebrand's disease or factor XI deficiency. *BJOG* 1998; **105**: 314–21.

71 Conti M, Mari D, Conti E, Muggiasca ML, Mannucci PM. Pregnancy in women with different types of von Willebrand disease. *Obstet Gynecol* 1986; **68**: 282–5.

72 Ramsoye BH, Davies SV, Dasani H, Pearson JF. Obstetric management in von Willebrand's disease: a report of 24 pregnancies and a review of the literature. *Haemophilia* 1995; **1**: 140–4.

73 Kujovich JL. von Willebrand Disease and pregnancy. *J Thromb Haemost* 2005; **3**: 246–53.

74 Rick ME, Williams SB, Sacher RA, McKeown LP. Thrombocytopenia associated with pregnancy in a patient with type IIB von Willebrand's disease. *Blood* 1987; **69**: 786–9.

75 Caliezi C, Tsakiris DA, Behringer H, Kuhne T, Marbet GA. Two consecutive pregnancies and deliveries in a patient with von Willebrand's disease type 3. *Haemophilia* 1998; **4**: 845–9.

76 James AH, Kouides PA, Abdul-Kadir R, *et al*. Von Willebrand disease and other bleeding disorders in women: Consensus on diagnosis and management from an international expert panel. *Am J Obstet Gynecol* 2009; **201**: 12.

77 Steer C, Campbell S, Davies M, Mason B, Collins W. Spontaneous abortion rates after natural and assisted conception. *BMJ* 1989; **299**: 1317–18.

78 Kouides P. Women and von Willebrand disease. In: Lee C, Berntorp E, Hoots K (eds.). *Textbook of Hemophilia*. 2nd edn. Wiley-Blackwell: Oxford, 2009, pp. 309–15.

79 Cohen AJ, Kessler CM, Ewenstein BM. Management of von Willebrand disease: a survey on the current clinical practice from the haemophilia centres of North America. *Haemophilia* 2001; **7**: 235–41.

80 Mannucci PM. How I treat patients with von Willebrands disease. *Blood* 2001; **97**: 1915–19.

81 Sanchez-Luceros A, Meschengieser SS, Turdo K, *et al*. Evaluation of desmopressin during pregnancy in women with a low plasmatic von Willebrand factor level and bleeding history. *Thromb Res* 2007; **120**: 387–90.

82 Castaman G, Tosetto A, Rodeghiero F. Pregnancy and delivery in women with von Willebrand disease and different von Willebrand factor mutations. Abstract As-Mo-029 XXII Congress. International Society on Thrombosis and Haemostasis, Boston, 2009.

83 Holmberg L, Nilsson IM, Borge L, Gunnarsson M, Sjorin E. Platelet aggregation induced by 1-desamino-8-arginine vasopressin (DDAVP) in type IIB von Willebrand's disease. *N Engl J Med* 1983; **309**: 816–21.

84 Dennis MW, Clough V, Toh CH. Unexpected presentation of type 2N von Willebrand disease in pregnancy. *Haemophilia* 2000; **6**: 696–7.

85 Chi C, Lee CA, England A, Hingorani J, Paintsil J, Kadir RA. Obstetric analgesia and anaesthesia in women with inherited bleeding disorders. *Thromb Haemost* 2009; **101**: 1104–11.

86 Varuguese J, Cohen AJ. Experience with epidural anaesthesia in pregnant women with von Willebrand disease. *Haemophilia* 2007; **13**: 730–3.

87 Marrache D, Mercier FJ, Boyer-Newmann C, Roger-Christoph S, Benhamou D. Epidural analgesia for patients with type 1 von Willebrand disease. *Int J Obstet Anesth* 2007; **16**: 231–5.

88 Greer IA, Lowe GD, Wailker JJ, Forbes CC. Haemorrhagic problems in obstetrics and gynaecology in patients with congenital coagulopathies. *Br J Obstet Gynaecol* 1991; **98**: 909–18.

89 Hanna W, McCarroll D, McDonald T, *et al*. Variant von Willebrand disease and pregnancy. *Blood* 1981; **58**: 873–9.

90 Roque H, Funai E, Lockwood CJ. von Willebrand disease and pregnancy. *J Matern Fetal Med* 2000; **9**: 257–66.

91 Kulkarni A, Riddell A, Lee CA, Kadir RA. Assessment of factor VIII and von Willebrand factor levels in cord blood. *6th International Scientific Meeting of the Royal College of Obstetricians and Gynaecologists, Cairo, Egypt*, 2005.

On the use of desmopressin in von Willebrand disease

Stefan Lethagen[1], Augusto B. Federici[2,3], and Giancarlo Castaman[4]

[1]Copenhagen Hemophilia Center, Thrombosis and Hemostasis Unit, Department of Hematology, Copenhagen University Hospital (Rigshopsitalet), Copenhagen, Denmark
[2]Division of Hematology and Transfusion Medicine, L. Sacco University Hospital, Milan, Italy
[3]Department of Internal Medicine, University of Milan, Milan, Italy
[4]Department of Cell Therapy and Hematology, Hemophilia and Thrombosis Center, San Bortolo Hospital, Vicenza, Italy

Summary

Desmopressin is an attractive hemostatic agent for the treatment of von Willebrand disease (VWD), mild hemophilia A, and several platelet disorders as it does not involve the risk of blood-borne diseases and is less costly than factor concentrates. In VWD, desmopressin acts by stimulating the endogenous release of von Willebrand factor (VWF) and factor VIII (FVIII). Desmopressin is used both for the treatment of bleeds and for prophylaxis in connection with surgery and other invasive procedures. The effect is virtually immediate, with on average two- to fourfold increases of VWF and FVIII levels. Although desmopressin has been used clinically in VWD for three decades, we still lack data from large prospective, controlled studies to scientifically prove its favorable clinical performance. Desmopressin responders should be selected with a test dose. Most patients with type 1 VWD are responders, whereas few with type 2 VWD and none with type 3 VWD will respond. Side-effects from desmopressin are usually mild; the most common is a facial flush and headache caused by the vasodilatory effect. Owing to the antidiuretic effect, fluid intake should be restricted. Desmopressin is administered parenterally (intravenously or subcutaneously) or intranasally (nasal spray). The subcutaneous and intranasal routes are useful for self-administration in the home setting.

History

Desmopressin was first synthesized as an analog of the native hormone vasopressin. The chemical structure, 1-desamino-8-D-arginine vasopressin, DDAVP, was derived by replacing the L-arginine with D-arginine in position 8 and by replacing the hemicysteine component at position 1 with β-mercaptopropionic acid, resulting in greater antidiuretic potency, decreased pressor activity, and prolonged duration (Figure 16.1) [1]. Thus, desmopressin has virtually no vasoconstrictive effect and does not contract the uterus or the gastrointestinal tract. The main sites of metabolic inactivation are the liver and kidney [2]. Being more resistant to enzymatic degradation, desmopressin is metabolized more slowly than vasopressin [3]. Desmopressin has mainly been used for its antidiuretic properties, for example in the treatment of diabetes insipidus and enuresis.

A systematic search for hemostatically active pharmacologic agents led to the discovery of desmopressin's hemostatic properties. Other substances, for example epinephrine [4,5], vasopressin and its synthetic analog, 8-lysine vasopressin, as well as different sympathomimetic amines, were known to affect hemostatic factors but also to cause vasoconstriction and other unacceptable side-effects [6,7].

Arginine vasopressin

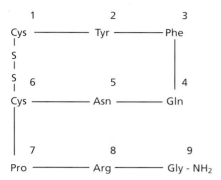

Desmopressin (1-desamino-8-D
arginine vasopressin, DDAVP)

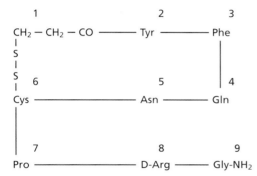

Figure 16.1 Chemical structure of the natural hormone vasopressin and its synthetic derivative desmopressin (DDAVP; 1-desamino-8-D-arginine vasopressin).

In the mid-1970s, two research groups [8,9] independently discovered that desmopressin had hemostatic effects (for a historical review, see references 10 and 11). When given in much higher dosage than those used in diabetes insipidus, desmopressin was found to increase plasma levels of FVIII, VWF, and tissue plasminogen activator (t-PA) in normal volunteers. Subsequently, the increases were found to be dose dependent [12]. There was, however, a ceiling limit to the response, possibly owing to saturation at receptor sites [13]. Similar effects were seen in patients with mild hemophilia A or VWD [14–17]. A major step forward was taken when surgical procedures could be safely performed under the cover of desmopressin in patients with hemophilia A and VWD without administration of blood products. This

proved that the endogenously released factors were functionally active [14,18–20]. Desmopressin has the advantages over factor concentrates of being less costly and of bearing no risk of transmitting blood-borne disorders. The use of desmopressin in VWD and hemophilia A has most certainly spared many patients from being infected with human immunodeficiency virus (HIV) and hepatitis virus [7].

Mechanism of action

The desmopressin-induced factor increase is so fast that it must by caused by release from endogenous reservoirs and not by increased synthesis. VWF is synthesized in endothelial cells and megakaryocytes, but plasma VWF is probably mainly released from endothelial cells [21–23]. In the endothelial cells, the high-molecular-weight multimers (HMWM) of VWF are packed in unique cell organelles, the Weibel–Palade bodies (WPBs), together with the VWF propeptide (VWFpp) and are released in a regulated manner upon stimulation by certain agonists such as thrombin, fibrin, and histamine [24]. The physiologic function of the regulated pathway may be to create a high local concentration of the large VWF multimers in order to enhance platelet adhesion at sites of vascular injury. VWF released by desmopressin contains HMWM, indicating that the release originates from the endothelial WPBs [25]. This is further strengthened by the observation that VWF and its propeptide are released in equimolar quantities [26]. Unstimulated endothelial cells probably direct much of the release from WPBs toward the subendothelium [27], which contains mainly the HMWM of the VWF [28]. An unregulated constitutive pathway with continuous release of lower molecular-weight multimers [29] may provide the VWF needed for FVIII binding in plasma. The cellular source of plasma FVIII is not yet completely determined. FVIII is mainly synthesized in sinusoid liver endothelial cells [30,31] and possibly hepatocytes [21,32,33]. FVIII production has also been identified in human microvascular lung endothelial cells [34].

The effect on FVIII levels is less understood. The desmopressin-induced FVIII release most likely does not originate from the hepatocyte, although this is assumed to be the most important site for FVIII synthesis. FVIII expression also has been demonstrated

187

in other tissues, especially in the kidneys, spleen, and lymph nodes, but the exact site of desmopressin-induced FVIII release remains an enigma [35]. It has been shown that intravenous infusion of VWF to a patient with type 3 VWD will stimulate an endogenous release of FVIII, which is much slower than that occurring after desmopressin [36]. As FVIII is released with the same dynamics as VWF after administration of desmopressin, this FVIII release cannot be explained as a secondary phenomenon to the VWF release. After liver transplantation, three hemophilic men showed VWF but no FVIII response to desmopressin. Conversely, both VWF and FVIII increased after desmopressin in a nonhemophilic liver transplant recipient. These, and other findings from studies of patients with severe VWD and severe hemophilia A, indicate that intracellular co-localization of FVIII and VWF may be necessary for *in vivo* secretion of FVIII after desmopressin [37,38]. However, a cell type that stores and secretes both factors has not yet been demonstrated.

There are two general classes of vasopressin receptors. V1 receptors (V1R) mediate smooth muscle contraction in the peripheral vasculature and glucose turnover in hepatocytes. V2 receptors (V2R) regulate water reabsorption in the collecting ducts of the kidney. Desmopressin is a strong V2R agonist but has no effect on V1R. Several findings confirm the receptor specificity. Patients with nephrogenic diabetes insipidus, who lack V2R, do not show any factor increases in response to desmopressin [39,40]. The effect is not mediated via V2R in the kidneys because anephric patients respond normally to desmopressin [9]. By contrast, patients with other rare forms of nephrogenic diabetes insipidus seem to manifest a normal clotting factor response to desmopressin [41,42].

It is known that the antidiuretic effect of vasopressin and desmopressin is caused by a cAMP-mediated translocation of the water channel aquaporin-2 from intracellular stores to the apical cell membrane in the kidney collecting ducts [43]. VWF is probably released from endothelial cell WPBs by way of a similar mechanism. Human umbilical vein endothelial cells (HUVECs), which do not normally express V2R, show a desmopressin-mediated release of VWF in a cAMP-dependent manner after transfection of V2R. Furthermore, desmopressin stimulates VWF release from human lung microvascular endothelial cells (HMVEC-Ls), which do express endogenous V2R [44]. Other theories for an indirect second messenger, either via the hypothalamus [45] or via platelet activating factor (PAF) [46] released by monocytes, have been disproven [35,47].

Desmopressin also releases t-PA, probably from endothelial cells [8,9]. There are data indicating that VWF and t-PA are collocalized in WPBs [48]. t-PA activates plasminogen, but most of the plasmin formed is bound to α-2-antiplasmin, which inhibits an increase of fibrinolytic activity in circulating blood [49]. In view of this, it is not necessary to give a fibrinolytic inhibitor (e.g., tranexamic acid or ε-aminocaproic acid) simultaneously with desmopressin in order to block this effect.

Desmopressin has a vasodilatory effect, which causes a facial flush and a slight decrease in blood pressure. The vasodilatory effect is probably secondary to V2R-mediated endothelial nitric oxide synthase activation [50].

Desmopressin also enhances the adhesion of platelets to the subendothelium [51] and to glass beads [52] in perfusion tests, without causing platelet aggregation [53]. The enhanced platelet retention after administration of desmopressin is not secondary to the increased VWF level in plasma, but appears to be dependent on the presence of platelet-VWF and the platelet receptor glycoprotein (GP) IIb/IIIa [54].

In addition to its antidiuretic and hemostatic effects, there are data indicating that desmopressin treatment may impair the spread of cancer cells and contribute to the encapsulation of tumor tissue [55]. Recent data suggest that desmopressin may contribute to the impaired aggressiveness of residual mammary tumors during chemotherapy [56].

Modes of administration and dosage

Desmopressin can be administered intravenously, subcutaneously, or intranasally (Table 16.1). Maximal (generally about two- to fourfold) FVIII and VWF release is reached with a dosage of 0.3 μg/kg intravenously in healthy volunteers [13,57]. An increase in factor levels is virtually immediate, with maximum activity 30–60 min after intravenous administration. A higher dose will not improve the response in spite of higher plasma levels of desmopressin [13].

Table 16.1 Recommended doses of desmopressin in von Willebrand disease.

Intravenous injection or infusion	0.3 µg/kg diluted in 10 ml saline and given as a slow injection over 15 min, or diluted in 50–100 ml saline and given as an infusion over 30 min
Subcutaneous injection	0.3 µg/kg
Intranasal spray	300 µg as nasal spray (150 µg if body weight is <30 kg)
Dose intervals	8- to 24-h intervals depending on the clinical situation and clearance of factors
Time to peak VWF and FVIII levels	30–60 min after intravenous injection or 90–120 min after subcutaneous injection or intranasal spray

VWF, von Willebrand factor.

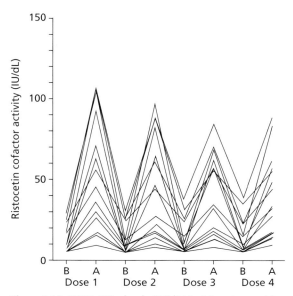

Figure 16.2 VWF:RCo levels (IU/dL) in 15 patients with type 1 von Willebrand disease after four doses of desmopressin (0.3 µg/kg intravenously) with 24 h intervals [61].

Subcutaneous administration will give a similar factor response to intravenous administration, but the factors peak after about 90–120 min [58]. The factor increases after intranasal administration with a high-dose spray, although even with a full dose of 300 µg the effect is marginally lower than that achieved with intravenous administration, and the factor levels peaks after about 90–120 min. The reproducibility of the spray effect is as good as that of intravenous administration [13,59].

Recommended doses of desmopressin are therefore 0.3 µg/kg intravenously or subcutaneously, or 300 µg intranasally with nasal spray. Desmopressin is usually given at intervals of 12–24 h, but, depending on the half-life of factor levels and the nature of the bleeding, the dose may be given with 8-h intervals in hospitalized patients. When repeated doses are given, the risk of hyponatremia [60] and tachyphylaxis [61] must be considered (see below). The duration of desmopressin treatment should normally not exceed 3 days, but it may be prolonged if factor levels and water balance (e.g. sodium levels) are monitored. Tachyphylaxis has been reported after several days of treatment (Figure 16.2). A test dose of desmopressin at the time of diagnosis is recommended to ensure that the response is sufficient for clinical use. Blood samples for the measurement of VWF and FVIII activity should be taken before administering desmopressin, and at least at 30 min (to identify the peak response) and 4 h (to identify patients with a fast clearance of VWF or FVIII) after the start of intravenous administration. More blood samples will add further information but may be difficult in clinical practice.

The target levels for VWF and FVIII depend on the clinical situation. In the case of major surgery, normal levels should be attained, but for minor bleeds lower levels may be sufficient. There are no controlled data determining which factor level is needed for different clinical situations. This probably also differs between patients. The definition of responders and nonresponders varies somewhat in different protocols. These definitions are usually based more on scientific than on clinical requirements. Recently, the Steering Committee of the European Study on Molecular and Clinical Markers for Diagnosis and Management of Type 1 VWD (MCMDM-1VWD) proposed the following definition of biologic response: complete responders, both VWF:RCo and FVIII:C ≥ 50 IU/dL after desmopressin; partial responders, VWF:RCo or FVIII:C < 50 IU/dL but increased at least threefold; nonresponders, none of these [62].

189

Table 16.2 General response to desmopressin in the different von Willebrand disease types.

VWD type	Response
Type 1	Most cases respond well. Response rate is lower in severe type cases
Types 2A and 2M	Some patients may respond, but most cases respond insufficiently owing to functional abnormalities
Type 2B	Contraindicated in most cases of classical type 2B because of thrombocytopenia. Patients with type Malmö/New York respond
Type 2N	Many cases respond, but FVIII half-life may be short
Type 3	No response

Experience of desmopressin in VWD

Biologic response

The response to desmopressin is dependent on the type and severity of VWD (Table 16.2). It has long been known that most patients with type 1 respond well, but the degree of biologic response, measured as increase of factor levels, varies significantly. The intra-individual response is, however, consistent from time to time. Therefore, the results of a test dose will predict the clinical utility of desmopressin in clinical situations.

Our knowledge about the cause of the response differences in patients with type 1 VWD has improved over past years. Data from the large European MCMDM-1VWD study showed that the response is dependent on the localization of mutations in the VWF gene and on differences in multimeric pattern. Data from 77 patients with type 1 VWD showed complete response in 83%, a partial response in 13%, and no response in 4%. According to study criteria there were fewer complete responders among patients with some abnormality of VWF multimeric pattern than those with a normal multimeric pattern. The presence of subtle multimeric abnormalities did not, however, hamper potential clinically useful responses. Median maximum relative VWF:RCo increases after desmopressin was 3.2-fold, but the range was huge: 1.3- to 53.7-fold. Most of the patients with more than a 10-fold increase had mutations at codons 1130 or 1205 in the D'-D3 domains, but they also

tended to have the shortest VWF survival with a VWF:RCo half-life usually of less than 4 h, indicating an increased clearance [62] (Figure 16.3). Patients with a reduced VWF survival phenotype may be identified by an increased ratio of steady-state VWFpp/VWF:Ag [63].

The response rate in a certain study is dependent both on the selection criteria for the study population and on the response criteria. Hence, a study with very strict inclusion criteria (type 1 VWD or type 2 VWD with a significant bleeding history and a bleeding time >15 min, VWF:RCo <10 IU/dL, or FVIII:C <20 IU/dL) and stringent response criteria (≥threefold increase of VWF:RCo and FVIII, ≥30 IU/dL, and a bleeding time ≤12 min) found a response rate of only 27% in patients with severe type 1 VWD [64] (Figure 16.4a).

Most patients with type 2 VWD will have a poor response because the released VWF is more or less dysfunctional. Thus, in the above-mentioned study only 7% of those with type 2A and 14% of those with type 2M were classified as responders (Figure 16.4a,c) [64]. Desmopressin is generally contraindicated in the classic form of type 2B VWD since the release of the abnormal VWF induces platelet aggregation and thrombocytopenia [65]. In the rare type 2B Malmö/New York variant, however, desmopressin does not cause platelet aggregation [66,67]. Patients with type 2N VWD may have a high relative FVIII response, but half-life is usually short (Figure 16.4d). Desmopressin may be useful in some patients with type 2N VWD provided that a desmopressin test has shown that adequate FVIII levels can be reached and maintained for a sufficient period of time [68].

Patients with type 3 VWD do not respond at all to desmopressin because they have a total lack of VWF. A subgroup of patients with severe recessive VWD with a unique mutation (C2362F) in compound heterozygosity or homozygosity may respond with normalization of FVIII, although there is no change in VWF:RCo [69].

Clinical response

There are several reports on the clinical efficacy of desmopressin in connection with bleeds or invasive procedures, but most of them are small, uncontrolled, and retrospective, and the patients were usually selected on the basis of earlier testing [14,18–20,70–73]. Presently, a large international prospective obser-

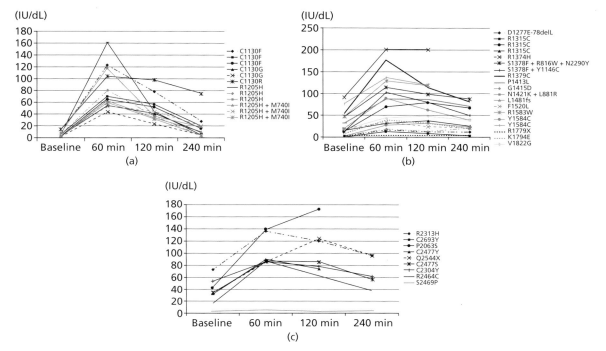

Figure 16.3 Data from the European study on Molecular and Clinical Markers for Diagnosis and Management of Type 1 von Willebrand Disease (MCMDM-1VWD). VWF:RCo levels (IU/dL) before and after administration of desmopressin at 0.3 μg/kg intravenously to patients with VWD with (a) mutations C1130F/G/R and R1205H; (b) mutations in domain A1-A3; and (c) mutations in domain D4-CK. This research was originally published in *Blood* [62] © the American Society of Hematology.

vational study, hosted by the International Society of Thrombosis and Haemostasis Scientific and Standardization Committee (ISTH-SSC) on VWF, evaluates the clinical efficacy of desmopressin in patients with type 1 VWD over 2 years and estimates if biologic response as measured with a desmopressin test can predict the clinical efficacy. This will hopefully tell us which biologic response criteria are adequate for clinical utility of desmopressin.

Administration of desmopressin as an intranasal spray or subcutaneous injection is suitable for home treatment. A questionnaire answered by 78 patients with mild hemophilia A ($n = 10$), VWD ($n = 46$), platelet disorders ($n = 20$), or other disorders ($n = 2$) who had used desmopressin intranasal spray as home treatment showed that these patients experienced decreased blood loss and shortened duration of epistaxis, menorrhagia, tissue bleeding, and bleeding in connection with minor surgery or tooth extraction. The use of VWF/FVIII concentrates was diminished,

as were the number of visits to outpatient care and absence from school or work. The main side-effects were a facial flush and warmth in 24% of cases and dizziness or headache in 13% of cases. Patients rated the efficacy of the spray to reduce bleeding on an analog scale, with "no effect" at the left and "very good effect" at the right. The ratings were scored from 0 to 100 (left to right), the median score being 82 (range 0–100). In general, the score could not be predicted by the biologic response, with at least one exception: one female patient with severe type 1 VWD (VWF, 2 IU/dL; FVIII, 10 IU/dL) who tried the spray for menstrual bleeds gave a score of only 2 [74]. In a prospective study of the use of subcutaneous administration of desmopressin in patients with hemophilia A or VWD, the effect was scored as excellent or good in 94% of cases (excluding menorrhagia) and 86% of menorrhagia treatments. Mild flushing, with or without headache, was the only consistent side-effect, reported in about 30% of cases [70].

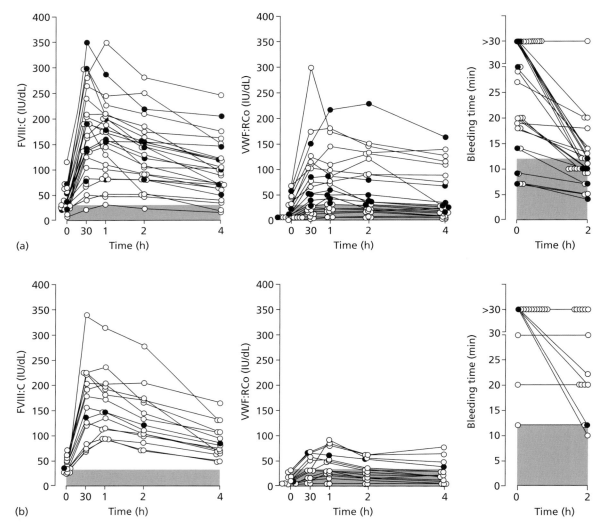

Figure 16.4 Biologic response to desmopressin (a) in 26 patients with type 1 von Willebrand disease; (b) in 15 patients with type 2A; (c) in 21 patients with type 2M; and (d) in four patients with type 2N [64].

Acquired von Willebrand syndrome

Desmopressin may also have a hemostatic effect in patients with acquired von Willebrand syndrome (aVWS), although the clinical effect may be limited by a short half-life of the released VWF. Bleeding was successfully controlled in 26 of 59 (44%) cases in an Italian study. A test dose of desmopressin should therefore also be given to patients with aVWS [75].

Adverse effects

Adverse effects of desmopressin include tiredness, headache, nausea, and temporary lowering of blood pressure with secondary tachycardia, facial flushing, fluid retention, hyponatremia, and seizures. Desmopressin was originally designed to have a potent antidiuretic effect with long duration. Maximal antidiuretic effect is achieved already at a low dose (2 mg

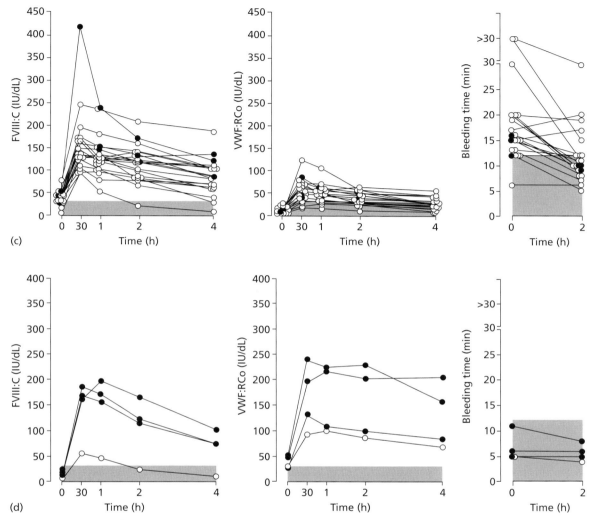

Figure 16.4 (*Continued*) DDAVP, 1-desamino-8-ᴅ-arginine vasopressin. ●, DDAVP responders; ○, DDAVP non-responders. This research was originally published in *Blood* [64] © the American Society of Hematology.

parenterally or 20 mg intranasally) [76]. The 10–20 times higher hemostatic dose will not give a stronger antidiuretic effect, but the duration is longer. Thus, the antidiuretic effect lasts for about 12 h after an antidiuretic dose and about 24 h after a single hemostatic dose (0.3 µg/kg intravenously or 300 µg intranasally). The antidiuretic effect is prolonged as long as the doses are repeated [60]. The risk of hyponatremia is small in healthy volunteers after a single desmo-

pressin dose if there is not an exaggerated water intake. Repeated doses will, however, induce a decrease in sodium levels, both in healthy individuals and in individuals with VWD; thus, sodium levels should be monitored (Figure 16.5) [60]. In patients with chronic renal failure, a single hemostatic dose of desmopressin increased urine osmolality significantly for 48 h. It did not cause fluid overload or electrolytic changes, but the clearance of desmopressin was

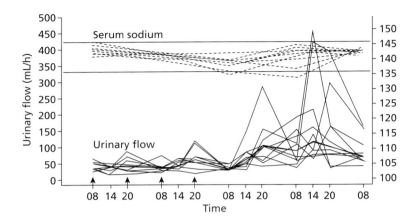

Figure 16.5 Urinary flow (mL/h) and serum sodium (mmol/L) in 10 healthy volunteers after four intranasal (i.n.) spray doses of 300 μg of desmopressin at 12-h intervals. The horizontal lines indicate the upper and lower limits of the normal reference range of serum sodium [60].

reduced to one-quarter and the half-life of desmopressin prolonged 2–3 times in those with VWD compared with healthy individuals [77]. There is no risk of fluid overload or congestive heart failure in uremic patients [78]. Although fluid overload is not a common feature connected with desmopressin treatment, several case reports have called attention to the risk of hyponatremia and seizures after administration of desmopressin. Most such cases have occurred in children, usually under the age of 5 years, after administration of frequent, repeated doses of desmopressin or in those receiving hypotonic intravenous fluids. It is therefore generally recommended that desmopressin be used with caution in small children or in patients with congestive heart failure and that hypotonic fluids be used sparingly [60].

Some case reports of thromboembolic events have been published, but extensive evaluations of clinical trials of desmopressin in conjunction with cardiac, orthopedic, and other major surgery did not demonstrate any risk of thrombosis [79,80].

Adjuvant therapy

Desmopressin is often given together with an antifibrinolytic agent, for example tranexamic acid or ε-aminocaproic acid. Antifibrinolytic agents are, however, not required because of the transient fibrinolytic activity induced by desmopressin, but they are given because of their beneficial effect inhibiting the fibrinolytic breakdown of formed clots. Tranexamic acid has the advantage over ε-aminocaproic acid of having fewer side-effects. Tranexamic acid has been

shown to be effective in connection with tooth extractions, menorrhagia, and gynecologic, cardiac, and orthopedic surgery. Antifibrinolytic agents may also be used alone for the treatment of mucous membrane bleeds and tooth extractions in patients with mild disorders. In females with menorrhagia, combined oral contraceptive pills, or intrauterine progesterone contraceptive devices may be beneficial.

Clinical use

Before desmopressin is used in connection with bleeds or invasive procedures, a test dose should be given to ensure that the response is sufficient (see above). It is enough to do this once, as the response is consistent from time to time. The test dose should preferably be given intravenously or subcutaneously in order to evaluate the maximum response of the particular patient.

Pregnancy

Data from more than 4000 deliveries in females with VWD, taken from the United States Nationwide Inpatient Sample (NIS) from the Healthcare Cost and Utilization Project of the Agency for Healthcare Research and Quality for the years 2000–2003, demonstrated a 10-fold increased risk of antepartum bleeding, a 1.5 times increased risk of postpartum bleeds and a fivefold increased risk of being transfused [81]. The hemophilia center should therefore be involved early in pregnancy and should present a plan for the hemostatic treatment in connection with delivery in cooperation with the obstetrician. The delivery should take place at an obstetric unit close to the hemophilia center. In all cases, treatment with tranexamic acid is commenced during labor and continued until 2 weeks post partum. In mild cases, one dose of desmopressin administered immediately after delivery is usually sufficient, but desmopressin may be repeated at 8- to 12-h intervals if needed.

However, as most cases of mild VWD show a FVIII and VWF normalization by the end of pregnancy, specific treatment is seldom required. Even though patients with the frequent VWD Vicenza (R1205H) and C1130F mutations show only a slight increase of these moieties during pregnancy, they can be successfully treated with desmopressin at delivery [82,83]. In general, patients with VWD should be monitored for VWF:RCo and FVIII:C levels at least during the third trimester of pregnancy and within 10 days of the expected delivery date.

Desmopressin has been used with caution in early pregnancy owing to a fear of side-effects. Desmopressin, however, does not contract the uterus and has no vasoconstrictive effect. Furthermore, desmopressin has safely been used during pregnancy in women with diabetes insipidus for many years, and the antidiuretic effect is not stronger with hemostatic dosages [60]. Mannucci [84] presented the use of desmopressin in early pregnancy in connection with chorion villus sampling or amniocentesis in 32 women with FVIII deficiency (27 with hemophilia A and five with type 1 VWD). The women were advised to avoid excessive fluid intake and to monitor their bodyweight. There were no side-effects except for facial flushing or headache and there was no increase in bodyweight [84]. In desmopressin nonresponders, treatment with a VWF concentrate is administered when the delivery starts and repeated when necessary. In mothers with severe VWD, treatment is continued with a VWF/FVIII concentrate about three times weekly for 2 weeks post partum.

Surgery

It is advisable to perform all major invasive procedures at a hospital with a specialized hemophilia center and a coagulation laboratory that can measure VWF and FVIII activities day and night. The FVIII activity level determines the risk of surgical and soft-tissue bleeds, whereas the VWF activity is more important for mucous membrane bleeds. In absence of generally agreed minimum factor levels in connection with surgery in VWD, recommended levels for FVIII in hemophilia A (http://www.wfh.org) can be used for guidance. During major surgery, FVIII:C levels should be kept at 80–100 IU/dL. Thereafter, the following rough levels are recommended: postoperative days 1–3, 60–80 IU/dL; postoperative days 4–6, 40–60 IU/dL; and postoperative days 7–14, 30–50 IU/dL.

The risk of water retention and tachyphylaxis may limit the usefulness of desmopressin. After major surgery, or in other situations in which a longer treatment period is needed, it may therefore be necessary to use a VWF/FVIII concentrate in addition to desmopressin.

It is often advantageous to give tranexamic acid as a synergistic therapy, especially if mucous membranes are involved (10 mg/kg intravenously or 20–25 mg/kg orally every 6–8 h).

Venous thromboprophylaxis is not generally recommended in VWD in connection with surgery, but may be considered in selected patients who receive high doses of a VWF/FVIII concentrate or undergo surgery associated with high risk of thrombosis [85].

Menorrhagia

Therapeutic alternatives for menorrhagia include tranexamic acid, desmopressin, VWF/FVIII concentrates, oral combined contraceptive pills, and intrauterine progesterone contraceptive devices. If the response to tranexamic acid and oral combined contraceptive pills is insufficient, desmopressin or a VWF concentrate may be required to control the menstrual bleed. Tranexamic acid, desmopressin, and concentrates are typically taken during the menstruation days, desmopressin often only during the first 1–3 days [74]. For home treatment, desmopressin is ideally administered subcutaneously or intranasally. The subcutaneous route for home treatment has shown an effective response in 86% of 43 self-treated cycles [70]. A similar figure (88%) was obtained by using the intranasal spray formulation [86] even though a crossover trial failed to demonstrate a substantial benefit with the use of desmopressin [87].

195

Conclusion

Desmopressin is an effective hemostatic agent in selected cases of VWD, hemophilia A, and several platelet disorders because of its hemostatic properties. Desmopressin increases plasma levels of VWF and FVIII and stimulates platelet adhesion. In inherited VWD, most patients with type 1 VWD respond, whereas only some with type 2 VWD and none with type 3 VWD respond. Desmopressin has a virtually immediate response and may therefore be used both for the treatment of bleeds and for prophylactic treatment in connection with invasive procedures. A test dose should be given to each patient to ensure a sufficient response. Desmopressin also has a strong antidiuretic effect, which must be taken into consideration, especially when repeated doses are given, as it may lead to hyponatremia if fluid intake is not limited. Desmopressin avoids the risk of blood-borne infectious agents, which accompany plasma-derived factor concentrates and other blood products. Historically, the use of desmopressin has probably saved many patients with hemophilia and VWD from blood-borne infections, for example hepatitis and HIV. With modern screening of blood donors and viral inactivation of concentrates, however, the risk of infection is today virtually negligible. Desmopressin still has the advantage over concentrates of being much less costly. For these reasons, it is advisable to use desmopressin as the first treatment of choice for patients who are responders. Although desmopressin has now been used successfully for the treatment of VWD for three decades, we still lack prospective studies that confirm the beneficial clinical experience.

References

1 Vavra I, Machova A, Holecek V, Cort JH, Zaoral M, Sorm F. Effect of a synthetic analogue of vasopressin in animals and in patients with diabetes insipidus. *Lancet* 1968; **1**: 948–52.

2 Walter R. Partial purification and characterization of post-proline cleaving enzyme: enzymatic inactivation of neurohypophyseal hormones by kidney preparations of various species. *Biochim Biophys Acta* 1976; **422**: 138–58.

3 Shimizu K Hoshino M, Kumagawa J, *et al.* Mechanism of the prolonged antidiuretic action of DDAVP and its metabolic features. In: Share L, Yoshida S, Yagi K (eds). *Antidiuretic Hormone*, pp.271–84. University Park Press: Baltimore, 1980.

4 Ingram GI. Increase in antihaemophilic globulin activity following infusion of adrenaline. *J Physiol* 1961; **156**: 217–24.

5 Egeberg O. Changes in the activity of antihemophilic A factor (F. Viii) and in the bleeding time associated with muscular exercise and adrenalin infusion. *Scand J Clin Lab Invest* 1963; **15**: 539–49.

6 Schneck SA, Von Kaulla KN. Fibrinolysis and the nervous system. *Neurology* 1961; **11**: 959–69.

7 Mannucci PM. Desmopressin (DDAVP) in the treatment of bleeding disorders: the first twenty years. *Haemophilia* 2000; **6** (Suppl. 1): 60–7.

8 Cash JD, Gader AM, da Costa J. Proceedings: The release of plasminogen activator and factor VIII to lysine vasopressin, arginine vasopressin, I-desamino-8-d-arginine vasopressin, angiotensin and oxytocin in man. *Br J Haematol* 1974; **27**: 363–4.

9 Mannucci PM, Aberg M, Nilsson IM, Robertson B. Mechanism of plasminogen activator and factor VIII increase after vasoactive drugs. *Br J Haematol* 1975; **30**: 81–93.

10 Mannucci PM. Desmopressin (DDAVP) and factor VIII: the tale as viewed from Milan (and Malmo). *J Thromb Haemost* 2003; **1**: 622–4.

11 Cash JD. DDAVP and factor VIII: a tale from Edinburgh. *J Thromb Haemost* 2003; **1**: 619–21.

12 Aberg M, Nilsson I, Vilhardt H. The release of fibrinolytic activator and factor VIII after injection of DDAVP. In: Davidson JF (ed). *Progress in Chemical Fibrinolysis and Thrombolysis*. Churchill Livingstone: Edinburgh, 1979, pp. 92–7.

13 Lethagen S, Harris AS, Sjorin E, Nilsson IM. Intranasal and intravenous administration of desmopressin: effect on F VIII/vWF, pharmacokinetics and reproducibility. *Thromb Haemost* 1987; **58**: 1033–6.

14 Mannucci PM, Ruggeri ZM, Pareti FI, Capitanio A. 1-Deamino-8-d-arginine vasopressin: a new pharmacological approach to the management of haemophilia and von Willebrands' diseases. *Lancet* 1977; **1**: 869–72.

15 Kobayashi I. Treatment of hemophilia A and von Willebrand's disease patients with an intranasal dripping of DDAVP. *Thromb Res* 1979; **16**: 775–9.

16 Nilsson IM, Holmberg L, Stenberg P, Henriksson P. Characteristics of the factor VIII protein and Factor XIII in various factor VIII concentrates. *Scand J Haematol* 1980; **24**: 340–9.

17 Nilsson IM, Vilhardt H, Holmberg L, Astedt B. Association between factor VIII related antigen and plasminogen activator. *Acta Med Scand* 1982; **211**: 105–12.

18 Warrier AI, Lusher JM. DDAVP: a useful alternative to blood components in moderate hemophilia A and von Willebrand disease. *J Pediatr* 1983; **102**: 228–33.

19 Mariani G, Ciavarella N, Mazzucconi MG, *et al.* Evaluation of the effectiveness of DDAVP in surgery and in bleeding episodes in haemophilia and von Willebrand's disease. A study on 43 patients. *Clin Lab Haematol* 1984; **6**: 229–38.

20 de la Fuente B, Kasper CK, Rickles FR, Hoyer LW. Response of patients with mild and moderate hemophilia A and von Willebrand's disease to treatment with desmopressin. *Ann Intern Med* 1985; **103**: 6–14.

21 Howard MA, Montgomery DC, Hardisty RM. Factor-VIII-related antigen in platelets. *Thromb Res* 1974; **4**: 617–24.

22 Nachman RL, Jaffe EA. Subcellular platelet factor VIII antigen and von Willebrand factor. *J Exp Med* 1975; **141**: 1101–13.

23 Nichols TC, Samama CM, Bellinger DA, *et al.* Function of von Willebrand factor after crossed bone marrow transplantation between normal and von Willebrand disease pigs: effect on arterial thrombosis in chimeras. *Proc Natl Acad Sci U S A* 1995; **92**: 2455–9.

24 Sporn LA, Marder VJ, Wagner DD. von Willebrand factor released from Weibel–Palade bodies binds more avidly to extracellular matrix than that secreted constitutively. *Blood* 1987; **69**: 1531–4.

25 Ruggeri ZM, Mannucci PM, Lombardi R, Federici AB, Zimmerman TS. Multimeric composition of factor VIII/von Willebrand factor following administration of DDAVP: implications for pathophysiology and therapy of von Willebrand's disease subtypes. *Blood* 1982; **59**: 1272–8.

26 Borchiellini A, Fijnvandraat K, ten Cate JW, *et al.* Quantitative analysis of von Willebrand factor propeptide release *in vivo*: effect of experimental endotoxemia and administration of 1-deamino-8-D-arginine vasopressin in humans. *Blood* 1996; **88**: 2951–8.

27 Sakariassen KS, Bolhuis PA, Sixma JJ. Human blood platelet adhesion to artery subendothelium is mediated by factor VIII-Von Willebrand factor bound to the subendothelium. *Nature* 1979; **279**: 636–8.

28 Tannenbaum SH, Rick ME, Shafer B, Gralnick HR. Subendothelial matrix of cultured endothelial cells contains fully processed high molecular weight von Willebrand factor. *J Lab Clin Med* 1989; **113**: 372–8.

29 Wagner DD, Marder VJ. Biosynthesis of von Willebrand protein by human endothelial cells: processing steps and their intracellular localization. *J Cell Biol* 1984; **99**: 2123–30.

30 Stel HV, van der Kwast TH, Veerman EC. Detection of factor VIII/coagulant antigen in human liver tissue. *Nature* 1983; **303**: 530–2.

31 Do H, Healey JF, Waller EK, Lollar P. Expression of factor VIII by murine liver sinusoidal endothelial cells. *J Biol Chem* 1999; **274**: 19587–92.

32 Wion KL, Kelly D, Summerfield JA, Tuddenham EG, Lawn RM. Distribution of factor VIII mRNA and antigen in human liver and other tissues. *Nature* 1985; **317**: 726–9.

33 Zelechowska MG, van Mourik JA, Brodniewicz-Proba T. Ultrastructural localization of factor VIII procoagulant antigen in human liver hepatocytes. *Nature* 1985; **317**: 729–30.

34 Jacquemin M, Neyrinck A, Hermanns MI, *et al.* FVIII production by human lung microvascular endothelial cells. *Blood* 2006; **108**: 515–17.

35 Kaufmann JE, Vischer UM. Cellular mechanisms of the hemostatic effects of desmopressin (DDAVP). *J Thromb Haemost* 2003; **1**: 682–9.

36 Lethagen S, Berntorp E, Nilsson IM. Pharmacokinetics and hemostatic effect of different factor VIII/von Willebrand factor concentrates in von Willebrand's disease type III. *Ann Hematol* 1992; **65**: 253–9.

37 Lamont PA, Ragni MV. Lack of desmopressin (DDAVP) response in men with hemophilia A following liver transplantation. *J Thromb Haemost* 2005; **3**: 2259–63.

38 Haberichter SL, Shi Q, Montgomery RR. Regulated release of VWF and FVIII and the biologic implications. *Pediatr Blood Cancer* 2006; **46**: 547–53.

39 Kobrinsky NL, Doyle JJ, Israels ED, *et al.* Absent factor VIII response to synthetic vasopressin analogue (DDAVP) in nephrogenic diabetes insipidus. *Lancet* 1985; **1**: 1293–4.

40 Bichet DG, Razi M, Lonergan M, *et al.* Hemodynamic and coagulation responses to 1-desamino[8-D-arginine] vasopressin in patients with congenital nephrogenic diabetes insipidus. *N Engl J Med* 1988; **318**: 881–7.

41 Brenner B, Seligsohn U, Hochberg Z. Normal response of factor VIII and von Willebrand factor to 1-deamino-8D-arginine vasopressin in nephrogenic diabetes insipidus. *J Clin Endocrinol Metab* 1988; **67**: 191–3.

42 Ohzeki T, Sunaguchi M, Tsunei M, *et al.* Coagulation factor responsiveness in nephrogenic diabetes insipidus. *J Pediatr* 1988; **113**: 790–1.

43 Oksche A, Rosenthal W. The molecular basis of nephrogenic diabetes insipidus. *J Mol Med* 1998; **76**: 326–37.

44 Kaufmann JE, Oksche A, Wollheim CB, Gunther G, Rosenthal W, Vischer UM. Vasopressin-induced von Willebrand factor secretion from endothelial cells involves V2 receptors and cAMP. *J Clin Invest* 2000; **106**: 107–16.

45 Cort JH, Fischman AJ, Dodds WJ, Rand JH, Schwartz IL. New category of vasopressin receptor in the central nervous system. Evidence that this receptor mediates the

release of a humoral factor VIII-mobilizing principle. *Int J Pept Protein Res* 1981; **17**: 14–22.

46 Hashemi S, Palmer DS, Aye MT, Ganz PR. Platelet-activating factor secreted by DDAVP-treated monocytes mediates von Willebrand factor release from endothelial cells. *J Cell Physiol* 1993; **154**: 496–505.

47 Budiansky S. Research fraud: false data confessed. *Nature* 1983; **301**: 101.

48 Huber D, Cramer EM, Kaufmann JE, *et al.* Tissue-type plasminogen activator (t-PA) is stored in Weibel–Palade bodies in human endothelial cells both *in vitro* and *in vivo*. *Blood* 2002; **99**: 3637–45.

49 Levi M, de Boer JP, Roem D, ten Cate JW, Hack CE. Plasminogen activation *in vivo* upon intravenous infusion of DDAVP. Quantitative assessment of plasmin-alpha 2–antiplasmin complex with a novel monoclonal antibody based radioimmunoassay. *Thromb Haemost* 1992; **67**: 111–16.

50 Kaufmann JE, Iezzi M, Vischer UM. Desmopressin (DDAVP) induces NO production in human endothelial cells via V2 receptor- and cAMP-mediated signaling. *J Thromb Haemost* 2003; **1**: 821–8.

51 Sakariassen KS, Cattaneo M, vd Berg A, Ruggeri ZM, Mannucci PM, Sixma JJ. DDAVP enhances platelet adherence and platelet aggregate growth on human artery subendothelium. *Blood* 1984; **64**: 229–36.

52 Lethagen S, Rugarn P, Aberg M, Nilsson IM. Effects of desmopressin acetate (DDAVP) and dextran on hemostatic and thromboprophylactic mechanisms. *Acta Chir Scand* 1990; **156**: 597–602.

53 Lethagen S, Rugarn P. The effect of DDAVP and placebo on platelet function and prolonged bleeding time induced by oral acetyl salicylic acid intake in healthy volunteers. *Thromb Haemost* 1992; **67**: 185–6.

54 Lethagen S, Nilsson IM. DDAVP-induced enhancement of platelet retention: its dependence on platelet-von Willebrand factor and the platelet receptor GP IIb/IIIa. *Eur J Haematol* 1992; **49**: 7–13.

55 Gomez DE, Ripoll GV, Giron S, Alonso DF. Desmopressin and other synthetic vasopressin analogues in cancer treatment. *Bull Cancer* 2006; **93**: E7–12.

56 Ripoll GV, Giron S, Krzymuski MJ, Hermo GA, Gomez DE, Alonso DF. Antitumor effects of desmopressin in combination with chemotherapeutic agents in a mouse model of breast cancer. *Anticancer Res* 2008; **28**: 2607–11.

57 Mannucci PM, Canciani MT, Rota L, Donovan BS. Response of factor VIII/von Willebrand factor to DDAVP in healthy subjects and patients with haemophilia A and von Willebrand's disease. *Br J Haematol* 1981; **47**: 283–93.

58 Kohler M, Hellstern P, Miyashita C, von Blohn G, Wenzel E. Comparative study of intranasal, subcutaneous and intravenous administration of desamino-D-arginine vasopressin (DDAVP). *Thromb Haemost* 1986; **55**: 108–11.

59 Lethagen S, Harris AS, Nilsson IM. Intranasal desmopressin (DDAVP) by spray in mild hemophilia A and von Willebrand's disease type I. *Blut* 1990; **60**: 187–91.

60 Lethagen S, Frick K, Sterner G. Antidiuretic effect of desmopressin given in hemostatic dosages to healthy volunteers. *Am J Hematol* 1998; **57**: 153–9.

61 Mannucci PM, Bettega D, Cattaneo M. Patterns of development of tachyphylaxis in patients with haemophilia and von Willebrand disease after repeated doses of desmopressin (DDAVP). *Br J Haematol* 1992; **82**: 87–93.

62 Castaman G, Lethagen S, Federici AB, *et al.* Response to desmopressin is influenced by the genotype and phenotype in type 1 von Willebrand disease (VWD): results from the European Study MCMDM-1VWD. *Blood* 2008; **111**: 3531–9.

63 Haberichter SL, Castaman G, Budde U, *et al.* Identification of type 1 von Willebrand disease patients with reduced von Willebrand factor survival by assay of the VWF propeptide in the European study: molecular and clinical markers for the diagnosis and management of type 1 VWD (MCMDM-1VWD). *Blood* 2008; **111**: 4979–85.

64 Federici AB, Mazurier C, Berntorp E, *et al.* Biologic response to desmopressin in patients with severe type 1 and type 2 von Willebrand disease: results of a multicenter European study. *Blood* 2004; **103**: 2032–8.

65 Holmberg L, Nilsson IM, Borge L, Gunnarsson M, Sjorin E. Platelet aggregation induced by 1-desamino-8-D-arginine vasopressin (DDAVP) in Type IIB von Willebrand's disease. *N Engl J Med* 1983; **309**: 816–21.

66 Holmberg L, Berntorp E, Donner M, Nilsson IM. von Willebrand's disease characterized by increased ristocetin sensitivity and the presence of all von Willebrand factor multimers in plasma. *Blood* 1986; **68**: 668–72.

67 Weiss HJ, Sussman, II. A new von Willebrand variant (type I, New York): increased ristocetin-induced platelet aggregation and plasma von Willebrand factor containing the full range of multimers. *Blood* 1986; **68**: 149–56.

68 Mazurier C, Goudemand J, Hilbert L, Caron C, Fressinaud E, Meyer D. Type 2N von Willebrand disease: clinical manifestations, pathophysiology, laboratory diagnosis and molecular biology. *Best Pract Res Clin Haematol* 2001; **14**: 337–47.

69 Castaman G, Lattuada A, Mannucci PM, Rodeghiero F. Factor VIII:C increases after desmopressin in a subgroup of patients with autosomal recessive severe von Willebrand disease. *Br J Haematol* 1995; **89**: 147–51.

70 Rodeghiero F, Castaman G, Mannucci PM. Prospective multicenter study on subcutaneous concentrated desmopressin for home treatment of patients with von Willebrand disease and mild or moderate hemophilia A. *Thromb Haemost* 1996; **76**: 692–6.

71 Nitu-Whalley IC, Griffioen A, Harrington C, Lee CA. Retrospective review of the management of elective surgery with desmopressin and clotting factor concentrates in patients with von Willebrand disease. *Am J Hematol* 2001; **66**: 280–4.

72 Revel-Vilk S, Schmugge M, Carcao MD, Blanchette P, Rand ML, Blanchette VS. Desmopressin (DDAVP) responsiveness in children with von Willebrand disease. *J Pediatr Hematol Oncol* 2003; **25**: 874–9.

73 Niessner H, Korninger C. 1-Deamino-8-D-arginine-vasopressin–an alternative in the management of mild haemophilia A and von Willebrand's disease. *Wien Klin Wochenschr* 1983; **95**: 753–7.

74 Lethagen S, Ragnarson Tennvall G. Self-treatment with desmopressin intranasal spray in patients with bleeding disorders: effect on bleeding symptoms and socioeconomic factors. *Ann Hematol* 1993; **66**: 257–60.

75 Federici AB, Rand JH, Bucciarelli P, *et al.* Acquired von Willebrand syndrome: data from an international registry. *Thromb Haemost* 2000; **84**: 345–9.

76 Tryding N, Sterner G, Berg B, Harris A, Lundin S. Subcutaneous and intranasal administration of 1-deamino-8-d-arginine vasopressin in the assessment of renal concentration capacity. *Nephron* 1987; **45**: 27–30.

77 Ruzicka H, Bjorkman S, Lethagen S, Sterner G. Pharmacokinetics and antidiuretic effect of high-dose desmopressin in patients with chronic renal failure. *Pharmacol Toxicol* 2003; **92**: 137–42.

78 Mannucci PM. Desmopressin: a nontransfusional form of treatment for congenital and acquired bleeding disorders. *Blood* 1988; **72**: 1449–55.

79 Mannucci PM, Lusher JM. Desmopressin and thrombosis. *Lancet* 1989; **2**: 675–6.

80 Mannucci PM, Carlsson S, Harris AS. Desmopressin, surgery and thrombosis. *Thromb Haemost* 1994; **71**: 154–5.

81 James AH, Jamison MG. Bleeding events and other complications during pregnancy and childbirth in women with von Willebrand disease. *J Thromb Haemost* 2007; **5**: 1165–9.

82 Castaman G, Eikenboom JC, Contri A, Rodeghiero F. Pregnancy in women with type 1 von Willebrand disease caused by heterozygosity for von Willebrand factor mutation C1130F. *Thromb Haemost* 2000; **84**: 351–2.

83 Castaman G, Federici AB, Bernardi M, Moroni B, Bertoncello K, Rodeghiero F. Factor VIII and von Willebrand factor changes after desmopressin and during pregnancy in type 2M von Willebrand disease Vicenza: a prospective study comparing patients with single (R1205H) and double (R1205H-M740I) defect. *J Thromb Haemost* 2006; **4**: 357–60.

84 Mannucci PM. Use of desmopressin (DDAVP) during early pregnancy in factor VIII-deficient women. *Blood* 2005; **105**: 3382.

85 Lethagen S, Kyrle PA, Castaman G, Haertel S, Mannucci PM. von Willebrand factor/factor VIII concentrate (Haemate P) dosing based on pharmacokinetics: a prospective multicenter trial in elective surgery. *J Thromb Haemost* 2007; **5**: 1420–30.

86 Leissinger C, Becton D, Cornell C, Jr., Cox Gill J. High-dose DDAVP intranasal spray (Stimate) for the prevention and treatment of bleeding in patients with mild haemophilia A, mild or moderate type 1 von Willebrand disease and symptomatic carriers of haemophilia A. *Haemophilia* 2001; **7**: 258–66.

87 Kadir RA, Lee CA, Sabin CA, Pollard D, Economides DL. DDAVP nasal spray for treatment of menorrhagia in women with inherited bleeding disorders: a randomized placebo–controlled crossover study. *Haemophilia* 2002; **8**: 787–93.

17 The use of plasma-derived concentrates

Pier Mannuccio Mannucci[1] and Massimo Franchini[2]

[1]Angelo Bianchi Bonomi Hemophilia and Thrombosis Center, Department of Medicine and Medical Specialties, University of Milan and IRCCS Maggiore Hospital, Mangiagalli and Regina Elena Foundation, Milan, Italy

[2]Immunohematology and Transfusion Center, Department of Pathology and Laboratory Medicine, University Hospital of Parma, Italy

Introduction

von Willebrand disease (VWD) is the most common genetic bleeding disorder, with a prevalence of approximately 1–2% according to population studies [1]. The severity of the bleeding tendency is usually proportional to the degree of the primary deficiency of von Willebrand factor (VWF) and to that of the deficiency of factor VIII (FVIII), secondary to the fact that VWF is the carrier of FVIII in plasma [2,3].

Inherited VWD has been classified into different types. Types 1 and 3 VWD reflect the partial or virtually complete quantitative deficiency of VWF, while type 2 VWD reflects qualitative defects. Type 1 is the most common form of VWD [2,3], transmitted as an autosomal dominant trait with incomplete penetrance. Type 1 VWD is characterized by a mild to moderately severe reduction in plasma levels of both VWF antigen (VWF:Ag) and ristocetin cofactor activity (VWF:RCo). In type 1 VWD, VWF is functionally normal, as is the pattern of plasma VWF multimers, and plasma levels of FVIII are usually reduced in proportion to VWF. Patients with type 1 present with a spectrum of mucocutaneous bleeding symptoms, the severity of which roughly correlates with the degree of VWF and FVIII deficiencies. Type 2A is the most frequent qualitative defect of VWF, inherited mainly with an autosomal dominant pattern.

The hallmark of type 2A VWD is a low VWF:RCo/VWF:Ag ratio (<0.7) with lack of large and intermediate size VWF multimers and impaired ristocetin-induced platelet agglutination (RIPA) in platelet-rich plasma. As for type 2A, the inheritance pattern of type 2B VWD is mainly autosomal dominant. The laboratory hallmark of the most typical and frequent forms of type 2B VWD is heightened RIPA, usually accompanied by mild to moderate thrombocytopenia, mildly reduced to normal FVIII and VWF:Ag, reduced VWF:RCo, and absence of large multimers in plasma, even though an intact multimeric pattern is seen in some patients (the so-called Malmö or New York variants) [4]. In type 2M VWD, the VWF multimeric distribution is normal but platelet-dependent VWF activities are reduced [2,3]. Type 2N VWD is characterized by normal levels of VWF:Ag and VWF:RCo and a normal multimeric pattern, but plasma levels of FVIII are low as a result of the increased clearance of this moiety, which cannot bind to VWF as a consequence of a qualitative abnormality of VWF. Type 2N VWD therefore resembles mild hemophilia A, but its inheritance pattern is autosomal recessive. Type 3 VWD is inherited as an autosomal recessive trait and is characterized by undetectable levels of VWF in plasma (and platelets) and very low but measurable levels (1–5 IU/dL) of FVIII. Therefore, patients with type 3 VWD have a severe bleeding tendency characterized not only by mucocutaneous hemorrhages but also by hemarthroses, as in moderately severe hemophilia.

In VWD the aim of therapy is to correct the dual defect of hemostasis, i.e. the abnormal platelet adhesion–aggregation as a result of low or dysfunc-

Von Willebrand Disease, 1st edition. Edited by Augusto B. Federici, Christine A. Lee, Erik E. Berntorp, David Lillicrap, Robert R. Montgomery. © 2011 Blackwell Publishing Ltd.

tional VWF and the abnormal intrinsic coagulation owing to low FVIII levels. The mainstays of treatment are autologous replacement therapy with desmopressin (1-deamino-8-D-arginine vasopressin, DDAVP) and allogeneic replacement therapy with virally inactivated plasma-derived concentrates. The latter may contain VWF and FVIII (VWF/FVIII concentrates) or VWF with only minimal amounts of FVIII. There are also adjunctive treatments that act upon VWF-mediated hemostasis, for example platelet transfusion and combined estrogen–progestogen drugs. Adjuvant therapies are antifibrinolytic amino acids, such as tranexamic acid and ε-aminocaproic acid, that improve hemostasis without affecting plasma VWF levels [5–8]. This chapter will focus on the use of plasma-derived concentrates.

VWF/FVIII concentrates

For those patients with VWD in whom DDAVP is either ineffective (inadequate response or prediction of prolonged treatments with the likelihood of tachyphylaxis) or contraindicated (type 2B VWD), VWF and FVIII levels can be restored to normal values by the infusion of virally inactivated plasma-derived concentrates containing both proteins. Several intermediate and high-purity products containing VWF/FVIII are available (Table 17.1). Yet only three of them (Haemate-P: CSL Behring, Marburg, Germany; Alphanate: Grifols, Los Angeles, CA, USA; Fanhdi: Grifols, Barcelona, Spain) have been extensively evaluated until now in large and numerous studies in terms of pharmacokinetics and efficacy [9–13].

Table 17.1 VWF/FVIII concentrates for the treatment of von Willebrand disease tested in prospective clinical studies.

Product	Manufacturer	Fractionation method	Viral inactivation	VWF:RCo/Ag[a] (ratio)	VWF:RCo/FVIII[a] (ratio)
Factor 8Y	BioProducts Laboratory	Heparin/glycine precipitation	Dry heat (80°C, 72h)	0.29	0.81
Alphanate	Grifols	Heparin ligand chromatography	S/D + dry heat (80°C, 72h)	0.47 ± 0.1	0.91 ± 0.2
Biostate	CSL Bioplasma	Heparin/glycine precipitation + gel filtration chromatography	S/D + dry heat (80°C, 72h)	0.87–0.95	2
Fanhdi	Grifols	Heparin ligand chromatography	S/D + dry heat (80°C, 72h)	0.47 ± 0.1	1.04 ± 0.1
Haemate-P	CSL Behring	Multiple precipitation	Pasteurization (60°C, 10h)	0.59 ± 0.1	2.45 ± 0.3
Immunate	Baxter	Ion-exchange chromatography	S/D + vapor heat (60°C, 10h)	0.47	1.1
Koate DVI	Talecris	Multiple precipitation + size exclusion chromatography	S/D + dry heat (80°C, 72h)	0.48	1.1
Wilate	Octapharma	Ion-exchange + size exclusion chromatography	S/D + dry heat (100°C, 2h)	—	0.9

VWF, von Willebrand factor; RCo, ristocetin cofactor; Ag, antigen; FVIII, factor VIII; S/D, solvent/detergent (TNBP/polysorbate 80).
[a] Mean ± SD for Alphanate, Fanhdi, and Haemate-P are derived from the analysis of 10 lots for each VWF/FVIII product. The analysis was independently done at the Milan Hemophilia Center using in-house methods. The other VWF/FVIII products (8Y, Immunate, Koate DVI, Biostate, and Wilate) so far have been less extensively evaluated than the aforementioned products for VWD management. The characteristics of these products were derived from the information provided by the manufacturers because these products were not made available for our independent analysis.

The first prospective study evaluating the pharmacokinetics and clinical efficacy in patients with VWD was published in 2002 [9]. This study included 53 patients who received treatment with a doubly virus-inactivated VWF/FVIII concentrate (Alphanate) for 87 bleeding episodes and 39 patients who received treatment before 71 surgical or invasive diagnostic procedures. For patients with type 3 VWD, the half-life of FVIII coagulant activity (FVIII:C) was approximately twice that of VWF:Ag (23.8 h vs. 12.9 h) owing to the endogenous production of FVIII. A good clinical response with this VWF/FVIII concentrate was observed in 86% of the spontaneous bleeding episodes and in 71% of surgical or invasive procedures. A smaller prospective study has also been performed using Fanhdi, a concentrate manufactured using a process very similar to that of Alphanate [10]. Fourteen patients received treatment for 30 bleeding episodes and before nine surgical procedures. An excellent/good hemostatic profile was achieved in 100% of the cases. The mean FVIII:C half-life was 33.4 h, that of VWF:Ag was 27.5 h.

The VWF/FVIII concentrate Haemate-P has been widely used in patients with VWD since the early 1980s and is characterized by a particularly high VWF content (VWF:RCo/FVIII ratio, 2.5) [14]. Two prospective studies have documented safety and efficacy in acute spontaneous bleeding (excellent/good results in 98% of the cases) and surgical events (excellent/good results in 100% of the cases) [11,12]. A prospective study that used pharmacokinetic analysis for the choice of dosages in the management of surgical patients [13] enrolled 29 individuals with VWD who were undergoing elective surgery and showed that Haemate-P, following a preoperative median VWF:RCo loading dose of 62.4 IU/kg chosen on the basis of a pharmacokinetic study, provided excellent or good hemostasis in 96% of cases on the day of surgery and 100% over the next few days. Notably, this study demonstrated for the first time that the incremental recovery of VWF:RCo is constant over a wide range of doses of VWF/FVIII concentrate (dose linearity relationship), and that the pretreatment pharmacokinetics results provide a reliable basis for subsequent dosing choices. A number of additional studies conducted retrospectively on Haemate-P, Alphanate, and Fanhdi matched the positive results of the aforementioned prospective studies [15–19]. The clinical efficacy of the double virus-inactivated VWF/FVIII concentrate Immunate was tested in a small prospective study conducted in 14 patients with VWD who were having acute bleeds or elective surgery [20]. Despite the occurrence of bleedings in three patients, the clinical efficacy was rated excellent or good in all cases. The mean FVIII:C half-life was 23.2 h, that of VWF:Ag was 19.2 h.

Successful surgical hemostasis was also achieved in patients with VWD after the infusion of the intermediate-purity VWF/FVIII concentrate Koate DVI (Talecris, Research Triangle Park, NC, USA) [21,22]. Another intermediate-purity VWF/FVIII concentrate, 8Y, has been reported to be effective and safe for the clinical management of patients with VWD [23,24]. The results of an open-label prospective multicenter study evaluating the high-purity plasma-derived double virus-inactivated VWF/FVIII concentrate Biostate in 23 patients with VWD have been recently published [25]. The hemostatic efficacy of Biostate was rated excellent or good in all major or minor surgery events, long-term prophylaxis, and in four of the six nonsurgical bleeding events.

Finally, a pooled analysis from four prospective clinical trials involving 44 patients with VWD on the safety and efficacy of the VWF/FVIII concentrate Wilate (Octapharma, Lachen, Switzerland) was recently published [26]. A total of 1095 spontaneous or post-traumatic bleeding episodes were treated with this plasma-derived concentrate, with an excellent or good clinical efficacy in 96% of cases.

On the whole, there is no evidence from retrospective or prospective clinical studies that the most extensively studied products (Alphanate, Fanhdi, Haemate-P, Wilate) differ with respect to hemostatic efficacy, because no head-to-head clinical study was ever carried out. Hence, the following recommendations apply to all (Table 17.2). Doses given once daily or every other day and spanning from 20 to 60 IU/kg of VWF:RCo/FVIII:C (depending on the risk and severity of bleeding) are hemostatically effective for treating spontaneous bleeding episodes or for preventing bleeding during surgical or invasive procedures in patients with severely reduced VWF levels (<10 IU/dL). However, a dosing pharmacokinetic study is advisable before major surgery, particularly for patients with type 3 VWD.

Patients with severe forms of VWD (i.e., FVIII:C levels <5 IU/dL) have sometime frequent hemarthroses

Table 17.2 Treatment of von Willebrand disease (VWD) with VWF/FVIII or von Willebrand factor (VWF) concentrates.

Clinical situation	Dose of VWF:RCo and/or factor VIII:C[a]	No. of infusions	VWF:RCo target plasma level[b]
Major surgery	40–60 IU/kg	Every 12 h initially, then once daily until wound healing is complete	50–100 IU/dL; maintain levels for 3–10 days
Minor surgery	30–50 IU/kg	Once daily (may require only 1–3 days)	>30 IU/dL
Dental extraction	20–30 IU/kg	Usually one dose only before procedure	>30 IU/dL for >12 h
Spontaneous bleeding	20–60 IU/kg	One daily dose until bleeding stops. Monitor clinically	>30 IU/dL
Delivery and puerperium	50 IU/kg	Once daily	>50 IU/dL; maintain levels for 3–4 days

[a]These dosages are indicated for patients with VWD with severely reduced FVIII:C/VWF:RCo levels (<10 IU/dL).
[b]Factor levels can be predicted based on pharmacokinetic data; 40–50 units/kg (VWF:RCO) will increase plasma VWF levels to 80–100% depending on the baseline levels and hematocrit.

and may therefore benefit from secondary long-term prophylaxis, which also should be considered in patients with recurrent gastrointestinal bleeding and in children with frequent epistaxis [6]. The largest experience on secondary prophylaxis in VWD has been collected in Sweden from 35 patients with severe VWD [27]. Secondary prophylaxis was also retrospectively evaluated in a cohort of 12 Italian patients with VWD [28] who underwent 17 secondary prophylaxis periods in order to prevent recurrent gastrointestinal or joint bleeding, with clinical responses rated as excellent or good in 100% of cases. Two prospective trials (PRO.WILL and VIP) are currently comparing the cost-effectiveness of prophylaxis with VWF/FVIII concentrates versus therapy given only at the time of bleeding [29].

Plasma-derived concentrates containing VWF are contraindicated in those rare patients with type 3 VWD who develop alloantibodies (i.e., those homozygous for gene deletions or nonsense mutations), because they often cause life-threatening anaphylactic reactions [30]. These patients can be effectively treated with VWF-free recombinant FVIII products, administered by continuous intravenous infusion, or with recombinant activated factor VII [31,32]. In pregnant women with type 3 VWD, the prophylactic treatment with VWF/FVIII concentrates is also required to cover vaginal delivery or cesarean section because VWF and FVIII do not increase during pregnancy in these women [33].

Thrombotic complications following VWF/FVIII concentrates

The accumulation of FVIII that is exogenously infused together with that endogenously synthesized and stabilized by the infused VWF may lead to very high FVIII:C concentrations in plasma (>150 IU/dL) when repeated and closely spaced infusions are given for severe bleeding episodes or to cover major surgery [34]. There is some concern that sustained high levels of FVIII:C may increase the risk of deep vein thrombosis in patients with VWD [35,36]. Therefore, when repeated infusions of VWF/FVIII concentrates are necessary, such as during major surgical procedures, plasma FVIII:C should be measured daily in order to avoid values in excess of 150 IU/dL, which is roughly recognized as the threshold for an increased risk of venous thromboembolism [37]. Treatment may also be monitored with VWF:RCo assays as a surrogate measure of VWF activity [13]. However, monitoring VWF:RCo alone may be not optimal during prolonged treatments because the plasma levels of this measurement fall relatively rapidly owing to its relatively short half-life while, as mentioned above, FVIII:C levels continue to rise as a result of endogenous FVIII production (plasma half-life of VWF:RCo, 8–10 h vs. plasma half-life of FVIII:C, 24–26 h) [9]. We recommend primary thromboprophylaxis with low-molecular-weight heparin or corresponding anticoagulants in patients with VWD who are undergoing replacement therapy for major surgery and procedures at high risk of venous thromboembolism, at the same doses and schedules that are adopted in at risk patients without VWD who are undergoing similar procedures.

VWF concentrates devoid of FVIII

Because patients with VWD have an intact endogenous production of FVIII, a highly purified plasma VWF concentrate containing very little FVIII has been developed for exclusive use in VWD (Wilfactin: LFB, Les Ulis, France) [38]. However, as postinfusion levels of FVIII:C rise slowly, reaching a peak only after 6–8 h, coadministration of a priming dose of FVIII is necessary when prompt hemostasis is required in patients with baseline FVIII:C levels of 30 IU/dL or lower. In a prospective study [39], 50 patients with clinically severe VWD (five type 1, 27 type 2, and 18 type 3) were treated with this VWF concentrate for a total of 139 spontaneous bleeding episodes and 108 surgical or invasive procedures, with an outcome judged as excellent or good in 89% and 100% of the cases, respectively. Only 38% of the spontaneous bleeding episodes and as few as 12% of the surgical/invasive procedures (i.e., emergency procedures) needed the coadministration of a priming dose of FVIII concentrate together with the first VWF infusion. Potential indications for VWF concentrates devoid of FVIII include elective major surgery, particularly when repeated infusions are foreseen in patients at high risk of thrombosis (old age, cancer surgery, orthopedic surgery) and also long-term prophylaxis (i.e., for target joints, gastrointestinal bleeding, recurrent epistaxis in children, etc). More studies on these possible indications are warranted.

Conclusions

Plasma-derived VWF/FVIII concentrates play a key role in the management of patients with VWD who are unsuitable for DDAVP. VWF concentrates devoid of FVIII may be considered for short-term prophylaxis in elective surgery or for long-term secondary prophylaxis. A VWF concentrate produced by means of recombinant DNA technology has recently initiated a phase I clinical study in humans. The new product provides an exciting technologic advance, particularly if one considers the size and structural complexity of a protein such as VWF. On the other hand, the record of safety of the available virus-inactivated plasma concentrates is impeccable, so it will be of interest to establish whether or not recombinant VWF is more efficacious than plasma-derived VWD. This is indeed a possibility, because recombinant VWF contains ultralarge VWF multimers not present in plasma concentrates that are hemostatically highly effective.

References

1 Rodeghiero F, Castaman G, Dini E. Epidemiological investigation of the prevalence of von Willebrand's disease. *Blood* 1987; **69**: 454–9.

2 Castaman G, Federici AB, Rodeghiero F, Mannucci PM. von Willebrand's disease in the year 2003: towards the complete identification of gene defects for correct diagnosis and treatment. *Haematologica* 2003; **88**: 94–108.

3 Sadler JE, Budde U, Eikenboom JC, *et al*. Update on the pathophysiology and classification of von Willebrand disease: a report of the Subcommittee on von Willebrand Factor. *J Thromb Haemost* 2006; **4**: 2103–14.

4 Holmberg L, Dent JA, Schneppenheim R, Budde U, Ware J, Ruggeri ZM. Willebrand factor mutation enhancing interaction with platelets in patients with normal multimeric structure. *J Clin Invest* 1993; **91**: 2169–77.

5 Mannucci PM. How I treat patients with von Willebrand disease. *Blood* 2001; **97**: 1915–19.

6 Mannucci PM. Treatment of von Willebrand's disease. *N Engl J Med* 2004; **351**: 683–94.

7 Mannucci PM. Hemostatic drugs. *N Engl J Med* 1998; **339**: 245–53.

8 Federici AB, Castaman G, Mannucci PM, Italian Association of Hemophilia Centers (AICE). Guidelines for the diagnosis and management of von Willebrand disease in Italy. *Haemophilia* 2002; **8**: 607–21.

9 Mannucci PM, Chediak J, Hanna W, Byrnes J, Marlies L, Ewenstein BM, and the Alphanate Study Group. Treatment of von Willebrand disease with a high-purity factor VIII/von Willebrand factor concentrate: a prospective, multicenter study. *Blood* 2002; **99**: 450–6.

10 Bello IF, Yuste VJ, Molina MQ, Navarro FH. Fanhdi, efficacy and safety in von Willebrand's disease: prospective international study results. *Haemophilia* 2007; **13** (Suppl. 5): 25–32.

11 Gill JC, Ewenstein BM, Thompson AR, Mueller-Velten G, Schwartz BA, Humate-P Study Group. Successful treatment of urgent bleeding in von Willebrand disease

with factor VIII/von Willebrand factor concentrate (Humate-P): use of the ristocetin cofactor assay (VWF: RCo) to measure potency and to guide therapy. *Haemophilia* 2003; **9**: 688–95.

12 Thompson AR, Gill JC, Ewenstein BM, Mueller-Velten G, Schwartz BA, Humate-P Study Group. Successful treatment for patients with von Willebrand disease undergoing urgent surgery using factor VIII/von Willebrand factor concentrate (Humate-P). *Haemophilia* 2004; **10**: 42–51.

13 Lethagen S, Kyrle PA, Castaman G, Haertel S, Mannucci PM, the Haemate P Surgical Study Group. Von Willebrand factor/factor VIII concentrate (Haemate P) dosing based on pharmacokinetics: a prospective multicenter trial in elective surgery. *J Thromb Haemost* 2007; **5**: 1420–30.

14 Berntorp E, Archey W, Auerswald G, *et al.* A systematic overview of the first pasteurised VWF/FVIII medicinal product, Haemate P/Humate-P: history and clinical performance. *Eur J Haematol Suppl* 2008; **70**: 3–35.

15 Lillicrap D, Poon M-C, Walker I, Xie F, Schwartz BA. Association of Hemophilia Clinic Directors of Canada. Efficacy and safety of the factor VIII/von Willebrand Factor concentrate, Haemate-P/Humate-P: ristocetin cofactor unit dosing in patients with von Willebrand disease. *Thromb Haemost* 2002; **87**: 224–30.

16 Federici AB, Castaman G, Franchini M, *et al.* Clinical use of Haemate P in inherited von Willebrand disease: a cohort study on 100 Italian patients. *Haematologica* 2007; **92**: 944–51.

17 Rivard GE, Aledort L, Alphanate Surgical Investigators. Efficacy of factor VIII/von Willebrand factor concentrate Alphanate in preventing excessive bleeding during surgery in subjects with von Willebrand disease. *Haemophilia* 2008; **14**: 271–5.

18 Federici AB, Baudo F, Caracciolo C, *et al.* Clinical efficacy of highly purified, doubly virus-inactivated factor VIII/von Willebrand factor concentrate (Fanhdi) in the treatment of von Willebrand disease: a retrospective clinical study. *Haemophilia* 2002; **8**: 761–7.

19 Hernandez-Navarro F, Quintana M, Jimenez-Yuste V, Alvarez MT, Fernandez-Morata R. Clinical efficacy in bleeding and surgery in von Willebrand patients treated with Fanhdi a highly purified, doubly inactivated FVIII/VWF concentrate. *Haemophilia* 2008; **14**: 963–7.

20 Auerswald G, Eberspacher B, Engl W, *et al.* Successful treatment of patients with von Willebrand disease using a high-purity double-virus inactivated factor VIII/von Willebrand factor concentrate (Immunate). *Semin Thromb Hemost* 2002; **28**: 203–14.

21 Srivastava A, Mathews V, Bhurani D, Baidya S, Chandy M. Successful surgical haemostasis in patients with von Willebrand disease following infusion of Koate DVI. *Thromb Haemost* 2002; **87**: 541–3.

22 Viswabandya A, Mathews V, Gorge B, *et al.* Successful surgical haemostasis in patients with von Wilebrand disease with Koate DVI. *Haemophilia* 2008; **14**: 763–7.

23 Cumming AM, Fildes S, Cumming IR, Wensley RT, Redding OM, Burn AM. Clinical and laboratory evaluation of National Health Service factor VIII concentrate (8Y) for the treatment of Von Willebrand's disease. *Br J Haematol* 1990; **75**: 234–9.

24 Pasi KJ, Williams MD, Enayat MS, Hill FGH. Clinical and laboratory evaluation of the treatment of Von Willebrand's disease patients with heat-treated factor VIII concentrate (BPL 8Y). *Br J Haematol* 1990; **75**: 228–33.

25 Dunkley S, Baker RI, Pidcock M, *et al.* Clinical efficacy and safety of the factor VIII/von Willebrand factor concentrate BIOSTATE in patients with von Willebrand's disease: a prospective multicentre study. *Haemophilia* 2010. [Epub ahead of print.]

26 Berntorp E, Windyga J, European Wilate Study Group. Treatment and prevention of acute bleedings in von Willebrand disease–efficacy and safety of Wilate, a new generation von Willebrand factor/factor VIII concentrate. *Haemophilia* 2009; **15**: 122–30.

27 Berntorp E, Petrini P. Long-term prophylaxis in von Willebrand disease. *Blood Coagul Fibrinolysis* 2005; **16**: S23–26.

28 Federici AB. Highly purified VWF/FVIII concentrates in the treatment and prophylaxis of von Willebrand disease. The PRO.WILL study. *Haemophilia* 2007; **13**: 15–24.

29 Federici AB. Highly purified VWF/FVIII concentrates in the treatment and prophylaxis of von Willebrand disease: the PRO.WILL Study. *Haemophilia* 2007; **13** (Suppl. 5): 15–24.

30 Mannucci PM, Tamaro G, Narchi G, *et al.* Life-threatening reaction to factor VIII concentrate in a patient with severe von Willebrand disease and alloantibodies to von Willebrand factor. *Eur J Hematol* 1987; **39**: 467–70.

31 Ciavarella N, Schiavoni M, Valenzano E, Mangini F, Inchingolo F. Use of recombinant factor VIIa (NovoSeven) in the treatment of two patients with type III von Willebrand's disease and an inhibitor against von Willebrand factor. *Haemostasis* 1996; **26**: 10–14.

32 Franchini M, Gandini G, Giuffrida A, De Gironcoli M, Federici AB. Treatment for patients with type 3 von Willebrand disease and alloantibodies: a case report. *Haemophilia* 2008; **14**: 645–6.

33 Foster PA. The reproductive health of women with von Willebrand Disease unresponsive to DDAVP: results of an international survey. On behalf of the Subcommittee on von Willebrand Factor of the Scientific and Standardization Committee of the ISTH. *Thromb Haemost* 1995; **74**: 784–90.

34 Franchini M. Surgical prophylaxis in von Willebrand's disease: a difficult balance to manage. *Blood Transfus* 2008; **6** (Suppl. 2): 33–8.

35 Makris M, Colvin B, Gupta V, Shields ML, Smith MP. Venous thrombosis following the use of intermediate purity FVIII concentrate to treat patients with von Willebrand's disease. *Thromb Haemost* 2002; **88**: 387–8.

36 Mannucci PM. Venous thromboembolism in von Willebrand disease. *Thromb Haemost* 2002; **88**: 378–9.

37 Kyrle PA, Minar E, Hirschl M, *et al.* High plasma levels of factor VIII and the risk of recurrent venous thromboembolism. *N Engl J Med* 2000; **343**: 457–62.

38 Goudemand J, Scharrer I, Berntorp E, *et al.* Pharmacokinetic studies on Wilfactin, a von Willebrand factor concentrate with a low factor VIII content treated with three virus-inactivation/removal methods. *J Thromb Haemost* 2005; **3**: 2219–27.

39 Borel-Derlon A, Federici AB, Roussel-Robert V, *et al.* Treatment of severe von Willebrand disease with a high-purity von Willebrand factor concentrate (Wilfactin): a prospective study of 50 patients. *J Thromb Haemost* 2007; **5**: 1115–24.

18 Prophylaxis in von Willebrand disease

Erik Berntorp

Malmö Centre for Thrombosis and Haemostasis, Lund University, Skåne University Hospital, Malmö, Sweden

Introduction

Regular or long-term prophylactic replacement therapy of congenital bleeding disorders is not a new concept. From the 1960s, and even earlier, it has been practiced in hemophilia with the aim of preventing bleeding and its sequelae. A current definition of prophylaxis for the treatment of hemophilia is given in Table 18.1. While there is general consistency among the definitions that have been used, minor differences do exist [1–3]. Prophylaxis can be given as primary prophylaxis, that is before joint destruction has started, or as secondary prophylaxis. Short-term prophylaxis can be used in situations where an increased risk of bleeding is anticipated.

The first long-term experience with prophylaxis in a large cohort of patients with hemophilia was published by Nilsson *et al.* in 1992 [4]. The results showed that it was possible to virtually prevent joint bleeds and arthropathy if treatment was started early at relatively high doses with short dosing intervals so that the factor trough levels remained measurable. When the era of prophylaxis began, treatment was used on a small scale and in few countries, but during the last decades it has become quite widespread. Nowadays, it is considered to be the state-of-the-art treatment in countries where cost and availability of factor concentrates do not hinder its use. In Europe, a number of cohort studies have shown the benefit of

prophylaxis in hemophilia [1,4–6] by using different dosing regimens. The strategy has been to either use a high and frequent dose from the onset of treatment, or to use lower doses and escalate the schedule according to the clinical response. In Canada, a dosing schedule that begins with once per week and is escalated by shortening the dose intervals, the so-called Canadian regimen [7], has been developed and tested. This treatment regimen may be better tailored to the individual than the more standardized regimens used in Europe, increasing convenience and cost-effectiveness. The need for ports to deliver the therapy may perhaps be reduced, although comparative studies to address this issue are lacking. In 2007, a randomized prospective study reported prophylaxis to be superior to enhanced on-demand treatment during acute joint bleeds [8] for the prevention of cartilage destruction in young boys with hemophilia. Finally, after 50 years of use of long-term prophylaxis, there is today no controversy as to whether it should be the preferred treatment, if affordable, for boys with severe hemophilia. Questions remain, however, concerning the optimum treatment schedule, including when to start, when (or if) to stop, dose, and dose interval. The use of prophylaxis in patients with hemophilia complicated by inhibitors is also under investigation [9,10].

Prophylaxis in VWD

In contrast to the situation in hemophilia, long-term prophylaxis is not commonly used in von Willebrand disease (VWD). There are multiple reasons for this:

Von Willebrand Disease, 1st edition. Edited by Augusto B. Federici, Christine A. Lee, Erik E. Berntorp, David Lillicrap, Robert R. Montgomery. © 2011 Blackwell Publishing Ltd.

Table 18.1 Definitions of prophylaxis in hemophilia [1].

Model	Definition
Primary prophylaxis determined by age	Long-term continuous[a] treatment started before the age of 2 years and before any clinically evident joint bleeding
Primary prophylaxis determined by first bleed	Long-term continuous[a] treatment started before the onset of joint damage (presumptively defined as having had no more than one joint bleed) irrespective of age
Secondary prophylaxis	Long-term continuous[a] treatment not fulfilling the criteria for primary prophylaxis
Short-term prophylaxis	Short-term treatment in anticipation of, and to prevent, bleeding

[a] With the intent of treating 52 weeks per year up to adulthood and receiving treatment for a minimum of 46 weeks per year.

(i) the vast majority of the patients do not experience severe bleeding symptoms; (ii) the hemostatic defect is mainly restricted to primary hemostasis with bleeding from mucous membranes such as epistaxis, gingival or gastrointestinal bleeding, and menorrhagia as the predominating symptoms. Although the bleeding associated with VWD may jeopardize quality of life, it does not as frequently result in the progressive and irreversible sequelae seen in hemophilic joint disease; (iii) treatment of VWD has been shadowed by the problems associated with replacement therapy in hemophilia such as blood-transmitted diseases and inhibitor development; and (iv) development of products for the treatment of VWD has had a low priority relative to product development for the treatment of hemophilia.

Because the von Willebrand factor (VWF) not only exerts a platelet function but also serves as a carrier of factor VIII (FVIII) in plasma, some VWD disease phenotypes also involve secondary derangements of FVIII. Patients with type 3 VWD, the least common and most severe type, lack essentially all VWF and have FVIII levels similar to those observed in moderate hemophilia, 1–5 IU/dL. As a result, individuals with type 3 VWD may experience significant joint bleeding in addition to mucosal bleeding. This was, in fact, reported in the first publication by Erik von Willebrand [11] and has since been well established. Thus, the prevalence of joint bleeding has been reported to range from 37% to 45% in type 3 VWD and 3% to 4% in type 1 and type 2 VWD, with an overall prevalence of 8% [12–14]. If the joint bleeds are not effectively prevented, patients may develop arthropathy, which results in significant impairment and disability and has an impact on quality of life. In particular, children with severe forms of VWD may have frequent mucosal bleeds without joint bleeds, resulting in anemia and interference in social and scholastic endeavors. Menorrhagia may also severely impact quality of life. A special entity is the symptom of gastrointestinal bleeding in patients with severe forms of VWD or those with functional defects, including types 2A and 2B VWD. Gastrointestinal bleeding may be very serious or life threatening and is associated with angiodysplasia in the gut [15,16].

From these data and other clinical experiences, it appears obvious that a substantial number of patients with VWD would benefit from prophylactic treatment with VWF-containing concentrates. However, experience with long-term prophylaxis in VWD is scarce, and rigorous studies designed to explore dosing schedules and document the results of treatment are lacking. In countries such as Sweden, with a long history of use of prophylaxis in hemophilia, there is also experience with long-term prophylaxis in VWD. Short-term prophylaxis using replacement therapy in connection with surgery, for example, is more widespread.

Experience in Sweden

In Sweden, an FVIII concentrate containing VWF was available in the 1950s [17,18] and studied in the treatment of VWD and hemophilia. As prophylaxis for the treatment of hemophilia began on a small scale in the 1950s and 1960s, it was logical to also treat severe forms of VWD with prophylaxis. Data from a Swedish cohort were compiled and reported in 2005 [19]. Of 48 individuals with VWF:RCo <8 IU/dL and FVIII:C <10 IU/dL, 35 were on long-term prophylaxis and 13 were treated on demand.

Prophylaxis was defined as treatment at least once per week for more than 45 weeks per year for at least 1 year. The study group included 18 females and 17 males ranging in age from 3 to 65 years. Most of the adults were on prophylaxis for more than 10 years, and 16 of the 18 children had been treated for more than 5 years. Thirty patients had type 3 VWD, four had type 2A or 2B, and one had type 1. The mean age at start of prophylaxis was 4 years in the cohort younger than 20 years of age. This is slightly older than the age at the start of prophylaxis in severe hemophilia [4]. In the cohort of patients older than 20 years, the mean age at the start of prophylaxis was considerably higher: 27 years old with a range of 3–57 years. The primary treatment indication was identified by the investigator, and a mixed indication was not uncommon. The two main indications for prophylaxis were nose/mouth bleeds and joint bleeds (Figure 18.1). The patients with type 2 VWD had frequent and severe gastrointestinal bleeding as their primary indication, and two patients were on prophylaxis because of menorrhagia. The indication varied with age at the start of treatment, with nose/mouth bleeds dominating in the very young and joint bleeds dominating in adolescents/adults. Until the mid-1980s, the concentrate used was fraction I-0 (AHF-Kabi) [20] and since then the main product has been Haemate/Humate-P (CSL Behring, Marburg,

Germany) [21]. The doses given and dose frequency were, in general, somewhat lower than those for hemophilia, ranging from 12 to 50 IU FVIII per kg of body weight with a mean of 24 IU given one to three times weekly. A more intensive schedule was used in patients with gastrointestinal bleeds. Also, older patients tended to have more frequent injections because of pre-existing joint problems. The overall results showed a substantial reduction in the number of bleeds, and in many patients symptoms virtually ceased. In children who started prophylaxis before the age of 5 years ($n=12$) in order to prevent nose or mouth bleeds, there were no reports of joint bleeds or signs of arthropathy. Using the nomenclature for hemophilia prophylaxis, these children received primary prophylaxis with an excellent outcome. Older patients who began prophylaxis after signs of joint disease were already present showed a substantial reduction in joint bleeds, decreasing to four or fewer events annually. In the few cases with gastrointestinal bleeds, the response to prophylaxis was not entirely satisfactory and two patients continued to require blood transfusions while on treatment.

Only four patients—two with histories of menorrhagia and two who were placed on the regimen because of joint symptoms—withdrew from treatment after 7–13 years. Side-effects were few. Notably, no events of thrombosis were reported. Three patients in the cohort developed inhibitors, one during prophylaxis and two before the initiation of prophylaxis. The authors concluded that long-term prophylactic treatment may be warranted in the majority of patients with type 3 VWD and in occasional patients with other subtypes, depending on the clinical phenotype.

Experience with prophylaxis in other cohorts

Federici et al. [22] reported on the experience of 12 patients with median age of 34.5 years (range 11–71 years), nine with type 3 VWD, who had been exposed to 17 long-term secondary prophylaxis regimens to prevent recurrent bleeding (47% in the gastrointestinal tract, 35% in joints). During the total 4358 days of prophylaxis (median 201 days; range 30–730 days), the patients received 1424 infusions of Haemate-P given either three times (53%) or twice

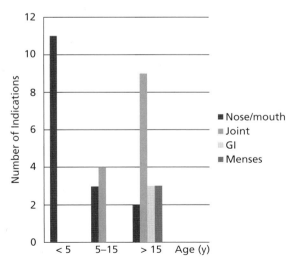

Figure 18.1 Indications for prophylaxis given by age at start of prophylaxis. GI, gastrointestinal; y, years.

(47%) each week. The doses per day were given as VWF:RCoIU/kg, and expressed as medians (ranges) were 60 IU/kg (24–96 IU/kg) for gastrointestinal bleeds; 72 IU/kg (69–72 IU/kg) for joint bleeds; and 86 IU/kg (72–96 IU/kg) for other bleeds. Doses in FVIII:C were not given but should be roughly half of those for VWF:RCo [21]. FVIII levels were measured at trough and peak and never exceeded 180 IU/dL. Clinical response was rated as excellent/good in 100% and no adverse events were reported.

Miners *et al.* [23] reported that bleeding frequency in VWD can be reduced with prophylaxis, but concentrate consumption is increased compared with treatment on demand.

In a compilation of data from European studies [24], 19 patients (age range 5–73 years), including six children, were treated with prophylaxis with Wilate (Octapharma, Vienna, Austria) for more than 3 months (mean 14.8 months; range 3–46 months) with a mean dose of 27.4 IU FVIII per kg and a mean frequency of 1.9 (median 1.7; range 0.8–3.4) infusions per week, a cumulative total of 27,861 infusions. Twelve of the patients had type 3 VWD, two had type 2A, two had type 2B, and one had type 1. A decrease in bleeding frequency from 4.5 to 1.4 bleeds per month was observed. No serious adverse events, including thrombosis, occurred.

Planned or ongoing studies

The VWD Prophylaxis Network (vWD PN) and the VWD International Prophylaxis (VIP) study

The vWD PN was formed to investigate the role of prophylaxis in clinically severe VWD that is nonresponsive to other treatments [25,26]. In a survey performed by the network, 74 investigators from centers in Europe and North America submitted data describing the population with VWD under their care. A total of 6208 patients were included in the census. Of these, 1085 were treated with plasma-derived products in the preceding 12 months. Only 102 patients were receiving prophylaxis, most commonly for joint bleeds. It was quite evident from the survey that only a small fraction of patients in potential need of prophylaxis were actually receiving the treatment. The vWD PN has since initiated the VWD International Prophylaxis (VIP) study. The VIP study includes a prospective and a retrospective study component. The

primary objectives of the study are (i) to examine the effect of prophylaxis on bleeding frequency, and (ii) to establish optimal treatment regimens for joint bleeding, gastrointestinal bleeding, epistaxis, and menorrhagia. Secondary objectives are to (i) determine how quality of life at baseline is related to bleeding history and whether changes in bleeding frequency are associated with changes in quality of life; (ii) identify the frequency of development of inhibitory antibodies to VWF; (iii) study the frequency and indications for hospitalizations; and (iv) evaluate the safety of prophylaxis.

The prospective component of the study is a nonrandomized dose-escalation study addressing the role of prophylaxis for the prevention of joint bleeds, gastrointestinal bleeding, epistaxis, and menorrhagia. Those considered for entry, provided that bleeding indication criteria are met, are those with type 1 VWD who have VWF:RCo ≤20 IU/dL and/or FVIII ≤20 IU/dL, and are nonresponsive to DDAVP (1-deamino-8-D-arginine vasopressin); those with type 2 VWD who are nonresponsive to treatment with DDAVP, or DDAVP contraindicated; and those with type 3 VWD. The treatment regimen allows for escalation depending on response, as used for hemophilia prophylaxis in Canada [27]. Any concentrates licensed for the treatment of VWD can be used. Treatment begins with 50 IU of RCo/kg administered once per week. In the event of bleeding recurrence, as defined for each indication, this escalates to two doses per week. If two doses per week are not sufficient to control bleeding, there is an escalation to three doses per week. Individuals enrolled in the menorrhagia study begin treatment at the level of one dose of 50 IU/kg on day 1 of menses for two cycles, and escalate to treatment on days 1 and 2 of menses or, at the final level, days 1–3 of menses. The primary outcome for the study is bleeding associated with VWD or, for menorrhagia, the pictorial blood assessment chart (PBAC) score [28]. Laboratory assessments in the prospective VIP study include VWF:RCo, VWF:Ag, FVIII:C, ABO blood group, and inhibitory antibodies to VWF. Musculoskeletal evaluation is done according to Gilbert [29] and radiologic assessment is conducted using the Pettersson classification [30]. The perceived health state is assessed using HRQOL-4 [31].

The retrospective studies examine the effect of prophylaxis on bleeding frequency in patients currently on a prophylactic regimen, and characterize the natural history of gastrointestinal bleeding in VWD. These studies are being conducted in parallel with the prospective study.

Enrollment has begun in both the prospective and retrospective arms of the VIP study.

PRO.WILL

In Italy, a prospective study (PRO.WILL) has been proposed. PRO.WILL is the shortened title of the project "Efficacy, safety and pharmaco-economic assessment of secondary long-term prophylaxis with highly purified, standardized, doubly virus inactivated VWF/FVIII concentrates in patients with severe, inherited VWD and frequent bleedings." In PRO. WILL, patients will be randomized between prophylaxis and treatment on demand [32]. The primary objective of the study is to evaluate whether long-term secondary prophylaxis with highly purified VWF/FVIII concentrates prevents spontaneous bleeding in patients with severe VWD who are unresponsive to DDAVP. Secondary objectives include safety parameters, cost, and health-related quality of life. Inclusion criteria require VWF:RCo <10 IU/dL, FVIII:C <20 IU/dL, and/or a bleeding time >15 min. The number of spontaneous bleeds requiring treatment with concentrates during the previous 12 months should be more than five in an anatomical site including epistaxis, or more than two gastrointestinal bleeds, or more than three hemarthroses in the same joint. Prophylaxis at a dose of 60 IU VWF:RCo per kg will be given every third day to patients with joint hemorrhages and every second day to patients with mucosal bleeding. Patients randomized to the on-demand arm will receive 60 IU VWF:RCo per kg at a dose frequency to maintain the VWF:RCo level at >30 IU/dL for mucosal bleeds and a FVIII:C level between 50–150 IU/dL for nonmucosal bleeds until bleeding stops. The duration of the treatment phase of the study is 12 months.

Wilcome

In the prospective Wilcome study (observational study, Octapharma), patients are treated prophylactically with Wilate and are followed for 12 months. Dosing is 30 IU of FVIII per kg body weight two to three times weekly or 40 IU per kg of bodyweight for gastrointestinal bleeds, which from other studies are known to require higher doses [24]. The primary study outcome is bleeding frequency. Other issues to be addressed include joint morbidity, absence from school and work, health-related quality of life, self-reported health status, treatment satisfaction, and treatment efficacy as well as drug tolerability. The enrollment goal is 20 patients.

The future of prophylaxis in VWD and recommendations

Prophylactic treatment of hemophilia is currently state-of-the-art for boys with severe hemophilia living in countries that can afford such costly care. This goal was achieved following the completion of a study that met the modern criteria for evidence-based medicine [8], which corroborated the superior effect of prophylaxis reported in previous cohort studies [4,5,33] conducted over several decades. The circumstances for VWD are somewhat similar to those for hemophilia, although there are differences. The phenotypic heterogeneity is greater in VWD. The bleeding pattern is usually milder than for severe hemophilia and irreversible sequelae are not as common. There is no question that there are patients with VWD who need prophylactic treatment and who derive substantial benefit from this treatment modality. However, it is important that rigorous studies are undertaken to ensure that recommendations can be offered both with respect to bleeding indication(s) and to the treatment regimen. Several such prospective studies have now been launched, of which the VIP study, within the framework of the vWD PN, is by far the largest. It can be predicted that long-term prophylaxis will be more common in VWD when data from these ongoing studies become available.

Recommendations must be based on published experience. The primary target for prophylaxis is type 3 VWD. A few patients with type 2 VWD and problematic gastrointestinal bleeds may also receive prophylaxis, but the search for the source of the bleed is important as local measures may improve the situation dramatically. In some cases, patients with type 1 VWD are in need of prophylaxis. The vast majority of these patients may, however, be managed on demand using DDAVP and/or antifibrinolytics, or occasionally be treated with VWF-containing concentrates.

211

Table 18.2 Long-term prophylaxis in VWD. Recommendations based on limited published data.

Indication	Main target group	Dose[a] FVIII IU/kg bodyweight	Doses per week	When to start
Joint	Type 3	10–50	1–3	After first bleed
Gastrointestinal	Type 2	20–50	2–4	After 2–3 severe bleeds per year[b]
Nose/mouth	Type 3	20–50	1–3	After 3–4 bleeds per year[c]
Menorrhagia	Type 3	20–50	3–4	If disabling (during menses)

[a] Dose refers to Haemate-P/Humate-P.
[b] Treatment at hospital.
[c] Anemia, impacting quality of life.

Prophylaxis in VWD is indicated for bleeding of such a severity and/or frequency that quality of life is substantially jeopardized. This includes chronic drops in hemoglobin or the occurrence of joint bleeds with the development of hemophilic arthropathy. Age at start of prophylaxis for VWD must be more individualized than for hemophilia, and a thorough clinical evaluation of bleeding symptoms should be performed before initiating prophylaxis because the bleeding phenotype is not as predictable as that in hemophilia. Prophylaxis may be stopped if there is an obvious decrease in bleeding risk, such as in the case of menorrhagia when the female reaches menopause, or for gastrointestinal bleeding following the successful treatment of causative telangiectasia. Proposed recommendations are provided in Table 18.2. The dosing schedule and interval can be individualized. A dose per kg of bodyweight of 20–40 IU of FVIII is recommended one to three times weekly, with patients who experience gastrointestinal bleeds usually requiring a more intensive schedule and sometimes even higher doses. Dosing according to VIII:C or VWF:RCo differs among treaters and countries, and when recommendations are given, the varying ratios between VIII:C and VWF:RCo among concentrate brands must be considered [34,35]. Most experience with prophylaxis in VWD has been acquired with Haemate-P/Humate-P, which constitutes the basis for the current recommendation. The plasma levels of VIII:C and VWF:RCo that are needed for effective prophylaxis in VWD in different types of bleeding are not well understood, and ongoing studies will provide further insight for guidance. Adverse events such as thromboembolic complications are extremely rare in VWD [21] and do not generally need to be considered during prophylaxis at the recommended dosing levels.

References

1 Berntorp E, Astermark J, Bjorkman S, *et al*. Consensus perspectives on prophylactic therapy for haemophilia: summary statement. *Haemophilia* 2003; **9** (Suppl. 1): 1–4.

2 Chambost H, Ljung R. Changing pattern of care of boys with haemophilia in western European centres. *Haemophilia* 2005; **11**: 92–9.

3 Ota S, McLimont M, Carcao MD, *et al*. Definitions for haemophilia prophylaxis and its outcomes: the Canadian consensus study. *Haemophilia* 2007; **13**: 12–20.

4 Nilsson IM, Berntorp E, Lofqvist T, Pettersson H. Twenty-five years' experience of prophylactic treatment in severe haemophilia A and B. *J Intern Med* 1992; **232**: 25–32.

5 van den Berg HM, Fischer K, van der Bom JG. Comparing outcomes of different treatment regimens for severe haemophilia. *Haemophilia* 2003; **9** (Suppl. 1): 27–31 (Discussion).

6 Steen Carlsson K, Hojgard S, Glomstein A, *et al*. On-demand vs. prophylactic treatment for severe haemophilia in Norway and Sweden: differences in treatment characteristics and outcome. *Haemophilia* 2003; **9**: 555–66.

7 Feldman BM, Pai M, Rivard GE, *et al*. Tailored prophylaxis in severe hemophilia A: interim results from the first 5 years of the Canadian Hemophilia Primary Prophylaxis Study. *J Thromb Haemost* 2006; **4**: 1228–36.

8 Manco-Johnson MJ, Abshire TC, Shapiro AD, *et al*. Prophylaxis versus episodic treatment to prevent joint disease in boys with severe hemophilia. *N Engl J Med* 2007; **357**: 535–44.

9 Berntorp E, Shapiro A, Astermark J, Blanchette VS, Collins PW, Dimichele D, *et al*. Inhibitor treatment in haemophilia A and B: summary statement for the 2006 international consensus conference. *Haemophilia* 2006; **12** (Suppl. 6):1–7.

10 Fischer K, Valentino L, Ljung R, Blanchette V. Prophylaxis for severe haemophilia: clinical challenges in the absence as well as in the presence of inhibitors. *Haemophilia* 2008; **14** (Suppl. 3):196–201.

11 von Willebrand EA. Hereditär pseudohämofili. *Finska Läkaresällskapets Handlingar* 1926; **LXVII**: 87–112.

12 Silwer J. Von Willebrand's disease in Sweden. *Acta Paediatr Scand Suppl* 1973; **238**: 1–159.

13 Lak M, Peyvandi F, Mannucci PM. Clinical manifestations and complications of childbirth and replacement therapy in 385 Iranian patients with type 3 von Willebrand disease. *Br J Haematol* 2000; **111**: 1236–9.

14 Federici AB. Clinical diagnosis of von Willebrand disease. *Haemophilia* 2004; **10** (Suppl. 4):169–76.

15 Fressinaud E, Meyer D. International survey of patients with von Willebrand disease and angiodysplasia. *Thromb Haemost* 1993; **70**: 546.

16 Ramsay DM, Buist TA, Macleod DA, Heading RC. Persistent gastrointestinal bleeding due to angiodysplasia in the gut in von Willebrand's disease. *Lancet* 1976; **2**: 275–8.

17 Nilsson IM, Blombäck M, Jorpes E, Blombäck B, Johansson SA. v. Willebrand's disease and its correction with human plasma fraction I-O. *Acta Med Scand* 1957; **159**: 179–88.

18 Blombäck M, Blombäck B, Nilsson IM. Response to fractions in von Willebrand's disease. In: Brinkhous KM (ed). *The Haemophilias*, pp.286–94. University North Carolina Press: Chapel Hill, 1964.

19 Berntorp E, Petrini P. Long-term prophylaxis in von Willebrand disease. *Blood Coagul Fibrinolysis* 2005; **16** (Suppl. 1): S23–6.

20 Berntorp E, Nilsson IM. Biochemical and *in vivo* properties of commercial virus-inactivated factor VIII concentrates. *Eur J Haematol* 1988; **40**: 205–14.

21 Berntorp E, Archey W, Auerswald G, *et al*. A systematic overview of the first pasteurised VWF/FVIII medicinal product, Haemate P/Humate-P: history and clinical performance. *Eur J Haematol Suppl* 2008; 3–35.

22 Federici AB, Castaman G, Franchini M, *et al*. Clinical use of Haemate P in inherited von Willebrand's disease: a cohort study on 100 Italian patients. *Haematologica* 2007; **92**: 944–51.

23 Miners AH, Sabin CA, Tolley KH, Lee CA. Assessing the effectiveness and cost-effectiveness of prophylaxis against bleeding in patients with severe haemophilia and severe von Willebrand's disease. *J Intern Med* 1998; **244**: 515–22.

24 Berntorp E, Wyndyga J. Treatment and prevention of acute bleedings in von Willebrand disease—efficacy and safety of Wilate, a new generation von Willebrand factor/factor VIII concentrate. *Haemophilia* 2009; **15**: 122–30.

25 Berntorp E, Abshire T. The von Willebrand disease prophylaxis network: exploring a treatment concept. *J Thromb Haemost* 2006; **4**: 2511–12.

26 Berntorp E, Abshire T. The von Willebrand disease prophylaxis network (vWD PN): exploring a treatment concept. *Thromb Res* 2006; **118** (Suppl. 1): S19–22.

27 Blanchette VS, Manco-Johnson M, Santagostino E, Ljung R. Optimizing factor prophylaxis for the haemophilia population: where do we stand? *Haemophilia* 2004; **10** (Suppl. 4): 97–104.

28 Higham JM, O'Brien PM, Shaw RW. Assessment of menstrual blood loss using a pictorial chart. *Br J Obstet Gynaecol* 1990; **97**: 734–9.

29 Gilbert MS. Prophylaxis: Musculoskeletal evaluation. *Semin Hematol* 1993; **30**: 3–6.

30 Pettersson H, Ahlberg A, Nilsson IM. A radiologic classification of hemophilic arthropathy. *Clin Orthop Relat Res* 1980: 153–9.

31 CDC. *Measuring Healthy Days*. Centers for Disease Control and Prevention, Atlanta, Georgia, 2000.

32 Federici AB. Highly purified VWF/FVIII concentrates in the treatment and prophylaxis of von Willebrand disease: the PRO.WILL Study. *Haemophilia* 2007: 15–24.

33 Petrini P, Chambost H, Nemes L. Towards the goal of prophylaxis: experience and treatment strategies from Sweden, France and Hungary. *Haemophilia* 2004; **10** (Suppl. 4): 94–6.

34 Lethagen S, Carlson M, Hillarp A. A comparative *in vitro* evaluation of six von Willebrand factor concentrates. *Haemophilia* 2004; **10**: 243–9.

35 Budde U, Metzner HJ, Muller HG. Comparative analysis and classification of von Willebrand factor/factor VIII concentrates: impact on treatment of patients with von Willebrand disease. *Semin Thromb Hemost* 2006; **32**: 626–35.

19

Pathophysiology, epidemiology, diagnosis, and treatment of acquired von Willebrand syndrome

Ulrich Budde[1], Augusto B. Federici[2,3] and Jacob H. Rand[4]

[1]Hemostaseology, Medilys Laborgesellschaft mbH, c/o Asklepios Klinik Altona, Hamburg, Germany

[2]Division of Hematology and Transfusion Medicine, L. Sacco University Hospital, Milan, Italy

[3]Department of Internal Medicine, University of Milan, Milan, Italy

[4]Hematology Laboratory, Department of Pathology, Montefiore Center, Bronx, NY, USA

General definition, history, and epidemiology

An apparently acquired form of von Willebrand disease (VWD) was first described in 1968 [1] and detailed a severe bleeding tendency in patients with systemic lupus erythematosus (SLE). Although that report preceded the development of quantitative von Willebrand factor (VWF) assays, the prolonged bleeding time, a normal platelet count, and reduced factor VIII (FVIII) activity were features similar to those found in patients with inherited VWD. To differentiate between the congenital and acquired forms, the term "acquired von Willebrand syndrome" (AVWS) is now accepted for this noninherited disorder. The following patients also had immunologic disease [2]. Between 1968 and 1998, 116 publications described several additional underlying clinical conditions associated with AVWS. Most of these studies were single case reports, as even large centers do not have sufficient patient numbers to provide a comprehensive description of this rare bleeding disorder. Despite numerous reviews of the etiology, pathophysiology, laboratory features, clinical manifestations, and outcome of treatment modalities of AVWS [3–6], there is no description of the prevalence of the disease

because most studies have relied on case reports for data; thus, most reviews have concluded that the prevalence is probably underestimated. Data from large prospective studies are not available, so the actual prevalence of AVWS in the general population is therefore unknown. In the only prospective study available, a prevalence of approximately 10% in 260 patients with hematologic disorders enrolled by a single institution was reported [7]. In 2000, data for 186 patients from a retrospective survey ("registry" in this chapter) conducted in 1998 and 1999 were published as an official communication of the Scientific and Standardization Committee (SSC) concerning the frequency of AVWS [8]. These data were critically compared with the data of the 288 patients described in the literature existing from 1968 to 1998 ("literature" in this chapter). This chapter, which describes the clinical conditions that may be associated with AVWS, will compare the data from the literature with those from the registry, those from 131 patients diagnosed in Hamburg, and those from a single-institution retrospective observational study from 1999 to 2005 [9]. The aim of the chapter is to increase awareness of this rare bleeding disorder.

Pathophysiologic mechanisms for the management of AVWS

In contrast to inherited VWD, VWF is synthesized in normal or even increased quantities in most patients

Von Willebrand Disease, 1st edition. Edited by Augusto B. Federici, Christine A. Lee, Erik E. Berntorp, David Lillicrap, Robert R. Montgomery. © 2011 Blackwell Publishing Ltd.

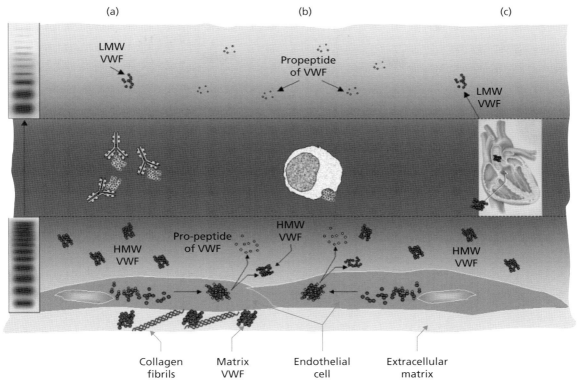

Figure 19.1 Pictorial representation of the three main pathogenetic mechanisms that cause acquired von Willebrand Syndrome (AVWS). Lower panel: Normal von Willebrand factor (VWF) biosynthesis and release from endothelial cells. Note that all the high-molecular-weight (HMW) multimers are present in the released VWF after the cleavage of VWF propeptide, which can be found in the circulation in equal amounts to native VWF. Middle panel: The three main mechanisms causing AVWS: (a) specific or nonspecific autoantibodies that inactivate VWF. These autoantibodies form circulating immune complexes with VWF and are cleared, together with VWF, by Fc-bearing cells; (b) adsorption of VWF onto malignant cell clones; and (c) loss of HMW VWF multimers under conditions of high shear stress occurring in heart valve abnormalities Upper panel: The effects of these three mechanisms on VWF structure and function. In the case of autoantibodies, mechanism (a), the entire native VWF normally secreted from the endothelial cells is usually removed from the circulation, resulting in very low concentrations of both VWF and antigen, but normal levels of VWF propeptide. When malignant cell clones, mechanism (b), and conditions of high shear stress, mechanism (c), cause AVWS, preferential removal of HMW VWF multimers occurs, resulting in reduced VWF activity with relatively normal VWF concentrations.

with AVWS. In these patients, low plasma VWF levels result from its accelerated removal from the plasma by three main pathogenetic mechanisms: (i) specific or nonspecific autoantibodies that form circulating immune complexes with and inactivate VWF (these complexes are cleared by Fc-bearing cells); (ii) adsorption of VWF by malignant cell clones; and (iii) loss of high-molecular-weight (HMW) VWF multimers under conditions of high shear stress (Figure 19.1).

The detailed mechanisms responsible for the quantitative and/or qualitative changes of VWF according to specific diseases are listed in Table 19.1. Compared with acquired hemophilia, which is always caused by autoantibodies against FVIII, the pathogenetic mechanisms underlying AVWS are more heterogeneous. None of the proposed mechanisms appear to be disease specific, and the same mechanism can be responsible for AVWS in different underlying disorders that

215

Table 19.1 List of the pathogenic mechanisms that operate in different disorders.

Specific autoantibodies or nonspecific autoantibodies that form circulating immune complexes and enhance the clearance of VWF
Lymphoproliferative disorders
Neoplastic diseases
Immunologic disorders

Adsorption of VWF on to malignant cell clones or other cell surfaces
Lymphoproliferative disorders
Neoplastic diseases
Myeloproliferative disorders
Enhanced shear stress

Increased proteolytic degradation of VWF
Specific
Myeloproliferative disorders
Enhanced shear stress
Uremia
Ciprofloxacin

Nonspecific (plasmin)
Primary hyperfibrinolysis
Secondary hyperfibrinolysis
Lysis therapy

Enhanced shear stress
Congenital cardiac defects
Aortic stenosis
Endocarditis
Malformation of vessels (Kasabach–Merritt syndrome)
Severe atherosclerosis
ß-thalassemia

Decreased synthesis
Hypothyroidism

Unknown
Valproic acid
Cefotaxime
Virus disease
Liver transplantation
Mixed cryoglobulinimia
AL amyloidosis
Glycogen storage disease type 1
Turner syndrome

VWF, von Willebrand factor.

are known to be associated with the syndrome. In some patients, however, the pathophysiologic mechanism cannot be determined. The clinical symptoms and management of AVWS will be discussed in the following paragraphs according to the underlying conditions associated with the syndrome.

Lymphoproliferative diseases

Lymphoproliferative diseases are a group of underlying disorders that accounts for a significant portion of patients (Table 19.2) with AVWS both in the literature (30%) and in the registry (48%). In a prospective study, Mohri et al. [7] enrolled 260 patients, 145 of whom presented with lymphoproliferative diseases. Eleven (7.5%) had AVWS, five of whom were classified as active bleeders (45%). Over a period of 10 years, Nitu-Whalley et al. [10] observed six patients with lymphoproliferative disorders who developed AVWS. In 2008, we observed 24 individuals in Hamburg with an underlying lymphoproliferative disease from a total of 131 patients with AVWS and 1124 with hereditary VWD (18%), and Tiede et al. [9] reported 11 patients (31%). In the registry, 87% of the patients were classified as bleeders. Before diagnosis, the 11 patients reported on by Tiede et al. experienced eight spontaneous bleeds (two severe), mostly epistaxis, gum bleeding (one severe), and gastrointestinal bleedings (one severe), and seven provoked bleeds (three severe), mostly postoperative (three severe) and after tooth extractions. All patients remained alive during the 2-year follow-up. The risk of new bleeds was 11% per year. Notably, 19% of the patients required surgery procedures within 1 year of diagnosis. Owing to the high risk of bleeding and the necessity for surgery in many patients, it is important to establish a firm diagnosis.

When patients suffer from severe bleeding episodes and even standard coagulation profiles such as the activated partial thromboplastin time (aPTT) show abnormal results, the diagnosis of AVWS can be easily made (Table 19.3). For these patients, VWF is clearly decreased (similarly to inherited type 2 VWD). In contrast, patients with a monoclonal gammopathy of unknown significance IgG type (MGUS-IgG) had AVWS similar to inherited type 1 VWD. It is important to determine whether the bleeding tendency started late in life. If only phenotypical data are avail-

Table 19.2 Main diseases associated with acquired von Willebrand syndrome.

Diseases	Registry ($n = 186$)	Literature ($n=266$)	Hamburg ($n=131$)
Lymphoproliferative	89 (48)	79 (30)	24 (18)
Monoclonal gammopathy of undetermined significance	43 (23)	37(14)	16 (12)
Multiple myeloma	16 (9)	19 (7)	3 (2)
M. Waldenström	8 (4)	5 (2)	3 (2)
Non-Hodgkin lymphoma	8 (4)	10 (4)	1
Hairy cell leukemia	0	1	0
Acute lymphocytic leukemia	1	0	1
Myeloproliferative	29 (15)	48 (18)	50 (38)
Essential thrombocythemia	21 (11)	17 (6)	37 (28)
Polycythemia vera	1	9 (3)	11 (8)
Chronic lymphoid leukemia	5 (3)	22 (8)	0
Myelofibrosis	2 (1)	0	2 (2)
Neoplasia	9 (5)	15 (6)	2 (2)
Wilms tumor	0	11 (5)	1
Carcinomas and solid tumors	9 (5)	3 (1)	1
Peripheral neuroectodermal tumor	0	1	0
Immune	4 (2)	15 (6)	0
Systemic lupus erythematosus	0	6 (2)	0
Autoimmune disease	4 (2)	6 (2)	0
Mixed connective tissue disease	0	1	0
Graft-versus-host disease	0	1	0
Ehlers–Danlos syndrome	0	1	0
Cardiovascular	39 (21)	31 (12)	48 (37)
Congenital and acquired cardiac defects			
Multiple or not defined	24 (13)	0	6 (5)
Ventricular septal defect	0	10 (4)	1
Atrial septal defect	2 (1)	1	0
Aortic stenosis	7 (4)	5 (2)	28 (21)
Mitral valve prolapse	2 (1)	10 (4)	0
Endocarditis	0	0	1
Cardiac assist device	0	0	12 (9)
Angiodysplasia	4 (2)	5 (2)	0
Miscellaneous	16 (9)	78 (28)	7 (5)
Drugs			
Ciprofloxacin	0	2 (1)	0
Griseofulvin	0	1	0
Valproic acid	1	19 (7)	2 (2)
Hydroxyethyl starch	0	11 (4)	0
Infectious diseases			
Hydatid cyst	0	1	0
Epstein–Barr virus infection	1	1	0
Hepatitis C	0	0	2 (2)

(*Continued*)

Table 19.2 (*Continued*)

Diseases	Registry (*n* = 186)	Literature (*n*=266)	Hamburg (*n*=131)
Other systemic diseases			
Hypothyroidism	3 (2)	21 (8)	0
Diabetes	0	7 (3)	0
Uremia	6 (3)	3 (1)	1
Hemoglobinopathies	2 (1)	10 (4)	0
Sarcoidosis	1	0	0
Teleangiectasia	1	0	0
Ulcerative colitis	1	0	0
Liver Cirrhosis	0	0	1
Idiopathic	1	1	1

able, some of the patients may easily be classified as having inherited type 2A VWD (subtype IIE) or severe type 1 VWD, as multimeric analysis provides very similar results in patients with MGUS-IgG (Figure 19.2). Patients with MGUS-IgM (phenotypically type 1 VWD) show an unmistakable multimeric pattern (Figure 19.3). This multimeric pattern can be explained by the giant VWF–IgM complexes that destroy the agarose during their passage through the gel and sometimes even leave holes. A brief inspection of the gels is thus sufficient for making a correct diagnosis.

Although the response to treatment with desmopressin (1-deamino-8-D-arginine vasopressin, DDAVP) or VWF/FVIII concentrates can be indicative of a circulating inhibitor, anti-VWF inhibitors can be identified only in a minority of patients. Mohri *et al.* [7] reported positive results in mixing assays for anti-VWF inhibitors in eight of 25 patients (32%). Mannucci *et al.* [11] had negative results in mixing assays in all seven patients studied. Laboley *et al.* [12] tested seven patients and detected anti-VWF inhibitors in all of them. In some lymphoproliferative disorders, such as multiple myeloma, VWF can be absorbed by plasma cells [13], which may explain why inhibitor assays of patients' plasmas will yield negative results. In the registry, 25% of patients showed positive results after a variety of tests, while Tiede *et al.* [9] reported positive ELISA (enzyme-linked immunosorbent assay) tests in two of 11 patients (29%), one of which was positive for IgG and one positive for IgM. Circulating antibodies

could not be detected in any of the nine patients in Hamburg. The standard method in Hamburg for detecting antibodies is analogous to the Bethesda assay for FVIII in hemophilia A, which uses VWF:Ag and VWF:CB ELISA methods (Table 19.4). Notably, such a VWF:CB test could detect circulating inhibitors in patients with inherited type 3 VWD who have a clinical risk of having alloantibodies against VWF. According to the data from the registry and the literature, patients with AVWS who have lymphoproliferative disorders show more severe bleeding symptoms than those with other underlying conditions associated with AVWS. For example, one patient with an underlying lymphoproliferative disease who developed AVWS experienced gastrointestinal bleeding that required more than 20 units of packed red blood cells per week. Another such patient, previously misdiagnosed with inherited severe type 1 VWD, experienced life-threatening bleeding complications during surgery that could be stopped only after a massive infusion of blood products, VWF/FVIII concentrates, and finally recombinant factor VIIa. Data from the registry showed that more than 60% of the patients did not benefit from any treatment options: 26 of 59 (44%) patients were treatable with DDAVP; VWF/FVIII concentrates were successful in 28 of 50 (56%) patients; 18 of 48 (38%) patients responded to high doses of intravenous immunoglobulin (IVIg); plasmapheresis was successful in six of 30 patients (20%); corticosteroids yielded a response in 10 of 31 (32%) patients; and immunosuppressive agents or chemotherapy showed a response in 17 of 47 (36%) patients.

Table 19.3 Laboratory findings in patients with acquired von Willebrand syndrome as identified in Hamburg.

	Lymphoproliferative	Myeloproliferative	Cardiovascular	Miscellaneous	Total
Case number (%)	24 (18)	50 (38)	48 (37)	9 (7)	131 (100)
VWF:Ag IU/dL, mean (range)	14.2 (4–33)	109 (59–205)	222 (60–664)	164 (41–544)	166 (4–644)
VWF:CB IU/dL, mean (range)	5.3 (<1–24)	72 (27–188)	136 (37–447)	98 (19–207)	109 (<1–447)
VWF:CB/VWF:Ag ratio mean (range)	0.35 (0.07–0.69)	0.65 (0.38–1.12)	0.70 (0.25–1.43)	0.72 (0.38–0.89)	0.69 (0.07–1.43)
Loss of HMW multimers (%)	88	96	100	87	95
Positive anti-VWF inhibitors vs. cases tested[a]	0/9	n.t.	n.t.	n.t.	0/9

[a]Measurement of residual VWF:Ag and VWF:CB after mixture with normal plasma.

HMW, heavy molecular weight; VWF, von Willebrand factor; n.t., not tested.

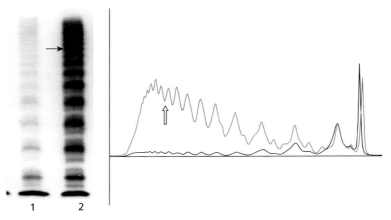

Figure 19.2 Comparison of von Willebrand factor multimers of a patient with monoclonal gammopathy of unknown significance (MGUS) of the IgG type (1) with those from normal pooled plasma (2). On the left side the multimers are shown, while on the right side the densito-metric tracings are presented (red, pooled plasma; black, patient plasma). The arrow shows the border between the intermediate (6–10) and large multimers (>10). In the patient sample, the large multimers are present but the concentration of these is greatly reduced.

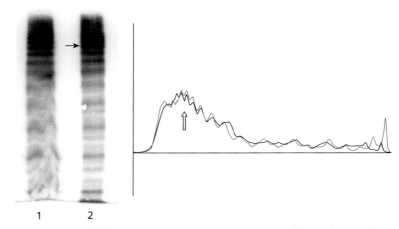

Figure 19.3 Comparison of the von Willebrand factor multimer of a patient with monoclonal gammopathy of unknown significance (MGUS) of the IgM type (1) with those from normal pooled plasma (2). On the left side the multimers are shown, while on the right side the densito-metric tracings are presented (red, pooled plasma; black, patient plasma). The arrow shows the border between the intermediate (6–10) and large multimers (>10). In the patient sample, the large multimers are present but the concentration of these is greatly reduced. All multimers are present (type 1 acquired von Willebrand syndrome). However, the greatly distorted band structure is a striking feature and is typical of an IgM paraprotein.

In the literature, the responses to DDAVP and VWF/FVIII concentrate infusions are always characterized by decreased recovery and rapid clearance of all VWF and FVIII activities within a few hours [20,21]. However, Tiede *et al.* [9] reported successful treat-ment in eight of 10 cases with higher doses of VWF/FVIII concentrates. In contrast to the usual poor response to the standard treatment of inherited VWD, the successful use of high doses of immunoglobulin (1–2 g/kg of body weight within 2–4 days) has been

Table 19.4 Laboratory tests for the diagnosis of AVWS.

Orienting procedures
Patient and family history
Bleeding time
Filter tests
Partial thromboplastin time (PTT)
Platelet count

Confirmatory tests
VWF : antigen (VWF : Ag)
Ristocetin cofactor activity (VWF : RCo)
Factor VIII activity (FVIII : C)
VWF collagen binding capacity (VWF : CB)

Tests performed by specialized laboratories
Ristocetin-induced platelet agglutination (RIPA)
VWF multimeric structure (low resolution gel)
Platelet VWF
VWF-pp (VWF : AgII)

Search for antibodies against the FVIII–VWF complex

Direct methods
Tests according to the Bethesda method for FVIII
    inhibitors (VWF : RCo, VWF : CB, VWF : Ag) [14]
Direct binding to immobilized VWF (high background for
    test with antihuman IgM and to lesser extent IgG,
    because blood group antigens are part of the VWF
    molecule even in patients with blood group O) [15,16]
Adsorption of the immune complex on a solid phase
    (protein A sepharose). Protein A binds VWF directly,
    thus spurious positive results are possible whenever the
    reaction is not verified by rigorous control mechanisms
    [17,18]
Acquired hemophilia A was has to be ruled out in all cases
    of AVWS by the absence of factor VIII autoantibodies in
    the Bethesda assay

Indirect measures
Response of the VWF to DDAVP and to factor VIII/VWF
    concentrate infusion and to high-dose intravenous
    gammaglobulin [19]
Analysis of the underlying mechanism causing AVWS.
    Correction of AVWS in response to appropriate
    treatment of the underlying disorder

AVWS, acquired von Willebrand syndrome; VWF, von
Willebrand factor.

reported several times since the first description by Horellou et al. [21–24]. A good response can be predicted in patients with monoclonal immunoglobulins of the IgG type. In cases where no monoclonal IgG is detectable, successful treatment is achieved in a much lower proportion of patients. The correction of the VWF and FVIII activities is transient and lasts between 15 and 21 days. By multimeric analysis of VWF, it can be shown that larger multimers reappear 24 h after immunoglobulin infusion and normal levels are reached about 48 h after the start of IVIg [21]. This normalization is followed by a progressive disappearance of the large and intermediate VWF multimers in the following 15–21 days. Therefore, AVWS cannot be cured by this therapy. On the other hand, the period of recovery was always sufficient for surgical intervention. With higher daily doses of immunoglobulin (1 g/kg of body weight) the time of 48 h until normalization can be shortened to about 24 h. Because IVIg normalizes the shortened half-life, in urgent cases an initial IVIg infusion followed by VWF/FVIII concentrates is a reasonable therapeutic option. The anti-CD20 monoclonal antibody rituximab showed no effect in the only patients for whom results have been published [25]. In patients with monoclonal immunoglobulins of the IgM type, IVIg had no effect [21]. Silberstein et al. [26] reported successful plasma exchange on 11 separate occasions in a patient with Waldenström macroglobulinemia. Following successful treatment of the primary disease, AVWS in lymphoproliferative diseases disappears, as reported for example in a case of non-Hodgkin lymphoma [27]. In situations where the other therapeutic options do not control severe bleedings, recombinant factor VIIa at the usual dose of 90 μg/kg of bodyweight or higher may be considered.

Cardiovascular diseases

Cases of cardiovascular diseases associated with AVWS have been found with increasing frequency over the last 20 years: from 12% in the literature (31 of 288 patients) and 21% in the registry (39 of 186 patients) to 37% in Hamburg (48 of 131 patients) and 46% (16 of 35 patients) reported by Tiede et al. [9]. AVWS in patients with congenital heart disease was described as early as 1986 by Gill et al. [28]. Recently, Arslan et al. [29] detected AVWS in six of 49 children (12.2%) who were investigated preoperatively. Besides complex inherited cardiac diseases, patent ductus arteriosus also may be accompanied by AVWS [30]. The association between aortic stenosis and gastrointestinal bleeding has been described since 1958 as "Heyde syndrome" [31]. In 1987, King *et al.* [32] confirmed this association by showing that gastrointestinal surgery could stop bleeding in only 5% of patients whereas aortic valve replacement was effective in 93%. The curative effect of aortic valve replacement was confirmed by Anderson *et al.* [33]. A form of AVWS in these patients has been described by many authors [34–38] and it has been shown that the pathophysiologic mechanism for the loss of large VWF multimers is the enhanced shear stress induced by the disturbed flow through the stenosed valve. Lopes *et al.* [39] described a loss of large multimers in patients with pulmonary hypertension. A very recent observation is that, with few exceptions, all patients on cardiac assist devices ("artificial hearts") show a severe loss of the large multimers (between 80% and 90% compared with normal plasma), which can be accompanied by severe bleeding symptoms (Figure 19.4). The loss of large

multimers starts within a few hours of implantation and continues as long as the device is in place [9,40,41].

In the registry (Table 19.2), the underlying conditions reported as being associated with AVWS were congenital cardiac defects, aortic stenosis, angiodysplasia, atrial septal defects and mitral valve prolapse, and gastrointestinal angiodysplasia. Of the patients with cardiovascular diseases who developed AVWS, 77% were classified as bleeders. In a recent retrospective study by Tiede *et al.* [9], the underlying conditions associated with AVWS were aortic valve stenosis, aortic valve replacement, aortic and mitral valve replacement, and cardiac assist devices. These authors reported that in the 16 patients tested, 10 had spontaneous bleeding (five severe), mostly epistaxis, gum bleeding, and gastrointestinal bleeds (three severe), and 11 experienced provoked bleeding episodes (nine severe), mostly postoperative (seven) and after tooth extractions (two severe). During the 2-year follow-up, 50% of the patients remained alive but none died as a result of bleeding: the risk of new bleeds was 19% per year. Notably, surgery procedures were required in 34% of the patients within 1 year of diagnosis.

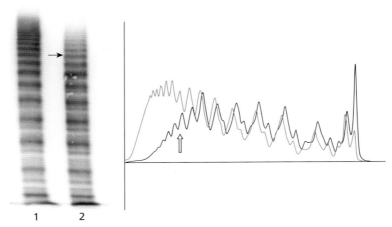

Figure 19.4 Comparison between von Willebrand factor (VWF) multimers in a patient with an implanted left ventricular cardiac assist device (2) and VWF multimers from normal pooled plasma (1). On the left side the multimers are shown, while on the right side the densitometric tracings are presented (red, pooled plasma; black, patient plasma). The arrow shows the border between the intermediate (6–10) and large multimers (>10). In the patient sample, the large multimers are present but the concentration of these is greatly reduced. The loss of the large multimers is clearly seen. Although VWF:Ag was greatly increased, the patient had severe bleeding symptoms.

Owing to the high risk of new bleeding episodes and the necessity for surgery in many patients, it is important to establish a firm diagnosis in these patients. Finally, in the Hamburg cohort (Table 19.2) the most common cardiovascular disorder was aortic stenosis, followed by use of a cardiac assist device, congenital cardiac defects, angiodyplasia, and endocarditis. During aortic surgery, the risk of bleeding is low and its relation to an AVWS is controversial [37,42]. On the other hand, 14 perioperative bleeding complications were observed in patients with aortic valve stenosis followed for 2 years. Four of the Hamburg patients suffering from endocarditis of the aortic valve experienced severe bleeding complications: In two patients, the aortic and mitral valve were both affected. In another patient, the shear stress-induced disturbances of hemostasis also induced thrombocytopenia, hemolytic anemia with schistocytes, and massive cerebral symptoms, suggesting a form of thrombotic thrombocytopenic purpura (TTP). Further investigation showed that the cerebral symptoms were the result of recurrent cerebral hemorrhage and not of microangiopathic thromboses. The clinical bleeding was controlled only after surgical removal of the affected valve. The shear stress-induced loss of large multimers seen in this patient was also observed in the remaining patients. Among the cohort of patients followed in Hamburg, nine patients (four women and five men) initially had unexplained bleeding complications during treatment with oral anticoagulants while the international normalized ratio was still in the target range. The most severe symptom was cerebral hemorrhage, which resulted in death or very severe handicap in five patients. The indication for the anticoagulant treatment was aortic valve replacement (two patients), pulmonary hypertension (one patient), and atrial fibrillation (two patients). As it is generally accepted that approximately 3% of the elderly population have clinically silent aortic stenosis, the number of these patients expected to be at risk of AVWS is very high. Although most cases of bleeding as a result of AVWS show a benign course, it is nevertheless surprising to us that little attention is paid to this mechanism and that the literature on this subject is rather limited. Children with congenital heart defects, especially those with shunt diseases and stenoses, are also at risk of bleeding. Even in the case of the patent ductus arteriosus, a prospective study found AVWS phenotypically similar to inherited type

2 VWD in 25% of patients [30]. In all cases, the pressure gradient was also particularly high and patients were usually diagnosed on auscultation alone.

The laboratory data (Table 19.3) show high levels for VWF:Ag, while VWF:CB and/or VWF:RCo are always lower but remain within the normal range. It is therefore apparent that the functional deficiency of VWF would be overlooked if multimeric analysis was not performed or if the ratios of VWF:CB and/or VWF:RCo to VWF:Ag were not considered. The functional defect of VWF in cardiovascular disorders arises as a result of an acquired loss of large multimers and therefore assays for multimeric analysis have the highest sensitivity to identify this peculiar form of AVWS [9]. The ratio of VWF:RCo and/or VWF:CB to VWF:Ag should provide the equivalent information because values below 0.6 are usually associated with the loss of HMW multimers. However, when VWF:RCo/VWF:Ag ratios can be measured, the large variability of VWF:RCo should be kept in mind, especially when at high levels: It is to be hoped that better reproducibility and sensitivity of VWF:RCo can be obtained by using the most specific VWF:RCo ELISA test [43]. The increased shear stress that arises as a result of these cardiovascular disorders can induce two chronic changes in VWF with opposite effects. On the one hand there is an increased concentration of VWF with a secondary increase of FVIII. On the other hand, the loss of large multimers induced by abnormal high shear stress possibly leads to a bleeding diathesis as a result of reduced platelet adhesion and aggregation. Often this silent VWF-dependent platelet defect can be associated with additional defects of secondary hemostasis. This is, for instance, the clinical situation for patients who require oral anticoagulation after heart valve replacement or after venous thrombosis who unexpectedly develop a life-threatening cerebral hemorrhage shortly after the start of anticoagulation. On the other hand, the high VWF observed in cardiovascular disorders is usually accompanied by a high FVIII level. Such high levels of FVIII are an established risk of venous thrombosis, while an increased risk factor for arterial thromboembolic complications as a result of high VWF levels is less well documented. Because the mechanism of AVWS associated with cardiovascular disorders is related to the loss of HMW multimers, it is not surprising that inhibitors were detected only in a minority of patients: Tiede et al. detected inhibitors in two of the 27 samples tested (7%) [9] and the registry detected inhibitors in two of the 39 samples tested (5%) [8].

Data from the registry [8] showed that the available treatment options were generally unsuccessful: three of 30 (10%) patients responded to DDAVP; four of 30 (13%) patients responded to VWF/FVIII concentrates; two of 25 (8%) patients showed a response to corticosteroids; while IVIg (10 patients) and plasmapheresis (two patients) showed no effect. In contrast to the registry data, Tiede *et al.* [9] reported a success rate of 70% in 10 patients treated with VWF/FVIII concentrates. DDAVP has theoretical advantages over VWF/FVIII concentrates in that the secretion of endogenous supranormal multimers and their immediate availability at the site of bleeding would be expected to improve local hemostasis potentially more than the exogenous VWF given with VWF/FVIII concentrates. Nevertheless, VWF/FVIII concentrates have been proven effective in many patients.

Thrombocythemia and other myeloproliferative disorders

Patients who have AVWS associated with essential thrombocythemia and other myeloproliferative disorders (MPDs) constituted 48 of the 288 (18%) patients described in the literature and 29 of the 186 (15%) described in the registry [8] (Table 19.2). Tiede *et al.* [9] reported just one such patient out of 35 (3%). In a study by Mohri *et al.* [7], 14 of 125 (11%) patients with MPDs showed AVWS and two were classified as active bleeders (14%). Among the 99 patients with AVWS from a study by Sanchez-Luceros *et al.* [44], MPDs were found in 75%. In the Hamburg cohort, 50 (38%) patients were found to have underlying MPDs. Most patients investigated were not actively bleeding but were tested to confirm the diagnosis or to plan for the best treatment in case of surgery or trauma. Thus, the higher patient number can be easily explained. Thrombosis and bleeding, in some instances occurring simultaneously, are frequent complications of MPDs. While thrombosis is the dominant feature in primary essential thrombocythemia, polycythemia vera and especially myelofibrosis primarily manifest with bleeding symptoms [45–47]. The sites and intensity of bleeding symptoms mimic those seen in inherited VWD. Gastrointestinal bleeding followed by soft-tissue bleeding and intra- or postoperative bleedings are the most common symptoms. The mean platelet count in 100 patients from the literature was $2050 \pm 1107 \times 10^9$/L at the time of bleeding. Whether a given patient suffers from a thromboembolism or bleeding is strongly dependent on the platelet count [6,48]. At platelet counts of between 400 and less than 1000×10^9/L, thromboembolism is the most common complication, while bleeding clearly predominates with platelet count above 1500×10^9/L. When platelet counts are between 1000 and 2000×10^9/L, both complications may occur and may even occur simultaneously. In the data from the registry [8], less than half of the patients (48%) were classified as bleeders. The VWF and FVIII activities show normal or elevated concentrations in most patients but VWF:RCo and VWF:CB are always lower than VWF:Ag [45,46,49] (Table 19.3) and the large multimers nearly always show an absolute or relative reduction [50] (Table 19.3). An AVWS with a phenotype similar to inherited type 1 VWD is rarely seen [51]. In medium resolution gels the outer sub-bands are increased. In congenital type 2A VWD this pattern is indicative of an increased proteolysis of VWF. An enhanced proteolysis was also demonstrated in patients with inherited VWD. Such an increased physiologic cleavage caused by expansion of the GPIb receptors was shown by using fragment-specific monoclonal antibodies [52] and was proven by Shim *et al.* [53]. In the retrospective study of Mohri *et al.* [7], inhibitors against VWF were detectable only in one of 14 (7%) patients and in the registry were detectable in only one patient of 26 (4%). Because no controlled studies evaluating pregnancy complications in women with an MPD have been published, recommendations can be based only on small studies and case reports. During pregnancy, the high platelet count usually decreases significantly compared with the count before pregnancy. Bangerter *et al.* [54] followed 17 pregnancies in nine patients with essential thrombocythemia. The rate of spontaneous first trimester abortion was high (35%). Three major and two minor bleeds were observed during pregnancy, all in patients with low-dose aspirin medication. One patient suffered from transient visual loss after stopping low-dose aspirin. Treatment with low-dose aspirin was correlated with a favorable outcome when birth versus abortion was compared.

Children only rarely experience MPDs, but these may be complicated by thrombotic and hemorrhagic events. In the Hamburg center, a 9-year-old male presented with severe headache, aggressive behavior, and migraine attacks. The cerebral symptoms did not recur while on low-dose aspirin therapy, but spontaneous soft-tissue bleeding developed. At that time, the platelet count was high (between 1500 and 2000×10^9/L) and essential thrombocythemia complicated by an AVWS was diagnosed. The infusion of VWF/FVIII concentrate stopped severe epistaxis immediately, an effect that lasted for several hours. Subsequent therapy with anagrelide resulted in normal platelet counts and relieved the bleeding symptoms. Data from the registry [8] showed that all treatment options were unsuccessful in most of the treated patients: three of 14 (21%) patients responded to DDAVP; two of 14 (14%) patients responded to VWF/FVIII concentrates; and immunosuppressants or chemotherapy achieved a response in five of 14 (36%) patients. Treatment with VWF/FVIII concentrates and DDAVP infusion will immediately stop bleeding complications. Normalization of VWF may, however, result in thromboembolic complications [45,55]. Moreover, once in the circulation, the newly secreted or infused normal VWF will become abnormal in a short time. Therefore, the correction lasts for a much shorter time than in congenital VWD. If severe bleeding complications occur, cytoreduction with hydroxyurea, anagrelide, or interferon alpha is indicated. Although the VWF level becomes normal and the hemorrhagic diathesis disappears after normalization of the platelet count, the functional impairment of platelets remains unchanged. This impairment in platelet function is of little clinical significance, and the typical abnormalities of platelet function are more diagnostic than prognostic [56]. In an acute case with essential thrombocythemia (in our case, the count was more than 6000×10^9/L), platelet apheresis can lower the platelet counts very rapidly and may be life saving [45]. The evaluation of postoperative outcomes in 105 patients with polycythemia vera and 150 patients with essential thrombocythemia [55] revealed that a high proportion of surgery was complicated by vascular occlusion (7.7%) or by major hemorrhage (7.3%). There was no correlation between the type of diagnosis, use of antithrombotic agents, type of surgery, and vascular or bleeding complications.

Neoplasms

Patients with solid tumors occasionally develop AVWS (Table 19.2). This cohort represents 6% of patients in the literature (15 of 288) and 5% of patients in the registry (nine of 186). AVWS was recently diagnosed in Hamburg in two patients, one with Wilms tumor and one with an ovarian carcinoma. AVWS in patients with cancer has been described most frequently in patients with Wilms tumor (nephroblastoma). It has been reported in 10 children [6], three of whom presented with mild symptoms while seven were asymptomatic. In a prospective study by Coppes et al. [57] of children with newly diagnosed Wilms tumors, only four of 50 (8%) consecutive patients were found to have asymptomatic AVWS at the time of presentation. Conversely, Baxter et al. [58] reported two children with severe bleeding complications who required ligation of the renal vessels. AVWS was only rarely seen in other types of neoplasm. In the cohort of patients diagnosed in Hamburg, there were only three patients with carcinomas and AVWS with mild symptoms. In the registry, 75% of the patients were classified as active bleeders [8] and a circulating inhibitor was detected in one of three (33%) patients tested. Data from the registry [8] showed that most treatment options were quite successful in most of the treated patients: three of four patients responded to DDAVP; six of six patients responded to VWF/FVIII concentrates; and two out of five patients responded to treatment with IVIg. Immunosuppressive agents or chemotherapy showed a response in one of two patients. Based on available reports, most patients with Wilms tumor do not bleed. The remaining 30% have only mild symptoms that can easily be controlled with DDAVP. AVWS was undetectable after successful treatment of the primary disease. Mild symptoms also predominate in patients with solid tumors and carcinomas—DDAVP is therefore the drug of choice. Although only few cases of AVWS with underlying thrombocythemias and MPDs have been reported, AVWS always disappeared following successful treatment of the primary disease.

Immunologic diseases

Although AVWS was first described in patients with SLE and autoantibodies to VWF, only 15 cases have been described in the literature, usually in association with SLE (six patients) and autoimmune diseases of another etiology (six patients) and very rarely in mixed connective tissue disease (one patient), graft-versus-host disease (one patient), and Ehlers–Danlos syndrome (one patient). One new patient with SLE has been described by Hong *et al.* [59]. The registry [8] contains only four patients with autoimmune diseases, none of which occurred in the cohort of patients from Hamburg. In the registry 75% of patients were classified as active bleeders. Although VWF is theoretically a target protein in immunologic diseases, autoantibodies to VWF are rare and were detected in two of eight patients in the registry (25%). Data from the registry [8] showed that the treatment options are not very successful in the few treated patients: one out of four patients was treatable with DDAVP (25%) and one out of two patients treated responded to IVIg (50%). Whenever an autoantibody has induced AVWS, the symptoms are severe. In these patients, VWF is very rapidly removed from the circulation and frequently both therapeutic options—DDAVP and IVIg—fail. Bleeding that cannot otherwise be controlled warrants consideration of recombinant FVIIa at the usual dose of 90 µg/kg of bodyweight or higher.

AVWS in patients with other diseases

Patients with other underlying diseases (Table 19.2) represent 28% of those in the literature (78 of 288), 9% of those in the registry (16 of 186) [8], and 20% (seven of 35) of those in the study by Tiede *et al.* [9]. In the cohort of patients diagnosed in Hamburg, we observed seven such patients (5%). Of the 16 patients from the registry, 57% were classified as bleeders. Before diagnosis, the seven patients from the study by Tiede *et al.* [9] experienced eight spontaneous bleedings (one severe): epistaxis (four cases), gum bleeding (two cases, one severe), menorrhagia (one case), and skin hematoma (two cases) and bleeding after surgery (three cases, one severe). During a 2-year follow-up, 78% of the patients remained alive. The risk of new bleeding episodes was 27% per year. Notably, surgical procedures were required within 1 year of diagnosis in 27% of the patients. Because of the high risk of new bleeds and the necessity for surgery in many patients, it is important to establish a firm diagnosis.

Four underlying disorders with 61 patients represent 78% of the cases of AVWS in the literature: a side-effect of treatment with valproic acid [60], a side-effect of treatment with hydroxyethyl starch [61], hypothyroidism [62], and hemoglobinopathies [63]. A prospective study by Koenig *et al.* [64] detected an AVWS in six of 23 (26%) children with epilepsy treated for longer than 6 months with valproic acid, while Eberl *et al.* [65] found a low incidence of this side-effect. Franchini *et al.* [66] diagnosed AVWS in 35 of 1342 (3%) consecutive patients with various thyroid diseases who were candidates for thyroid surgery. Of these patients, 33 presented with AVWS similar to inherited type 1 VWD and two with AVWS similar to inherited type 2 VWD. AVWS in uremia [67], liver cirrhosis, and with no detectable underlying disease was diagnosed in single patients. More recently, new disease associations with AVWS have been described (usually in single cases) in essential mixed cryoglobulinimia by Pasa *et al.* [68], in immunoglobulin light chain amyloidosis (four cases, two with abnormal multimers) by Kos *et al.* [69], after treatment with the third-generation cephalosporin, Cefotaxime [70], in six out of 10 patients with glycogen storage disease type 1a [71], and in Turner syndrome [72].

The laboratory data for patients with other underlying disorders (Table 19.3) show slightly decreased to high levels for VWF:Ag while VWF:CB and/or VWF:RCo are usually in the normal range, although sometimes moderately decreased. Thus, the functional defects of VWF may be overlooked, as in cardiovascular diseases, if multimeric analysis is not performed or if the ratio of VWF:CB and/or VWF:RCo to VWF:Ag is not considered. Inhibitors were detected in only a minority of patients: in the registry, one of 14 (7%) patients tested for displayed inhibitors. Data from the registry showed that all treatment options were unsuccessful in most of the treated patients: two patients of nine were treatable with DDAVP or VWF/FVIII concentrates (22%), but IVIg (one patient), corticosteroids (six patients), and immunosuppressants or chemotherapy (three patients) failed. In contrast to this, Tiede *et al.* [9] reported good responses in all five patients treated with VWF/FVIII concentrates. Pasa *et al.* [68] reported a good response to rituximab in their patient with essential mixed cryoglobulinimia. Although the bleeding symptoms are mild in AVWS in patients who are on valproate therapy, treatment may be needed in some instances. DDAVP can trigger seizures and therefore should be avoided in patients who are at risk; VWF/ FVIII concentrates are a preferred modality for treating these patients. In hypothyroidism, DDAVP has been shown to have an excellent therapeutic effect; however, treatment with DDAVP is needed only rarely because the administration of thyroxine as treatment of the primary disease leads to complete normalization. Dialysis results in a normalization of hemostasis in uremic patients with AVWS even though it is not always sufficient. Because of the usually high VWF levels, in most patients there is an unfavorable ratio between the patient's endogenous VWF and infused exogenous VWF, which results in high demands on the VWF/FVIII concentrates. Thus, DDAVP is more effective than VWF/FVIII concentrates. Conjugated estrogens (e.g. Presomen; Wyeth Pharmaceuticals, Münster, Germany and Solvay Pharmaceuticals, Hanover, Germany) have also been repeatedly described as a hemostyptic agent in these patients. Otherwise, for uncontrollable bleeding, clinicians may consider using recombinant FVIIa (NovoSeven; Novo Nordisk Ltd, Bagsvaerd, Denmark) at the usual dosage of 90 μg/kg of bodyweight or higher. In hepatic diseases the same criteria apply as for patients with uremia. However, Presomen has not been shown to be effective in patients with hepatic diseases and is not recommended.

Current issues and future perspectives on AVWS

Compared with acquired hemophilia, AVWS is remarkably heterogeneous and its basic mechanisms remain undefined in many cases. An updated version of the International Registry on AVWS has been established online (http://www.intreavws.com) to promote direct registration of new cases. The aim is to gain a better understanding of the basic mechanisms of AVWS (through the use of new assays), the limits of standard therapies, and the efficacy of novel and experimental therapeutic approaches. The contribution of the three main underlying clinical conditions associated with AVWS, namely lympho- and myeloproliferative, immunologic, and cardiovascular disorders, will also be established. Experts on AVWS should work with relevant specialists to design appropriate screening algorithms for patients at risk of bleeding. New, interesting cases should be enrolled into this online registry to promote this international investigator-driven prospective study on AVWS organized on behalf of the VWF Subcommittee of the International Society on Thrombosis and Haemostasis Scientific and Standardization Committee. The use of more sensitive and specific assays should be encouraged to determine the role of anti-VWF autoantibodies in AVWS: a working party on the standardization of these assays has recently started with the task of promoting the best diagnostic approach to identify and characterize these anti-VWF inhibitors. Management of bleeding in AVWS relies mainly on DDAVP, VWF concentrates, and high-dose IVIg, but no single approach is effective for all AVWS cases. As bleeding episodes are sometimes life threatening and require prolonged hospitalization with the infusion of large doses of blood products, the organization of large prospective multicenter studies of patients with AVWS will be required to definitively answer these questions.

References

1 Simone JV, Cornet JA, Abildgaard CF. Acquired von Willebrand's syndrome in systemic lupus erythematodes. *Blood* 1968; **31**: 806–11.

2 Ingram GIC, Kingston PJ, Leslie J, Bowie EJW. Four cases of acquired von Willebrand's syndrome. *Br J Haematol* 1971; **21**: 189–99.

3 Jakway JL. Acquired von Willebrand's disease in malignancy. *Sem Thromb Hemost* 1992; **18**: 434–9.

4 Rinder MR, Richard RE, Rinder HM. Acquired von Willebrand's disease: a concise review. *Am J Hematol* 1997; **54**: 139–45.

5 Kumar S., Pruthi RK, Nichols WL. Acquired von Willebrand's syndrome: A single institution experience. *Am J Hematol* 2003; **72**: 243–7.

6 Michiels JJ, Budde U, van Genderen PJJ, *et al.* Acquired von Willebrand Syndromes: Clinical features, etiology, pathophysiology, classification and management. *Best Pract Res Clin Haematol* 2001; **14**: 401–36.

7 Mohri H, Motomura S, Kanamori H, *et al.* Clinical significance of inhibitors in acquired von Willebrand syndrome. *Blood* 1998; **91**: 3623–9.

8 Federici AB, Rand JH, Bucciarelli P, *et al.* Acquired von Willebrand syndrome: Data from an international registry. *Thromb Haemost* 2000; **84**: 345–9.

9 Tiede A, Priesack J, Werwitzke S, *et al.* Diagnostic workup of patients with acquired von Willebrand

syndrome: a retrospective single-centre cohort study. *J Thromb Haemost* 2008; **6**: 569–76.

10 Nitu-Whalley IC, Lee CA. Acquired von Willebrand syndrome—report of 10 cases and review of the literature. *Haemophilia* 1999; **5**: 318–26.

11 Mannucci PM, Lombardi R, Bader R, *et al.* Studies of the pathophysiology of acquired von Willebrand disease in seven patients with lymphoproliferative disorders or benign monoclonal gammopathies. *Blood* 1984; **64**: 614–21.

12 Laboley V, Zabraniecki L, Sie P, Pourrat J, Fournie B. Myeloma and monoclonal gammopathy of uncertain significance associated with acquired von Willebrand syndrome. Seven new cases with a literature review. *Joint Bone Spine* 2002; **69**: 62–7.

13 Richard C, Cuadrado MA, Pieto M, *et al.* Acquired von Willebrand disease in multiple myeloma secondary to absorption of von Willebrand facor by plasma cells. *Am J Hematol* 1990; **35**: 114–17.

14 van Genderen PJJ, Vink T, Michiels JJ, Vantveer MB, Sixma JJ, van Vliet HHDM. Acquired von Willebrand disease caused by an autoantibody selectively inhibiting the binding of von Willebrand factor to collagen. *Blood* 1994; **84**: 3378–84.

15 Stewart MW, Etches WS, Shaw ARE, Gordon PA. VWF inhibitor detection by competitive ELISA. *J Immunol Meth* 1997; **200**: 113–19.

16 Siaka C, Rugeri L, Caron C, Goudemand J. A new ELISA assay for diagnosis of acquired von Willebrand syndrome. *Haemophilia* 2003; **9**: 303–8.

17 Zettervall O, Nilsson IM. Acquired von Willebrand's disease caused by monclonal antibody. *Acta Med Scand* 1978; **204**: 521–8.

18 Hartleib J, Köhler N, Dickinson RB, *et al.* Protein A is the von Willebrand factor binding protein on Staphylococcus aureus. *Blood* 2000; **96**: 2149–56.

19 Luboshitz J, Lubetsky A, Schliamser L, Kotler A, Tamarin I, Inbal A. Pharmacokinetic studies with FVIII/von Willebrand factor concentrate can be a diagnostic tool to distinguish between subgroups of patients with acquired von Willebrand syndrome. *Thromb Haemost* 2001; **85**: 806–9.

20 Van Genderen PJJ, Terpstra W, Michiels JJ, Kapteijn L, van Vliet HHDM. High-dose intravenous immunoglobulin delays clearance of von Willebrand factor in acquired von Willebrand disease. *Throm Haemost* 1995; **73**: 891–2.

21 Federici AB, Stabile F, Castaman G, Canciani MT, Mannucci PM. Treatment of acquired von Willebrand syndrome in patients with monoclonal gammopathy of uncertain significance: comparison of three different therapeutic approaches. *Blood* 1998; **92**: 2707–11.

22 Horellou MH, Baumelou E, Sitbon N, *et al.* Quatre cas de deficit acquis en facteur Willebrand associés a une dysgubulinémie monoclonale. *Ann Med Int* 1983; **143**: 707–12.

23 Michiels JJ, Berneman Z, Gadisseur A, *et al.* Immune mediated etiology of acquired von Willebrand syndrome in systemic lupus erythematosus and in benign monoclonal gammopathy: therapeutic implications. *Semin Thromb Hemost* 2006; **32**: 577—88.

24 Yamamoto K, Takamatsu J, Saito H. Intravenous immunoglobulin therapy for coagulation inhibitors: a critical review. *Int J Hematol* 2007; **85**: 287–93.

25 Grimaldi D, Bartolucci P, Gouault-Heilmann M, Martin-Toutain I, Khellaf M, Godeau B. Rituximab failure in a patient with monoclonal gammopathy of undetermined significance (MGUS)-associated acquired von Willebrand syndrome. *Thromb Haemost* 2008; **99**: 782–3.

26 Silberstein LE, Abrahm J, Shattil SJ. The efficacy of intensive plasma exchange in acquired von Willebrand's disease. *Transfusion* 1987; **27**: 234–37.

27 Tran TC, Mannucci PM, Schneider P, Federici AB, Bachmann F. Profound alterations of the multimeric structure of von Willebrand factor in a patient with malignant lymphoma. *Br J Haemost* 1985; **61**: 307–14.

28 Gill JC, Wilson AD, Endres-Brooks J, Montgomery RR. Loss of the largest von Willebrand factor multimers from plasma of patients with congenital cardiac defects. *Blood* 1986; **67**: 758–61.

29 Arslan MT, Ozyurek R, Kavakli K, *et al.* Frequency of acquired von Willebrand's disease in children with congenital heart disease. *Acta Cardiol* 2007; **63**: 403–8.

30 Rauch R, Budde U, Girisch M, Klinge J, Hofbeck M. Acquired von Willebrand disease in an infant. Resolution by interventional occlusion of patent ductus arteriosus. *Thromb Res* 2001; **102**: 407–9.

31 Heyde EC. Gastrointestinal bleeding in aortic stenosis. *N Engl J Med* 1958; **259**: 196.

32 King RM, Pluth JR, Giuliani ER. The association of unexplained bleeding with calcific aortic stenosis. *Ann Thorac Surg* 1987; **44**: 514–16.

33 Anderson RP, McGrath K, Street A. Reversal of aortic stenosis, bleeding gastrointestinal angiodysplasia, and von Willebrand syndrome by aortic valve replacement. *Lancet* 1996; **347**: 689–90.

34 Warkentin TE, Moore JC, Morgan DG. Aortic stenosis and bleeding gastrointestinal angiodysplasia—Is acquired von Willebrands disease the link? *Lancet* 1992; **340**: 35–7.

35 Knobloch W, Hauser E, Niehues R, Schiele T, Metzger G, Jacksch R. Calcifying aortic valve stenosis and cryptogenic gastrointestinal bleeding (Heyde syndrome): report of two cases. *Zeitschr Kardiol* 1999; **88**: 448–53.

36 Veyradier A, Balian A, Wolf M, *et al.* Abnormal von Willebrand factor in bleeding angiodyplasias of the digestive tract. *Gastroenterology* 2001; **120**: 346–53.

37 Vincentelli A, Susen S, Le Touneau T, *et al.* Acquired von Willebrand syndrome in aortic stenosis. *N Engl J Med* 2003; **349**: 343–9.

38 Pareti FI, Lattuada A, Bressi C, *et al.* Proteolysis of von Willebrand factor and shear stress-induced platelet aggregation in patients with aortic valve stenosis. *Circulation* 2000; **102**: 1290–5.

39 Lopes AAB, Maeda NY, Aiello VD, Ebaid M, Bydlowski SP. Abnormal multimeric and oligomeric composion is associated with enhanced endothelial expression of von Willebrand factor in pulmonary hypertension. *Chest* 1993; **104**: 1455–60.

40 Velik-Salchner C, Eschertzhuber S, Streif W, Hangler H, Budde U, Fries D. Acquired von Willbrand syndrome in cardiac patients. *J Thorac Vasc Anesth* 2008; **22**: 719–24.

41 Geisen U, Heilmann C, Beyersdorf F, *et al.* Non-surgical bleeding in patients with ventricular assist devices could be explained by acquired von Willebrand disease. *Eur J Cardiothorac Surg* 2008; **33**: 679–84.

42 Weinstein M, Ware JA, Troll J, Salzman E. Changes of the von Willebrand factor during cardiac surgery: effect of desmopressin acetate. *Blood* 1988; **71**: 1648–55.

43 Federici AB, Canciani MT, Forza I, *et al.* A sensitive ristocetin cofactor activity assay with recombinant glycoprotein Ib alpha for the diagnosis of patients with low von Willebrand factor levels. *Haematologica* 2004; **89**: 77–85.

44 Sanchos-Luceros A, Meschengieser SS, Woods AI, *et al.* Acquired von Willebrand factor abnormalities in myeloproliferative disorders and other hematologic diseases: a retrospective analysis by a single institution. *Haematologica* 2002; **87**: 264–70.

45 Budde U, Schäfer G, Müller N, *et al.* Acquired von Willebrand's disease in the myeloproliferative syndrome. *Blood* 1984; **64**: 981–5.

46 Budde U, Scharf RE, Franke P, Hartmann-Budde K, Dent J, Ruggeri ZM. Elevated platelet count as a cause of abnormal von Willebrand factor multimer distribution in plasma. *Blood* 1993; **82**: 1749–57.

47 Van Genderen PJJ, Michiels JJ. Erythromelalgic, thrombotic and hemorrhagic thrombocythemia. *Press Med* 1994; **23**: 73–7.

48 Michiels JJ, Berneman Z, Finazzi G, Budde U, van Vliet HH. The paradox of platelet activation and impaired function: platelt-von Willebrand factor interactions, and the etiology of thrombotic and hemorrhagic manifestations in essential thrombocythemia and polycythemia vera. *Semin Thromb Hemost* 2006; **32**: 589–604.

49 Fabris F, Casonato A, Del Ben MG, De Marco L, Girolami A. Abnormalities of von Willebrand factor in myeloproliferative disease: A relationship with bleeding diathesis. *Br J Haematol* 1986; **63**: 75–83.

50 Van Genderen PJJ, Budde U, Michiels JJ, van Strik R, van Vliet HHDM. The reduction of large von Willebrand factor multimers in patients with essential thrombocythemia is related to the platelet count. *Br J Haematol* 1996; **93**: 962–5.

51 Casonato A, Fabris F, Zancan L, Girolami A. Acquired type I von Willebrand's disease in a patient with essential thrombocytosis. *Acta Haematol (Basel)* 1986; **75**: 188–9.

52 Budde U, Dent JA, Berkowitz SD, Ruggeri ZM, Zimmerman TS. Subunit composition of plasma von Willebrand factor in patients with the myeloproliferative syndrome. *Blood* 1986; **68**: 1213–17.

53 Shim K, Anderson PJ, Tuley EA, Wiswall E, Sadler E. Platelet–VWF complexes are preferred substrates of ADAMTS13 under fluid shear stress. *Blood* 2008; **111**: 651–7.

54 Bangerter M, Güthner C, Beneke H, Hildebrand A, Grünewald M, Grieshammer M. Pregnancy in essential thrombocythaemia: treatment and outcome of 17 pregancies. *Eur J Haematol* 2000; **65**: 165–9.

55 Ruggeri M, Rodegiero F, Tosetto A, *et al.*, Groppo Italiano Malatie Ematologiche dell Adulto (GIMEMA) Chronic Myeloproliferateve Diseases Working Party. Postsurgery outcomes in patients with polycythemia vera and essential thrombocythemia: a retrospective study. *Blood* 2008; **111**: 666–71.

56 Finazzi G, Budde U, Michiels JJ. Bleeding time and platelet function in essential thrombocythemia and other myeloproliferative syndromes. *Leuk Lymphoma* 1996; **22** (Suppl. 1): 71–8.

57 Coppes MJ, Zandvoort SWH, Sparling CR, Poon AO, Weitzman S, Blanchette VS. Acquired von Willebrand disease in Wilm's tumor paients. *J Clin Oncol* 1992; **10**: 422–7.

58 Baxter PA, Nuchtern JG, Guillerman RP, *et al.* Acquired von Willebrand syndrome and Wilms tumor: not always benign. *Pediatr Blood Cancer* 2009; **52**: 392–4.

59 Hong S, Lee J, Chi H, *et al.* Systemic lupus erythematosus comlicated by acquired von Willebrand Syndrome. *Lupus* 2008; **17**: 846–8.

60 Kreuz W, Linde R, Funk M, *et al.* Induction of von Willebrand disease type 1 by valproic acid. *Lancet* 1990; **335**: 178–84.

61 Strauss RG, Stump DC, Henriksen RA. Hydroxyethyl starch accentuates von Willebrand's disease. *Transfusion* 1985; **25**: 235–7.

62 Dalton RG, Dewar MS, Savidge GF, *et al.* Hypothyroidism as a cause of acquired von Willebrand's disease. *Lancet* 1987; **8540**: 1007–9.

63 Benson PJ, Peterson LC, Hasegawa DK, Smith CM. Abnormality of von Willebrand factor in patients with hemoglobin E-ß thalassemia. *Am J Clin Pathol* 1990; **93**: 395–9.

64 Koenig S, Gerstner T, Keller A, Teich M, Longin E, Dempfle CE. High incidence of valproate-induced coagulation disorders in children receiving valproic acid: a prospective study. *Blood Coagul Fibrinolysis* 2008; **19**: 375–82.

65 Eberl W, Budde U, Bentele K, *et al*. Acquired von Willebrand syndrome as side effect of valproic acid therapy in chidren is rare. *Hämostaseologie* 2009; **29**: 137–42.

66 Franchini M, Zugni C, Veneri D, *et al*. High prevalence of acquired von Willebrand's syndrome in patients with thyroid diseases undergoing thyroid surgery. *Haematologica* 2004; **89**: 1341–6.

67 Gralnick HR, McKeown LP, Williams SB, Shafer BC. Plasma and platelet von Willebrand factor: defects in uremia. *Am J Med* 1988; **85**: 806–10.

68 Pasa S, Altinta A, Cil T, Danis R, Ayyildiz O, Muftuoglu E. A case of essential mixed cryoglobulinemia and associated acquired von Willebrand disease treated with rituximab. *J Thromb Thrombolysis* 2008; **27**: 220–2.

69 Kos CA, Ward JE, Malek K, *et al*. Association of acquired von Willebrand syndrome with AL amyloidosis. *Am J Hematol* 2007; **82**: 363–7.

70 Haj MA, Murch N, Bowen DJ, *et al*. Cefotaxime as the potential cause of transient acquired von Willebrand syndrome. *Eur J Haematol* 2006; **76**: 440–3.

71 Mülhausen C, Schneppenheim R, Budde U, *et al*. Decreased plasma concentration of von Willebrand factor antigen (VWF:Ag) in patients with glycogen storage disease type Ia. *J Inherited Metab Dis* 2005; **28**: 945–50.

72 Sokol L, Stueben ET, Jaikishen JP, Lamarche MB. Turner syndrome associated with acquired von Willebrand syndrome, primary biliary cirrhosis, and inflammatory bowel disease. *Am J Hematol* 2002; **70**: 257–9.

20 Gene therapy for von Willebrand disease

Marinee K.L. Chuah[1,2], *Inge Petrus*[1], *and Thierry VandenDriessche*[1,2]

[1]Flanders Institute for Biotechnology (VIB), Vesalius Research Center, University of Leuven, Leuven, Belgium

[2]Faculty of Medicine and Pharmacy, Free University of Brussels (VUB), Brussels, Belgium

Introduction

von Willebrand disease

von Willebrand disease (VWD) is the most common inherited bleeding disorder in humans, caused by a defective (types 1 and 3 VWD) or dysfunctional (type 2 VWD) von Willebrand factor (VWF) protein. The phenotype of VWF deficiency varies with the mutations in the VWF gene. Most forms of the disease are inherited as dominant traits, whereas type 3 VWD is recessive. In mild cases, problems with abnormal homeostasis develop only after trauma or surgery. In more severe cases, spontaneous bleeding can develop from the nasal, oral, gastrointestinal, and genitourinary mucosa, and joint bleeding can also develop [1].

The VWF is an adhesive multimeric glycoprotein that plays an important role in primary and secondary hemostasis [2]. In primary hemostasis, VWF functions as a bridge between subendothelial structures such as collagen and platelets, allowing them to adhere to sites of vascular injury in high shear conditions. In secondary hemostasis, VWF functions as a carrier protein for coagulation factor VIII (FVIII). The lack of these two functions in VWD results in bleeding problems. Current options for the treatment of VWD are relatively limited. Usually, therapy is based on infusion of desmopressin (DDAVP, 1-deamino-8-D-arginine vasopressin) that induces secretion of VWF from endothelial cells [3]. In general, the result-

ing high plasma concentration of VWF/FVIII lasts for several hours, so desmopressin needs to be administered multiple times depending on the severity of the bleeding episode. However, repeated treatment at short intervals mostly results in a decreased response to desmopressin therapy [4]. The most commonly encountered side-effects are tachycardia, headache, facial flushing, and risk of seizures. As ultralarge, highly active VWF multimers are also released, the use of desmopressin has been associated with myocardial infarction and arterial thrombosis [5,6]. Although treatment with desmopressin is effective in most patients with type 1 VWD, it is not applicable in type 3 or for most of the patients with type 2 VWD. For those patients who are unresponsive to desmopressin, the replacement of the deficient protein with plasma concentrates containing VWF or VWF in conjugation with FVIII is the current treatment of choice. Multiple administrations are needed, and these preparations do not contain the largest and more active multimers of VWF. Moreover, because these products are derived from blood, the risk of contamination with blood-borne viruses cannot be excluded. Type 3 VWD is an attractive candidate for gene therapy because it is caused by a single gene defect and results in a recessive loss-of-function phenotype that could potentially be corrected by *de novo* expression of VWF following gene therapy. Most of the gene therapy approaches described herein focus on type 3 VWD. Moreover, as VWF is secreted in the circulation, it may not be necessary to target specific organs or tissues if gene transfer in the desired target cells results in adequate post-translational processing and multimerization of VWF. Gene therapy for VWD can

Von Willebrand Disease, 1st edition. Edited by Augusto B. Federici, Christine A. Lee, Erik E. Berntorp, David Lillicrap, Robert R. Montgomery. © 2011 Blackwell Publishing Ltd.

231

potentially provide constant, sustained VWF synthesis within the patient, thereby obviating the risk of spontaneous bleeding, the need for repeated injections with VWF, and the risk of viral infections associated with plasma-derived VWF. Gene therapy for VWD could, at least theoretically, provide a cure for this disease. The present review focuses on the current approaches and possible future directions toward the development of effective and safe gene therapy for VWD.

Gene therapy

It is widely anticipated that improved gene therapy approaches will yield new treatments and cures for a plethora of diseases including bleeding disorders such as VWD and hemophilia. Convincing evidence continues to emerge from clinical trials supporting the fact that gene therapy is effective for patients suffering from a wide range of diseases and results in long-term therapeutic effects [7–13]. Long-term clinical benefits have been obtained following gene therapy in over 40 children suffering from otherwise lethal hereditary disorders, and they are now essentially leading normal lives. The first successes have also been achieved recently in treating chronic degenerative disorders, such as Parkinson disease [14], with gene therapy. Despite these successes, gene therapy has also faced a number of setbacks and there have been concerns regarding the safety of some gene delivery approaches. Whereas multiple factors appear to determine the success of a gene therapy trial, the major limiting mechanisms identified today are insertional mutagenesis by integrating vectors, inappropriate expression of the transgene in unwanted cell types or conditions, and immune activation against the vector or the transgene product [15–17]. The consequences of these events range from the failure to establish stable transgene expression or elimination of the gene-modified cells [16,17] to the triggering of acute systemic toxicity [18] and even transformed cell growth and oncogenesis [15]. Fortunately, these hurdles are not insurmountable and the success of gene therapy warrants the continuous development of improved gene transfer technologies. It thus appears that our efforts toward perfecting gene transfer should aim to substantially improve our control on the fate of the genetic material that is stably introduced in the cells and on its expression.

Gene delivery approaches

Ex vivo and in vivo gene therapy

Ex vivo and *in vivo* approaches are being pursued for gene therapy of VWD. *Ex vivo* gene therapy involves the isolation of cells from the patient followed by expansion and genetic modification in culture with vectors expressing VWF and subsequent readministration of the engineered cells to the patient. The main advantage of *ex vivo* gene delivery is that the VWF gene is directly transferred into the desired cell type, obviating inadvertent gene expression in ectopic nontarget cells that may result in inappropriate posttranslational processing of VWF. Another advantage of *ex vivo* gene therapy is that the immune system is not directly confronted with the gene delivery vector, which obviates the risk of inducing immune responses that are directed against the vectors, particularly if viral vectors are employed.

Successful *ex vivo* gene therapy requires efficient engraftment of the engineered cells in order to lead to sustained VWF production in the circulation. One of the main challenges of *ex vivo* gene therapy in general is that most cell types engraft relatively poorly after readministration unless the recipient is subjected to some type of conditioning or injury. Engraftment of hematopoietic stem cells (HSCs) typically requires myeloablative or nonmyeloablative conditioning treatment to create "niches" in the bone marrow. Since myeloablative conditioning represents a relatively harsh conditioning regimen associated with significant toxicities and side-effects, the use of milder conditioning regimens, such as busulfan treatment, is desired [9,19–21].

However, milder conditioning regimens typically result in lower engraftment efficiencies of gene-engineered HSCs. The efficiency and duration of cellular engraftment of nonhematopoietic cells depends on several confounding variables, including the cell type, cell viability and clearance rate *in vivo*, and the injection site. Augmenting cell engraftment efficiencies may require approaches that are typically employed in the tissue engineering field and are based on biocompatible scaffolds derived from collagen or other extracellular matrix components [22–24].

In vivo gene delivery involves the administration of a gene transfer vector encoding VWF directly to the patient, which leads to *in situ* genetic modification of the target cells. Intravenous administration of a VWF vector would provide a more cost-effective treatment than *ex vivo* protocols that involve *ex vivo* expansion of the target cells, which requires the appropriate good manufacturing practice/good laboratory practice (GMP/GLP) facilities. Moreover, *in vivo* gene delivery in a long-lived target cell overcomes some of the intrinsic engraftment challenges of *ex vivo* gene delivery approaches. However, the main disadvantage of *in vivo* gene therapy, especially when based on viral vectors, is that a host immune response toward the viral vector would preclude vector readministration if more than one injection was required to achieve therapeutic VWF levels. Instead, repeated administration of *ex vivo* engineered cells would be possible. Finally, unlike most *ex vivo* gene therapy approaches, direct *in vivo* VWF gene transfer can lead to the inadvertent transduction of antigen-presenting cells depending partly on the type of vector used, which could in turn trigger an immune response directed against the transduced cells and/or the VWF protein itself.

Gene therapy for VWD requires the use of a gene delivery system that is efficient, safe, nonimmunogenic, and allows for long-term gene expression. Most importantly, gene therapy for VWF must compare favorably with existing protein replacement therapies. The availability of animal models of VWD, including VWF-knockout mice [25] and dogs [26,27], that mimic human clinical symptoms significantly facilitated preclinical efficacy and safety studies of gene therapy strategies.

Viral and nonviral vectors

The development of gene therapy for VWD has been hampered by the considerable length of the VWF cDNA (8.4 kb) and the inherent complexity of the VWF protein, which requires extensive post-translational processing including glycosylation and multimerization [28]. Both viral vectors and nonviral vectors have been considered for the development of gene therapy of VWD. In general, viral vector-mediated gene transfer is far more efficient than nonviral gene transfer and has therefore been adopted as the method of choice for many gene therapy applications. Different types of viral vectors have been developed, each with their own advantages and limitations. The most commonly used viral vectors in gene therapy are the retroviral and lentiviral vectors—adenoviral and adeno-associated viral (AAV) vectors. All of these vectors have resulted in robust and long-term therapeutic effects and/or long-term gene expression in both small and large animal models. They have also been used extensively in phase I/II and III clinical trials for a variety of diseases.

Despite the typical robust gene transfer with most viral vectors, there are several reasons why an alternative nonviral gene therapy treatment would also be desirable. Nonviral vectors can be assembled in cell-free systems from well-defined components and have the potential to be less immunogenic than viral vectors. Moreover, there is no typical size restriction as in the case of viral vectors, implying that a large insert such as the VWF cDNA could readily be accommodated in a nonviral, plasmid-based vector gene delivery paradigm.

Retroviral and lentiviral vectors

Moloney murine leukemia virus (MoMLV)-based γ-retroviral vectors are the first and most commonly used vectors for clinical trials and offer the potential for long-term gene expression by virtue of their stable chromosomal integration and lack of viral gene expression [29,30]. Their integration allows passage of the transgene to all progeny cells. However, a disadvantage of γ-retroviral vectors is that cell division is required for transduction and integration, thereby limiting γ-retroviral-mediated gene therapy to actively dividing target cells. To our knowledge, there have been no reports to date of VWF gene delivery using MoMLV-based γ-retroviral vectors, so it is not certain whether it is possible to use γ-retroviral vectors for VWF gene delivery given the packaging constraints of MoMLV-based vectors. In order to overcome the need for active cell division to achieve efficient transduction, retroviral vectors have been developed from lentiviruses with human immunodeficiency virus (HIV) as the prototype [31–34]. The lentivirus life cycle differs from that of MoMLV retroviruses in that the preintegration complex is readily transported across an intact nuclear membrane via the nuclear pores into the nucleus and requires no disassembly of the nuclear membrane. This intrinsic property of lentiviral vectors enables efficient transduction of nondividing cells. Moreover, even in dividing cells, gene transfer with lentiviral vectors is more efficient than with MoMLV-based γ-retroviral vectors [26]. An additional advantage of lentiviral vectors over MoMLV-based γ-retroviral vectors is that they seem to be less sensitive to positional silencing after integrating into the chromosome. They contain fewer CpG dinucleotides, which via cytosine methylation contribute to histone deacetylation and chromatin condensation-mediated vector silencing. To ensure minimal risk of silencing, lentiviral vectors may contain *cis*-elements such as chromosomal insulators, locus control regions (LCR), and scaffold/matrix attachment regions (S/MAR) [35].

As HIV-1 is a human pathogen, it is critically important to ensure that the corresponding lentiviral vectors are replication defective and therefore cannot yield functional wild-type HIV virus. The current lentiviral vector technology has several built-in safety features that preclude the generation of replication of competent wild-type human HIV-1 recombinants. While present efforts are aimed at the generation of stable packaging cell lines and safe, clinically acceptable vectors [34], the attributes of the lentiviral vector system may be well suited for the treatment of VWD by gene therapy. The latest generation lentiviral vector packaging system relies on a self-inactivating (SIN) HIV-derived vector backbone that does not contain any HIV-1 genes but only the *cis*-acting elements necessary for integration, reverse transcription, and expression. To increase gene transfer and expression efficiency, additional regulatory *cis*-acting elements are routinely incorporated into the vector. The woodchuck hepatitis virus post-transcriptional regulatory element (WPRE) [36] stimulates transgene expression post-transcriptionally by augmenting 3'-end processing and polyadenylation. Finally, it has been shown that the central polypurine tract (cPPT) facilitates nuclear translocation of the pre-integration complex and consequently increases lentiviral transduction [37,38].

Typically, lentiviral vectors can accommodate larger transgenes (up to ~10 kb) than γ-retroviral vectors, although vector titers tend to decrease with larger inserts. We have previously shown that functional lentiviral vectors can be generated that express the human VWF cDNA from an internal human cytomegalovirus (CMV) promoter, which allows for efficient transduction and VWF expression in various cell types [26,39]. In principle, the expression of VWF cDNA can be driven from any internal cell type-specific or ubiquitously expressed promoter provided that the expression cassette does not exceed the packaging capacity of the lentiviral vector. The VWF lentiviral vector that we generated showed only a modest

decrease in vector titer compared with similar lentiviral vectors that expressed other transgenes. This could be attributed to the size of the VWF cDNA and/or the lack of WPRE, which was intentionally omitted from the VWF lentiviral vectors to accommodate the VWF cDNA. Nevertheless, this modest decrease in vector titer could easily be overcome by concentrating the vector by ultrafiltration. The ability to deliver functional VWF using lentiviral vectors has now been independently confirmed by other groups.

Although genomic integration is essential to obtain stable expression of the gene of interest following lentiviral transduction of dividing cells (e.g., following hematopoietic reconstitution), it is a double-edged sword that may potentially contribute to insertional oncogenesis. Indeed, it is now well established that the integration of a γ-retroviral vector that encodes the IL-2Rγ_c gene in proximity of the *LMO2* proto-oncogene contributed to the deregulated LMO2 expression and ultimately to the leukemiogenesis observed in several patients enrolled in a clinical trial for SCID-X1 [40]. Consequently, the risk of leukemiogenesis prompted several investigations into the safety consequences of using integrating vectors for gene therapy. One of the main potential safety concerns related to the use of lentiviral vectors in clinical applications relates to its intrinsic ability to integrate into the target cell genome and, to a much lesser extent, to the HIV-1 pathogenicity of the wild-type virus from which they are derived. To reduce the risk of insertional oncogenesis, the long terminal repeat (LTR) promoters/enhancers of the lentiviral vectors have been modified to generate a so-called self-inactivating lentiviral vector. In the SIN vector configuration, a 400 bp sequence is removed from the LTR region, including the TATA box [41], that consequently abolishes the transcriptional activity of the LTR regions. This SIN configuration reduces the likelihood that cellular coding sequences located adjacent to the vector integration site will be aberrantly expressed, either as a result of promoter activity of the 3' LTR or through an enhancer effect, and therefore further improves the vector safety. The SIN lentiviral VWF vector that we have generated contains this built-in safety feature.

The intrinsic genotoxicity of γ-retroviral versus lentiviral vectors is currently being compared in several preclinical models to further address this safety issue. In general it can be stated that lentiviral or γ-retroviral vectors exhibit semirandom insertion profiles with varying degrees of preference for actively described genes and distinct *cis*-regulatory regions such as CpG islands and DNase I hypersensitive sites [42,43]. Both γ-retroviral and lentiviral vectors show an integration bias into transcriptional units, which indicates that integration is not random *per se*. Nevertheless, the integration pattern of γ-retroviral vectors seems to differ from that of lentiviral vectors. γ-retroviral vectors have a predilection toward integrating in the immediate proximity of transcription start sites (TSS) and a small window around DNase I hypersensitive sites, whereas lentiviral vectors are more likely to integrate further away from the TSS [35,44]. To assess the relative oncogenicity/genotoxicity of lentiviral vectors, HSC gene transfer studies are being conducted in a tumor-prone mouse models (i.e., Cdkn2a$^{-/-}$ mice) [45]. These studies uncovered the low genotoxicity of lentiviral vector integration compared with that of γ-retroviral vector integration. However, in these studies a SIN lentiviral vector design was compared with a non-SIN γ-retroviral vector, and it would be worthwhile to compare the intrinsic genotoxicity/oncogenicity of SIN lentiviral vectors with SIN retroviral vectors, as recent studies clearly indicate that SIN γ-retroviral vectors have a much more favorable safety profile than their non-SIN counterparts [46].

Lentiviral integration profiles and/or oncogenic risks may depend on several confounding variables including the vector copy number, the target cell type, the proliferation and/or activation status of the target cells, the nature of the transgene itself, the vector design (SIN vs. non-SIN, choice of promoters/enhancers), underlying disease and possible selective advantages of rapidly growing cells, protocol-specific cofactors, and finally the intrinsic genotypic variation of the model animals and the treated patients. Most importantly, expression of VWF following lentiviral transduction is not likely to confer any selective growth advantage to the transduced target cells, which decreases the risk of insertional oncogenesis. In contrast, the strong selective pressure on the IL-2Rγ$_c$-expressing cells in the context of hematopoietic reconstitution in SCID-X1 patients intrinsically carried a much greater risk of insertional oncogenesis because high expression of IL-2Rγ$_c$ conferred a selective growth advantage to the gene-engineered cells.

Adenoviral vectors

Most adenoviral vectors are derived from human adenovirus serotypes 2 and 5 and are rendered replication-deficient by the removal of essential viral regulatory genes (e.g., the *E1* gene) [47]. However, these vectors still contain residual viral genes that can be expressed at low levels even in the absence of *E1*, presumably as a result of activation by cellular E1-like proteins. Inflammatory responses and toxicity have been observed in animal models and in clinical trials, which prompted the development of high-capacity adenoviral (HC-Ad) vectors that are devoid of all viral genes and have reduced inflammatory properties. The HC-Ad vectors have a very large cloning capacity (>30 kb) and can therefore readily accommodate the VWF cDNA. Since HC-Ad vectors have been used successfully to deliver large transgene cassettes *in vivo* [48,49], they are potentially useful for VWF gene delivery in mouse models of VWD, but this has not yet been validated. The main advantages of HC-Ad vectors are their broad host range and their ability to transduce dividing as well as nondividing cells, unlike MoMLV-based γ-retroviral vectors. The adenoviral genome remains episomal in the transduced cells, implying that there is virtually no risk for neoplastic transformation as a result of insertional mutagenesis. Although HC-Ad vectors have a significantly improved safety profile compared with early generation adenoviral vectors, a nonlinear threshold effect was apparent in mouse models that is probably at least partly due to the uptake and degradation of viral particles by antigen-presenting cells (APCs) [48,49]. Since the interaction of HC-Ad vectors with APCs could trigger a rapid innate immune reaction, it is important to devise strategies (e.g., by vector capid modifications or localized gene delivery) that further minimize the interaction of the HC-Ad vectors with APCs [50]. Nevertheless, HC-Ad vectors have recently been shown to result in prolonged transgene expression in nonhuman primates [51].

Adeno-associated vectors

Some of the most promising vectors for gene therapy have been derived from AAV vectors. AAV vectors can efficiently transduce nondividing cells, including hepatocytes, *in vivo* and are capable of achieving long-term transgene expression in mouse and large animal models [52–54]. They have recently been used to partially correct congenital blindness [13] and yield transient therapeutic clotting factor IX (FIX) levels in humans following liver-directed gene delivery [16]. At high vector doses, however, a T cell immune response curtailed long-term gene expression consistent with the apparent loss of transduced hepatocytes. Nevertheless, the use of alternative AAV serotypes, more robust AAV vectors, and/or transient immuno-suppressive regimens may eventually overcome this limitation. One drawback of most AAV vectors is their limited cloning capacity (<5 kb), which at first glance indicates that AAV vectors could not be used for gene therapy of VWD. It has been possible to overcome the size constraints of AAV vectors by using two different AAV vectors that span either the 5' or 3' end of the transgene expression cassette and that recombine *in vivo* through head-to-tail dimerization [55]. This strategy may potentially work for VWF gene delivery as well. However, a single vector approach would still be preferred. Recent data suggest that alternative AAV serotypes derived from AAV5 have a larger cloning capacity that was initially assumed and can accommodate large genomes of up to 8.9 kb. Although this resulted in a decrease in vector titer, it was still possible to efficiently deliver large therapeutic genes and demonstrate phenotypic correction of congenital blindness in mouse models [56]. Hence, the use of AAV5 may represent an attractive novel approach for *in vivo* gene delivery of VWF but awaits further validation in mouse models of VWD. Since AAV5 can result in efficient hepatic gene delivery in dog and nonhuman primate models, this avenue may be worth pursuing.

Nonviral approaches

The use of nonviral delivery approaches may overcome some of the immune complications associated with some viral vectors. Plasmid-based vectors are easier and less expensive to manufacture and can be produced in bacteria such as *Escherichia coli*. This important advantage overcomes some of the regulatory hurdles associated with viral vector production and consequently should greatly facilitate the implementation of clinical trials. However, the efficiency of naked DNA delivery is generally low because the mammalian cell membrane is not penetrable to electrically charged large molecules. In developing nonviral gene delivery, the most important challenge is to design a system that simultaneously achieves high efficiency, prolonged gene expression, and low toxic-

ity. From a technical perspective transfection is a relatively simple method whereby the DNA is mixed with a carrier molecule that facilitates its entry into the cells. These carriers are compounds, polymers, or cationic lipids that can shield the negative electric charge of the cargo to be delivered. In addition to neutralizing the negative charge on the DNA, many reagents compact the size of the cargo (DNA condensing agents) to facilitate delivery into cells. The most sophisticated carrier molecules try to induce endocytosis to take up the complex. Polyethylenimine (PEI)-based reagents couple the carrier molecule to ligands for specific receptors, thereby targeting specific cell types. The DNA entry can also be facilitated by electroporation or nucleofection, whereby cells that are suspended in specific buffers are exposed to high-voltage pulses of electricity that create transient holes in the cell membrane, promoting DNA transfer. Magnetofection associates DNA with cationic magnetic nanoparticles and utilizes magnetic force to transport DNA into cells [57].

Most of these methods can be used for *ex vivo* gene delivery and usually result in adequate transient transfection efficiencies. However, expression from plasmid-based vectors typically rapidly declines in the days following transfection, particularly in dividing cells, unless the plasmid vector integrates by nonhomologous recombination, which is very inefficient, and selective pressure is applied to select for these rare integrants (typically $<10^{-5}$ for stable integrants/transfected cells). Transposon-based gene delivery can overcome this limitation, leading to a substantial improvement over classic plasmid-based nonviral delivery approaches that results in long-term and efficient transgene expression by virtue of their ability to stably integrate the gene of interest into the target cell genome. The advantages of transposons as nonviral systems include their reduced immunogenicity compared with viral vectors, no strict limitation of the size of expression cassette [58], and potentially improved safety/toxicity profiles. We have recently developed and validated a very robust transposon-based gene delivery system derived from the so-called "Sleeping Beauty" transposon that allows, for the first time, efficient and stable nonviral gene transfer in $CD34^+$ hematopoietic stem/progenitor cells that retain their ability for functional immune reconstitution in immunodeficient mice with gene-engineered cells [59]. This novel transposon-based gene delivery technology may therefore represent an attractive paradigm for VWF gene delivery into different cell types, including endothelial cells, endothelial precursor cells, and HSCs. Moreover, these hyperactive Sleeping Beauty transposons do not show a biased integration pattern into genes, unlike γ-retroviral and lentiviral vectors.

One challenge of the current nonviral gene delivery in general is that direct *in vivo* transfection remains relatively inefficient. Hence, it is particularly challenging to obtain therapeutically relevant VWF levels with the current nonviral vector technology. However, there is one notable exception, which is the hydrodynamic transfection method [60]. This nonviral gene delivery approach is based on the principle of rapid, high-pressure gene delivery with large volumes of an aqueous DNA solution. Hydrodynamic gene delivery can result in relatively efficient hepatic gene delivery and long-term expression of the gene of interest in mice. With specific modifications it can even be adapted to achieve localized gene transfer in isolated liver lobes [61] or muscle groups in large animal models. Although this approach results in acute and transient liver toxicity, it is possible to reduce these side-effects by carefully controlling the injection rate [61].

Gene correction

Gene correction by homologous recombination is a promising gene therapy modality for the treatment of monogenic diseases that allows for *in situ* correction of a defective gene. Gene correction has several advantages: (i) it avoids the potential risks associated with (quasi)random genomic integration and, in particular, insertional oncogenesis; (ii) it preserves the natural expression pattern of the corrected gene and consequently avoids the potential complications that are associated with ectopic expression of the gene of interest; and (iii) it allows for the correction of genes that result in recessive and dominant phenotypes. This could potentially constitute an attractive modality for treating some forms of VWD that are the consequence of dominantly inherited gain-of-function mutations. However, in general, the overall efficiency of homologous recombination is extremely low, which hampers clinical applications; it is possible to overcome this limitation by introducing DNA double-strand breaks (DSBs) in the desired target gene that needs to be corrected, which results in a dramatic increase in efficiency of homologous recombination with several orders of magnitude.

Introducing a DSB into the target DNA increases the interaction between the host and an exogenous homologous DNA sequence by mobilizing the homologous recombination repair mechanism [62]. Engineered zinc-finger nucleases (ZFNs) are attractive molecular tools for achieving more precise and efficient gene correction at the targeted locus [63]. Typically, ZFNs are modular and correspond to a C2H2 class of zinc-finger DNA binding domains that is specifically engineered to recognize the DNA sequence of interest and is fused to the nuclease domain of the FokI endonuclease. By virtue of the specificity of the designer zinc-finger proteins, the FokI endonuclease is then "recruited" to the target locus where it catalyzes the DSB and subsequently allows the exogenous homologous DNA to correct the cognate-defective sequence. Since FokI must dimerize to be able to induce DSBs, two different ZFNs that bind the DNA at palindromic sequences of the complementary DNA strands need to be delivered into the cells of interest along with the exogenous DNA sequence. However, the efficiency of gene correction is dependent on several confounding variables, including the targeted locus, the transduction efficiency, and the target cell type. One key issue that needs to be addressed further is the potential "off target" effect, whereby DSBs are introduced in other loci besides the desired locus and which may contribute to ZFN cytotoxicity [44]. Although promising, the technology warrants further optimization in terms of efficiency and safety.

To repair mutant VWF mRNA, it may also be possible to use spliceosome-mediated RNA trans-splicing (SMaRT) [64]. To achieve this, a pre-trans-splicing molecule (PTM) needs to be delivered to the cells using viral or nonviral vectors to achieve correction at the transcriptional level. This approach has successfully produced sufficient functional FVIII to correct endogenous FVIII mRNA in FVIII knockout mice with the hemophilia A phenotype.

Target cells

In most animals, including humans, VWF synthesis and storage occurs in endothelial cells and megakaryocytes and their platelet progeny. The precise contributions of the endothelial versus platelet VWF compartment in thrombotic and hemostatic processes are still not completely clear and may be species specific. For instance, in the canine model, VWF synthesis and storage is limited to endothelial cells and does not occur in megakaryocytes and platelets [39]. There are several outstanding questions that await further study and it is not clear whether VWF needs to be expressed in the vascular endothelium to achieve optimal phenotypic correction or whether it is sufficient to supply multimerized VWF from transduced cells to the plasma. Moreover, it is not clear whether VWF expression from platelets would be important for optimal therapeutic benefit. Nevertheless, as VWF infusion in humans is therapeutically beneficial, the amount and quality of VWF secreted into the circulation may be the most critical factor in determining the therapeutic efficacy following gene therapy.

Endothelial cells

Endothelial cells are attractive target cells for gene therapy of VWD as they naturally express VWF. Several approaches have been developed to augment gene transfer into endothelial cells that line the blood vessels. Some of these approaches are potentially amenable for *in vivo* VWF gene delivery. Although several viral vectors can be retargeted to the vascular endothelium [65–67], it has been particularly challenging to prevent transduction of other non-target cell types, particularly hepatocytes. In addition, although endothelial cell-specific retargeting is possible, *in vivo* transduction of the blood vessel endothelium is still relatively inefficient. However, alternative endothelial cell sources are attractive targets for VWF gene transfer, including circulating endothelial progenitor cells and endothelial cells that can be expanded from the blood (originally defined as blood outgrowth endothelial cells, BOECs, by R. Hebbel) [24,26,68,69]. The precise physiologic role of the cells that give rise to these BOECs is not known, but it is plausible that they may act as endothelial precursors that play a role in tissue repair and primary hemostasis. In that case, BOECs may be well suited to deliver the VWF protein to the site of injury, but this needs to be proven.

Endothelial cells from dogs with type 3 VWD do not express VWF and do not contain Weibel–Palade bodies, which are the storage granules of VWF. Nucleofection of endothelial cells with VWF expression plasmids obtained from aortic veins of dogs with VWD resulted in *de novo* VWF expression and subsequent restoration of Weibel–Palade body biogenesis. This pioneering study by Montgomery and colleagues [70] provided proof of concept that VWF gene transfer in endothelium has the potential to correct VWD. Nevertheless, it would be difficult to procure a source of such endothelial cells in a practical manner that could be used as a potential clinically relevant strategy for gene therapy of VWD. Moreover, under these conditions VWF expression was transient. To overcome these limitations, we used BOECs as an alternative endothelial cell source as they can readily be obtained from the peripheral blood and can be enriched and expanded *in vitro* [26] (Figure 20.1). Transduction of these BOECs with lentiviral vectors expressing VWF resulted in >90% stable gene transfer. These relatively robust, stable lentiviral transduction efficiencies obviated the need for elaborate selection schemes to enrich for gene-engineered BOECs, unlike when nonviral transfections were employed. Lentiviral transduction resulted in *de novo* expression of functional VWF in the VWD BOECs. The secreted VWF is capable of normal binding to GPIbα and collagen, consistent with a normal multimerization pattern including high-molecular-weight (HMW) multimers. Moreover, VWF expressed by the transduced VWD BOECs was capable of binding to factor VIII. *De novo* expression of VWF also resulted in the formation of VWF-positive Weibel–Palade bodies, further confirming the role of VWF in the biogenesis of these endothelial cell-specific secretory granules. This confirms that BOECs are attractive targets for gene therapy of VWD as they are equipped with the necessary post-translational machinery to generate fully functional VWF. Recent studies suggest that stably selected BOECs transfected with FVIII plasmids can result in the sustained expression of FVIII following transplantation into NOD-SCID mice. Similarly, when BOECs transduced with FVIII lentiviral vectors were implanted subcutaneously in matrigel scaffolds, therapeutic FVIII levels could be obtained in hemophilic mice. In those mice that had been tolerized to FVIII, expression was sustained for several months but eventually declined to basal levels consistent with the disappearance of the implanted cells. Whether injection of VWF-transduced BOECs would provide therapeutic VWF levels *in vivo* requires additional study but based on the FVIII studies it is

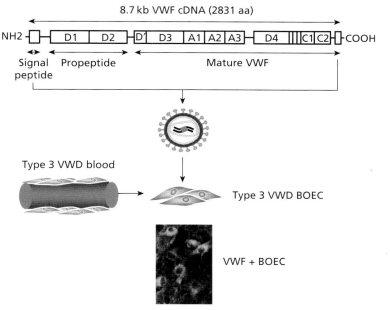

Figure 20.1 Gene therapy for type 3 von Willebrand disease (VWD). The von Willebrand factor (VWF) cDNA 8.7 kb encodes a 2831 amino acid (aa) polypeptide that contains different functional domains (indicated as D1, D2, D', D3, A1, A2, A3, D4, C1, C2) that are essential for its function. The signal-peptide and propeptide are cleaved to yield a mature VWF. To develop an effective gene therapy approach it is necessary to clone a full-length VWF cDNA into a gene delivery vector that can either be viral or nonviral. In this schematic representation, a lentiviral vector is depicted that accommodates the full-length VWF cDNA driven from a ubiquitously expressed CMV (cytomegalovirus). Blood outgrowth endothelial cells (BOECs) can be isolated and expanded from the blood of dogs with type 3 VWD and, upon transduction with the lentiviral VWF vector, express high functional levels of fully multimerized VWF capable of stabilizing FVIII and binding to collagen and GPIbα. Adapted from De Meyer *et al.* [26], with permission.

possible that matrigel or collagen scaffolds may be required to improve the long-term engraftment of the VWF-transduced cells [22,24,71].

These studies suggest that the endothelial compartment is not only a useful target for VWF gene transfer as a potential gene therapy for type 3 VWD, but also represents an attractive paradigm for FVIII gene delivery and gene therapy of hemophilia A. The recent observations that FVIII is normally also produced by endothelial cells in addition to hepatocytes further supports this notion [72,73]. Moreover, several studies have demonstrated that expression of FVIII in endothelial cells results in localized storage of VWF and FVIII in Weibel–Palade bodies, which constitutes a releasable pool of FVIII [74]. It was originally proposed that FVIII-regulated storage is secondary to VWF storage and results from a high-affinity VWF–FVIII interaction early in the secretory pathway [74–76]. However, recent studies challenge that notion by demonstrating cotargeting of FVIII and VWF to secretory granules even in the absence of such high-affinity interactions, such as in the case of type 2N VWD [77,78]. These data also explain why DDAVP results in a concomitant release of FVIII and VWF in patients with type 2N VWD.

Hematopoietic cells

Since megakaryocytes and their platelet progeny also store and secrete VWF, this makes the hematopoietic compartment particularly attractive for gene therapy of VWD. To direct expression of VWF in the

239

megakaryocytes and platelets, it would be necessary to deliver the VWF gene into the HSCs and, ideally, use a megakaryocyte-specific promoter (e.g., GPIIb) to restrict VWF expression to the megakaryocyte/platelet lineage. This approach has not yet been validated for VWD. A similar strategy was devised recently using either lentiviral vector or transgenic approaches to direct expression of FVIII in the megakaryocyte lineage, which resulted in phenotypic correction of the bleeding diathesis in hemophilic FVIII-deficient mice. Remarkably, a therapeutic effect could be achieved even in the face of high-titer FVIII-specific neutralizing antibodies, suggesting that localized release of FVIII by the platelets inside the platelet plug was somehow protected from neutralization by these inhibitory antibodies. Ectopic expression of FVIII in the megakaryocytes/platelets resulted in the co-localized storage of FVIII and VWF in the α-granules, which constitutes a releasable pool of FVIII. This paradigm is reminiscent of the FVIII cotargeting into the Weibel–Palade bodies of endothelial cells [75,76].

Gene transfer into HSCs has also been explored recently with a view toward developing an effective and safe gene therapy for thrombotic thrombocytopenic purpura (TTP) [79]. TTP is a potentially fatal syndrome resulting from genetic or acquired deficiency of plasma ADAMTS13. ADAMTS13 is a metalloprotease primarily synthesized in liver and endothelial cells that cleaves VWF at the central A2 domain, thereby reducing the sizes of circulating VWF multimers. Transplantation of HSCs transduced *ex vivo* with a lentiviral vector encoding ADAMTS13 into myeloablated ADAMTS13($^{-/-}$) mice resulted in detectable ADAMTS13 antigen and proteolytic activity in plasma that sufficed to eliminate the ultralarge VWF multimers. Consequently, this resulted in systemic protection against ferric chloride-induced arterial thrombosis. This success may provide the basis for the development of a novel therapeutic strategy to cure hereditary TTP in humans.

Hepatocytes

As infusion of VWF is therepeutically beneficial to patients with type 3 VWD, it may be possible to achieve phenotypic correction of VWD following expression in ectopic cell types. The liver remains an attractive target for many gene therapy applications, including for VWD, because of its ability to efficiently produce and secrete therapeutically relevant proteins into the blood. Long-term liver-directed gene expression has been accomplished after systemic administration of retroviral [80], lentiviral [38,81], AAV [82], and "gutless" adenoviral vectors [48]. In addition, liver-directed gene transfer can be achieved by nonviral hydrodynamic gene delivery of expression plasmids [83].

To test the hypothesis that ectopic VWF expression in the liver can be hemostatically effective, we and others transfected different VWF expression constructs into hepatocytes of VWF-deficient mice by hydrodynamic gene delivery [84–87]. This resulted in hepatocyte-specific VWF gene expression that corrected the bleeding phenotype of mice with VWD. Ectopic VWF expression in transfected hepatocytes also resulted in increased circulating FVIII levels. Furthermore, we showed that the type of promoter used is critically important and that hepatocyte-specific promoters/enhancers yield more prolonged and higher VWF expression levels (>10-fold) than when viral promoters (CMV) are used. Liver-expressed VWF was fully multimerized, including the HMW molecules, and able to restore proper platelet plug formation in severe VWD. Although VWF expressed in hepatocytes is biologically active, the low-molecular-weight multimers were more abundant than the HMW multimers compared with normal wild-type plasma VWF or VWF expressed from VWF-transduced BOECs. This is consistent with a lower activity-to-antigen ratio based on collagen and GPIb-binding assays compared with wild-type plasma-derived VWF. These apparent qualitative differences in VWF expressed ectopically may reflect differences in the post-translational processing machinery in hepatocytes versus endothelial cells or megakaryocytes/platelets. Nevertheless, the liver-expressed VWF contains more HMW multimers than the majority of recombinant VWF products that are commonly used for the treatment of VWD. Interestingly, VWF mutants with impaired multimerization as a result of a mutation in the D' region (Arg799 instead of Cys799) failed to achieve effective correction of the bleeding diathesis in mice with VWD. VWF mutants with impaired binding to GPIIbIIIa and collagen also resulted in a correction of bleeding time, whereas GPIb binding mutants of

VWF continued to bleed, although blood loss was decreased.

Conclusions and perspectives

The continued development of improved gene delivery approaches has greatly benefited the field of gene therapy in general, and gene therapy for VWD in particular. Most of the gene therapy efforts have focused on type 3 VWD, but the ongoing development of *in situ* gene correction approaches based on ZFN-technology may ultimately pave the way toward gene therapy of the autosomal dominant VWD subtypes. The use of lentiviral vectors is well suited for *ex vivo* gene delivery into endothelial or endothelial progenitor cells, resulting in fully functional VWF. However, it is still necessary to develop approaches that result in robust and sustained engraftment of the VWF-expressing cells while allowing for continued VWF secretion *in vivo*. The use of HSCs as targets for gene therapy of VWD has not yet been explored, but also holds promise as an alternative gene therapy strategy for VWD, particularly since megakaryocytes and platelets normally express VWF. Although ectopic cell types, like hepatocytes, do not possess the necessary post-translational machinery to produce VWF with an identical multimerization pattern as natural plasma-derived VWF, hepatocyte-derived VWF can still prevent bleeding in VWD mouse models. This opens new avenues for gene therapy of VWD using clinically relevant viral vectors that are known to result in stable and/or efficient gene delivery into hepatocytes. However, it will be desirable to demonstrate effective, safe, and long-term correction of the bleeding disorder in large animal models before exploring the use of gene therapy in clinical trial for the treatment of patients suffering from severe VWD. Finally, the lessons learned from other ongoing and planned gene therapy trials for various genetic diseases, and hemophilia in particular, will be critically important in ultimately paving the way toward clinical gene therapy trials for VWD.

Acknowledgements

We thank V.I.B., F.W.O., and I.W.T. for financial support. I.P. is an I.W.T. fellow.

References

1 Sadler JE, Mannucci PM, Berntorp E, *et al.* Impact, diagnosis and treatment of von Willebrand disease. *Thromb Haemost* 2000; **84**: 160–74.

2 Ruggeri ZM. Von Willebrand factor. *Curr Opin Hematol* 2003; **10**: 142–9.

3 Kaufmann JE, Oksche A, Wollheim CB, Gunther G, Rosenthal W, Vischer UM. Vasopressin-induced von Willebrand factor secretion from endothelial cells involves V2 receptors and cAMP. *J Clin Invest* 2000; **106**: 107–16.

4 Mannucci PM, Bettega D, Cattaneo M. Patterns of development of tachyphylaxis in patients with haemophilia and von Willebrand disease after repeated doses of desmopressin (DDAVP). *Br J Haematol* 1992; **82**: 87–93.

5 Bond L, Bevan D. Myocardial infarction in a patient with hemophilia treated with DDAVP. *N Engl J Med* 1988; **318**: 121.

6 Byrnes JJ, Larcada A, Moake JL. Thrombosis following desmopressin for uremic bleeding. *Am J Hematol* 1988; **28**: 63–5.

7 Aiuti A, Slavin S, Aker M, *et al.* Correction of ADA-SCID by stem cell gene therapy combined with nonmyeloablative conditioning. *Science* 2002; **296**: 2410–13.

8 Aiuti A, Vai S, Mortellaro A, *et al.* Immune reconstitution in ADA-SCID after PBL gene therapy and discontinuation of enzyme replacement. *Nat Med* 2002; **8**: 423–5.

9 Aiuti A, Cattaneo F, Galimberti S, *et al.* Gene therapy for immunodeficiency due to adenosine deaminase deficiency. *N Engl J Med* 2009; **360**: 447–58.

10 Kohn DB, Candotti F. Gene therapy fulfilling its promise. *N Engl J Med* 2009; **360**: 518–21.

11 Cavazzana-Calvo M, Hacein-Bey S, de Saint Basile G, *et al.* Gene therapy of human severe combined immunodeficiency (SCID)-X1 disease. *Science* 2000; **288**: 669–72.

12 Ott MG, Schmidt M, Schwarzwaelder K, *et al.* Correction of X-linked chronic granulomatous disease by gene therapy, augmented by insertional activation of MDS1-EVI1, PRDM16 or SETBP1. *Nat Med* 2006; **12**: 401–9.

13 Bainbridge JW, Smith AJ, Barker SS, *et al.* Effect of gene therapy on visual function in Leber's congenital amaurosis. *N Engl J Med* 2008; **358**: 2231–9.

14 Kaplitt MG, Feigin A, Tang C, *et al.* Safety and toleraesybility of gene therapy with an adeno-associated virus (AAV) borne GAD gene for Parkinson's disease: an open label, phase I trial. *Lancet* 2007; **369**: 2097–105.

15 Hacein-Bey-Abina S, Von Kalle C, Schmidt M, *et al.* LMO2-associated clonal T cell proliferation in two

patients after gene therapy for SCID-X1. *Science* 2003; **302**: 415–19.

16 Manno CS, Pierce GF, Arruda VR, *et al.* Successful transduction of liver in hemophilia by AAV-Factor IX and limitations imposed by the host immune response. *Nat Med* 2006; **12**: 342–7.

17 Mingozzi F, Maus MV, Hui DJ, *et al.* CD8(+) T-cell responses to adeno-associated virus capsid in humans. *Nat Med* 2007; **13**: 419–22.

18 Raper SE, Chirmule N, Lee FS, *et al.* Fatal systemic inflammatory response syndrome in a ornithine transcarbamylase deficient patient following adenoviral gene transfer. *Mol Genet Metab* 2003; **80**: 148–58.

19 Chang AH, Stephan MT, Lisowski L, Sadelain M. Erythroid-specific human factor IX delivery from *in vivo* selected hematopoietic stem cells following nonmyeloablative conditioning in hemophilia B mice. *Mol Ther* 2008; **16**: 1745–52.

20 Kuramoto K, Follman D, Hematti P, *et al.* The impact of low-dose busulfan on clonal dynamics in nonhuman primates. *Blood* 2004; **104**: 1273–80.

21 Moayeri M, Hawley TS, Hawley RG. Correction of murine hemophilia A by hematopoietic stem cell gene therapy. *Mol Ther* 2005; **12**: 1034–42.

22 Thorrez L, Shansky J, Wang L, *et al.* Growth, differentiation, transplantation and survival of human skeletal myofibers on biodegradable scaffolds. *Biomaterials* 2008; **29**: 75–84.

23 Thorrez L, Vandenburgh H, Callewaert N, *et al.* Angiogenesis enhances factor IX delivery and persistence from retrievable human bioengineered muscle implants. *Mol Ther* 2006; **14**: 442–51.

24 Matsui H, Shibata M, Brown B, *et al.* Ex vivo gene therapy for hemophilia A that enhances safe delivery and sustained *in vivo* factor VIII expression from lentivirally engineered endothelial progenitors. *Stem Cells* 2007; **25**: 2660–9.

25 Denis C, Methia N, Frenette PS, *et al.* A mouse model of severe von Willebrand disease: defects in hemostasis and thrombosis. *Proc Natl Acad Sci U S A* 1998; **95**: 9524–9.

26 De Meyer SF, Vanhoorelbeke K, Chuah MK, *et al.* Phenotypic correction of von Willebrand disease type 3 blood-derived endothelial cells with lentiviral vectors expressing von Willebrand factor. *Blood* 2006; **107**: 4728–36.

27 Nichols TC, Bellinger DA, Reddick RL, *et al.* The roles of von Willebrand factor and factor VIII in arterial thrombosis: studies in canine von Willebrand disease and hemophilia A. *Blood* 1993; **81**: 2644–51.

28 Mendolicchio GL, Ruggeri ZM. New perspectives on von Willebrand factor functions in hemostasis and thrombosis. *Semin Hematol* 2005; **42**: 5–14.

29 Miller AD. Retroviral vectors. *Curr Top Microbiol Immunol* 1992; **158**: 1–24.

30 Miller AD, Miller DG, Garcia JV, Lynch CM. Use of retroviral vectors for gene transfer and expression. *Methods Enzymol* 1993; **217**: 581–99.

31 Naldini L, Blomer U, Gage FH, Trono D, Verma IM. Efficient transfer, integration, and sustained long-term expression of the transgene in adult rat brains injected with a lentiviral vector. *Proc Natl Acad Sci USA* 1996; **93**: 11382–8.

32 Naldini L, Blomer U, Gallay P, *et al. In vivo* gene delivery and stable transduction of nondividing cells by a lentiviral vector. *Science* 1996; **272**: 263–7.

33 Blomer U, Naldini L, Kafri T, Trono D, Verma IM, Gage FH. Highly efficient and sustained gene transfer in adult neurons with a lentivirus vector. *J Virol* 1997; **71**: 6641–9.

34 Zufferey R, Nagy D, Mandel RJ, Naldini L, Trono D. Multiply attenuated lentiviral vector achieves efficient gene delivery *in vivo*. *Nat Biotechnol* 1997; **15**: 871–5.

35 Sinn PL, Sauter SL, McCray PB, Jr. Gene therapy progress and prospects: development of improved lentiviral and retroviral vectors–design, biosafety, and production. *Gene Ther* 2005; **12**: 1089–98.

36 Zufferey R, Donello JE, Trono D, Hope TJ. Woodchuck hepatitis virus posttranscriptional regulatory element enhances expression of transgenes delivered by retroviral vectors. *J Virol* 1999; **73**: 2886–92.

37 Follenzi A, Ailles LE, Bakovic S, Geuna M, Naldini L. Gene transfer by lentiviral vectors is limited by nuclear translocation and rescued by HIV-1 pol sequences. *Nat Genet* 2000; **25**: 217–22.

38 VandenDriessche T, Thorrez L, Naldini L, *et al.* Lentiviral vectors containing the human immunodeficiency virus type-1 central polypurine tract can efficiently transduce nondividing hepatocytes and antigen-presenting cells *in vivo*. *Blood* 2002; **100**: 813–22.

39 Montgomery RR. A package for VWD endothelial cells. *Blood* 2006; **107**: 4580–1.

40 Hacein-Bey-Abina S, Garrigue A, Wang GP, *et al.* Insertional oncogenesis in 4 patients after retrovirus-mediated gene therapy of SCID-X1. *J Clin Invest* 2008; **118**: 3132–42.

41 Zufferey R, Dull T, Mandel RJ, *et al.* Self-inactivating lentivirus vector for safe and efficient *in vivo* gene delivery. *J Virol* 1998; **72**: 9873–80.

42 Schroder AR, Shinn P, Chen H, Berry C, Ecker JR, Bushman F. HIV-1 integration in the human genome favors active genes and local hotspots. *Cell* 2002; **110**: 521–9.

43 Trono D. Virology. Picking the right spot. *Science* 2003; **300**: 1670–1.

44 Baum C. Insertional mutagenesis in gene therapy and stem cell biology. *Curr Opin Hematol* 2007; **14**: 337–42.

45 Montini E, Cesana D, Schmidt M, *et al.* Hematopoietic stem cell gene transfer in a tumor-prone mouse model

uncovers low genotoxicity of lentiviral vector integration. *Nat Biotechnol* 2006; **24**: 687–96.

46 Cornils K, Lange C, Schambach A, et al. Stem cell marking with promotor-deprived self-inactivating retroviral vectors does not lead to induced clonal imbalance. *Mol Ther* 2009; **17**: 131–43.

47 Berkner KL. Development of adenovirus vectors for the expression of heterologous genes. *Biotechniques* 1988; **6**: 616–29.

48 Chuah MK, Schiedner G, Thorrez L, et al. Therapeutic factor VIII levels and negligible toxicity in mouse and dog models of hemophilia A following gene therapy with high-capacity adenoviral vectors. *Blood* 2003; **101**: 1734–43.

49 Brown BD, Shi CX, Powell S, Hurlbut D, Graham FL, Lillicrap D. Helper-dependent adenoviral vectors mediate therapeutic factor VIII expression for several months with minimal accompanying toxicity in a canine model of severe hemophilia A. *Blood* 2004; **103**: 804–10.

50 Kreppel F, Kochanek S. Modification of adenovirus gene transfer vectors with synthetic polymers: a scientific review and technical guide. *Mol Ther* 2008; **16**: 16–29.

51 Brunetti-Pierri N, Stapleton GE, Law M, et al. Efficient, long-term hepatic gene transfer using clinically relevant HDAd doses by balloon occlusion catheter delivery in nonhuman primates. *Mol Ther* 2009; **17**: 327–33.

52 Xiao X, Li J, Samulski RJ. Efficient long-term gene transfer into muscle tissue of immunocompetent mice by adeno-associated virus vector. *J Virol* 1996; **70**: 8098–108.

53 Kaplitt MG, Leone P, Samulski RJ, et al. Long-term gene expression and phenotypic correction using adeno-associated virus vectors in the mammalian brain. *Nat Genet* 1994; **8**: 148–54.

54 Snyder RO, Miao CH, Patijn GA, et al. Persistent and therapeutic concentrations of human factor IX in mice after hepatic gene transfer of recombinant AAV vectors. *Nat Genet* 1997; **16**: 270–6.

55 Chao H, Sun L, Bruce A, Xiao X, Walsh CE. Expression of human factor VIII by splicing between dimerized AAV vectors. *Mol Ther* 2002; **5**: 716–22.

56 Allocca M, Doria M, Petrillo M, et al. Serotype-dependent packaging of large genes in adeno-associated viral vectors results in effective gene delivery in mice. *J Clin Invest* 2008; **118**: 1955–64.

57 Mykhaylyk O, Zelphati O, Hammerschmid E, Anton M, Rosenecker J, Plank C. Recent advances in magnetofection and its potential to deliver siRNAs *in vitro*. *Methods Mol Biol* 2009; **487**: 111–46.

58 Zayed H, Izsvak Z, Walisko O, Ivics Z. Development of hyperactive sleeping beauty transposon vectors by mutational analysis. *Mol Ther* 2004; **9**: 292–304.

59 Chuah M, Mates L, Belay E, et al. Molecular evolution of a novel hyperactive sleeping beauty transposase enables robust stable gene transfer in vertebrates. *Nat Genet* 2009; **41**: 753–61.

60 Knapp JE, Liu D. Hydrodynamic delivery of DNA. *Methods Mol Biol* 2004; **245**: 245–50.

61 Kamimura K, Suda T, Xu W, Zhang G, Liu D. Image-guided, lobe-specific hydrodynamic gene delivery to swine liver. *Mol Ther* 2009; **17**: 491–9.

62 Porteus MH, Carroll D. Gene targeting using zinc finger nucleases. *Nat Biotechnol* 2005; **23**: 967–73.

63 Lombardo A, Genovese P, Beausejour CM, et al. Gene editing in human stem cells using zinc finger nucleases and integrase-defective lentiviral vector delivery. *Nat Biotechnol* 2007; **25**: 1298–306.

64 Chao H, Mansfield SG, Bartel RC, et al. Phenotype correction of hemophilia A mice by spliceosome-mediated RNA trans-splicing. *Nat Med* 2003; **9**: 1015–19.

65 White SJ, Nicklin SA, Buning H, et al. Targeted gene delivery to vascular tissue *in vivo* by tropism-modified adeno-associated virus vectors. *Circulation* 2004; **109**: 513–19.

66 Work LM, Buning H, Hunt E, et al. Vascular bed-targeted *in vivo* gene delivery using tropism-modified adeno-associated viruses. *Mol Ther* 2006; **13**: 683–93.

67 Nettelbeck DM, Miller DW, Jerome V, et al. Targeting of adenovirus to endothelial cells by a bispecific single-chain diabody directed against the adenovirus fiber knob domain and human endoglin (CD105). *Mol Ther* 2001; **3**: 882–91.

68 Lin Y, Chang L, Solovey A, Healey JF, Lollar P, Hebbel RP. Use of blood outgrowth endothelial cells for gene therapy for hemophilia A. *Blood* 2002; **99**: 457–62.

69 Milbauer LC, Enenstein JA, Roney M, et al. Blood outgrowth endothelial cell migration and trapping *in vivo*: a window into gene therapy. *Transl Res* 2009; **153**: 179–89.

70 Haberichter SL, Merricks EP, Fahs SA, Christopherson PA, Nichols TC, Montgomery RR. Re-establishment of VWF-dependent Weibel–Palade bodies in VWD endothelial cells. *Blood* 2005; **105**: 145–52.

71 Van Damme A, Thorrez L, Ma L, et al. Efficient lentiviral transduction and improved engraftment of human bone marrow mesenchymal cells. *Stem Cells* 2006; **24**: 896–907.

72 Shi Q, Fahs SA, Kuether EL, Cooley BC, Weiler H, Montgomery RR. Targeting FVIII expression to endothelial cells regenerates a releasable pool of FVIII and restores hemostasis in a mouse model of hemophilia A. *Blood* 6 July 2010. [Epub ahead of print]

73 Shahani T, Lavend'homme R, Luttun A, Saint-Remy JM, Peerlinck K, Jacquemin M. Activation of human endothelial cells from specific vascular beds induces the release of a FVIII storage pool. *Blood* 2010; **115**: 4902–9.

74 Rosenberg JB, Greengard JS, Montgomery RR. Genetic induction of a releasable pool of factor VIII in human

endothelial cells. *Arterioscler Thromb Vasc Biol* 2000; **20**: 2689–95.

75 Yarovoi HV, Kufrin D, Eslin DE, *et al.* Factor VIII ectopically expressed in platelets: efficacy in hemophilia A treatment. *Blood* 2003; **102**: 4006–13.

76 Shi Q, Wilcox DA, Morateck PA, Fahs SA, Kenny D, Montgomery RR. Targeting platelet GPIbalpha transgene expression to human megakaryocytes and forming a complete complex with endogenous GPIbbeta and GPIX. *J Thromb Haemost* 2004; **2**: 1989–97.

77 van den Biggelaar M, Meijer AB, Voorberg J, Mertens K. Intracellular cotrafficking of factor VIII and von Willebrand factor type 2N variants to storage organelles. *Blood* 2009; **113**: 3102–9.

78 Haberichter SL. VWF and FVIII: the origins of a great friendship. *Blood* 2009; **113**: 2873–4.

79 Laje P, Shang D, Cao W, *et al.* Correction of murine ADAMTS13 deficiency by hematopoietic progenitor cell-mediated gene therapy. *Blood* 2009; **113**: 2172–80.

80 VandenDriessche T, Vanslembrouck V, Goovaerts I, *et al.* Long-term expression of human coagulation factor VIII and correction of hemophilia A after *in vivo* retroviral gene transfer in factor VIII-deficient mice. *Proc Natl Acad Sci USA* 1999; **96**: 10379–84.

81 Follenzi A, Battaglia M, Lombardo A, Annoni A, Roncarolo MG, Naldini L. Targeting lentiviral vector expression to hepatocytes limits transgene-specific immune response and establishes long-term expression of human antihemophilic factor IX in mice. *Blood* 2004; **103**: 3700–9.

82 Snyder RO, Miao C, Meuse L, *et al.* Correction of hemophilia B in canine and murine models using recombinant adeno-associated viral vectors. *Nat Med* 1999; **5**: 64–70.

83 Ye P, Thompson AR, Sarkar R, *et al.* Naked DNA transfer of Factor VIII induced transgene-specific, species-independent immune response in hemophilia A mice. *Mol Ther* 2004; **10**: 117–26.

84 Pergolizzi RG, Jin G, Chan D, *et al.* Correction of a murine model of von Willebrand disease by gene transfer. *Blood* 2006; **108**: 862–9.

85 Lenting PJ, de Groot PG, De Meyer SF, *et al.* Correction of the bleeding time in von Willebrand factor (VWF)-deficient mice using murine VWF. *Blood* 2007; **109**: 2267–8.

86 De Meyer SF, Vandeputte N, Pareyn I, *et al.* Restoration of plasma von Willebrand factor deficiency is sufficient to correct thrombus formation after gene therapy for severe von Willebrand disease. *Arterioscler Thromb Vasc Biol* 2008; **28**: 1621–6.

87 Marx I, Lenting PJ, Adler T, Pendu R, Christophe OD, Denis CV. Correction of bleeding symptoms in von Willebrand factor-deficient mice by liver-expressed von Willebrand factor mutants. *Arterioscler Thromb Vasc Biol* 2008; **28**: 419–24.

Index

Page numbers in *italics* denote figures, those in **bold** denote tables.

Von Willebrand Disease, 1st edition. Edited by Augusto B. Federici, Christine A. Lee, Erik E. Berntorp, David Lillicrap, Robert R. Montgomery. © 2011 Blackwell Publishing Ltd.